MORE THAN GOLD
IN CALIFORNIA

MORE THAN GOLD IN CALIFORNIA

The Life and Work of Dr. Mary Bennett Ritter

MARY BENNETT RITTER, MD

INTRODUCTION BY GESA E. KIRSCH

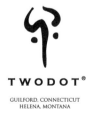

TWODOT®

GUILFORD, CONNECTICUT
HELENA, MONTANA

A · T W O D O T® · B O O K

An imprint and registered trademark of Rowman & Littlefield

Distributed by NATIONAL BOOK NETWORK

British Library Cataloguing-in-Publication Information Available

Library of Congress Cataloging-in-Publication Data available

ISBN 978-1-4930-2651-7 (paperback)
ISBN 978-1-4930-2652-4 (e-book)

∞™ The paper used in this publication meets the minimum requirements of American National Standard for Information Sciences—Permanence of Paper for Printed Library Materials, ANSI/ NISO Z39.48-1992.

Printed in the United States of America

For **Deborah A. Day,** longtime archivist at the Scripps Institution of Oceanography, who early on recognized the importance of Dr. Mary Bennett Ritter's legacy and has made her materials widely available to scholars and interested readers.

For **Ruth Bennett Cody,** Dr. Ritter's niece, who greatly admired her aunt Mary and wrote, after hearing her present a lecture to the La Jolla Woman's Club about a trip to Japan: *"I remember how I listened filled with awe that I should know and be related to one who had had such strange and wondrous adventures."*

For **Cindy Melter,** great-grandniece of Dr. Ritter, a pioneering spirit in her own right, forging a path for women software engineers in Silicon Valley.

Contents

A Note to Readers

To preserve the tone, style, and historical character of this memoir, original spelling, punctuation, and phrases common at the time of the book's publication in 1933 have been retained. Readers will notice that some words now commonly spelled as a single word are hyphenated or paired, sometimes inconsistently (e.g., "week-end," "country-side," "school teacher," "head strong," "worth while"); unusual spellings of medical terms (e.g., "anaestetic," "haemoglobin") and geographical places (e.g., "Tia Juana"); and several terms used by Mr. Ritter that describe his scientific approach (e.g., "philosophico-biological"), an approach we might describe as "ecological" or "holistic" today.

The original publication of *More than Gold in California* contains an opening section that is *not* included in this book. That section is distinctly different in tone and style from the rest of the book. It is not based on firsthand experience; rather, Dr. Ritter reconstructs the details of her family's migration from stories she heard as a child and from family letters, diaries, and published historical accounts. It was written at the request of Dr. Ritter's nieces as she notes in her foreword. In it, she chronicles the history of her paternal and maternal lines (the Bennett and Noble families) and describes their expeditions to California via steamship and railroad during the Gold Rush period, their exploration of California land and business opportunities, and their farming in the San Jose area. While this section is likely to be of interest to readers of California history and culture, it stands in contrast to the vivid firsthand account Dr. Ritter presents here. I refer interested readers to the original publication, copies of which can be found in a good number of California libraries and requested via interlibrary loan.

ACKNOWLEDGMENTS

I want to thank colleagues at the Interdisciplinary Humanities Center, University of California, Santa Barbara (UCSB), especially Susan Derwin and Emily Zinn, for hosting me as a visiting scholar during my sabbatical and providing me with an office, access to libraries and resources, and an opportunity to present my work in a stimulating environment. Many thanks go to Shelby Miller for assistance with digital images and to colleagues in the writing program, Linda Adler-Kassner, Patricia Fancher, and Karen Lunsford, for welcoming me to UCSB.

I am grateful to Bentley University for supporting a sabbatical leave and several trips to conduct archival research, and to my colleagues in the English and Media Studies Department for their interest and support of my work.

Many thanks go to the Humanities Center at Syracuse University for inviting me to serve as the Jeannette K. Watson Distinguished Visiting Professor in the Humanities and giving me the opportunity to share my research on nineteenth-century medical women with an interdisciplinary audience. Lois Agnew, Patrick Berry, and Brice Nordquist were wonderful hosts during my visits to Syracuse.

I appreciate the access, information, and resources provided by many special collections, archives, libraries, and historical societies that have allowed me to access primary sources and deepen my knowledge of the life and times of Dr. Mary Bennett Ritter. These include the Stanford Medical History Center, Lane Medical Library, Stanford University, with special thanks to Drew Bourn, historical curator and former archivist Patty French; the Bancroft Library, University of California, Berkeley, with thanks to Crystal Miles and her colleagues; and the Special Collections and Archives at the University of California, San Diego, with thanks to Heather Smedberg. I have also benefited from visits to the Berkeley Historical Society; the La Jolla Historical Society; the archives at Denison Library, Scripps College, Claremont, California; the Countway Library of Medicine, Harvard Medical School; and the Office of Medical History and Archives, Lamar Soutter Library, University of Massachusetts Medical School.

I am grateful to Erin Turner, editorial director, TwoDot Books, for her enthusiasm, support, and guidance with this project.

Many colleagues have provided helpful comments, questions, and feedback as I conducted archival research, presented talks, and wrote articles about medical women in the nineteenth century. Many thanks to Maureen Goldman, astute reader and wonderful friend; Gail Hawisher, longtime friend and colleague; Jabari Mahiri, dear friend and colleague who hosted me during visits to Berkeley; Ellen More, who has generously shared her insights, contacts, and deep knowledge of medical history; Liz Rohan, friend, colleague, and coeditor with a shared interest in archival research; Jacqueline Jones Royster, esteemed mentor, coauthor, and friend; and many others who have inspired and encouraged me along the way.

Finally, my heartfelt thanks go out to wonderful friends and family who enrich my life in so many ways, most especially, to Tony Schreiner, for his love, friendship, and playfulness all these years.

INTRODUCTION

More than Gold in California:
The Life and Work of Dr. Mary Bennett Ritter

Gesa E. Kirsch

More than Gold in California is a fascinating memoir written by Dr. Mary Elizabeth Bennett Ritter, a physician, women's rights advocate, and civic leader working in California at the turn of the last century. It tells the story of a farmer's daughter who defies all conventions to pursue her passion: to receive medical training and become a physician. It is filled with adventures and drama—house calls via horse and buggy rides through the darkened streets of Berkeley, a spurned lover's suicide, a near drowning at Pacific Grove beach, one of the first automobile rides across rugged California dirt roads, intercontinental rail travel, and voyages to the Far East. As Dr. Ritter tells her story, readers encounter the movers and shakers of their times—University of California presidents and families of wealth and influence, including the Scrippses, the Hearsts, and the Rockefellers.[1]

More than Gold in California is set in the late nineteenth century after the Gold Rush had brought waves of pioneers and fortune seekers to California (1849), the University of California was established (1868), and Chinese laborers had built the railroads (1860s). Women's rights were limited, and modern medicine was still emerging (pathogens were poorly understood, penicillin and antibiotics had yet to be discovered, and the use of vaccines and X-rays were still emerging). Women physicians were small in number but increasing rapidly, estimated from a few hundred at the middle of the century to several thousand by century's end.[2] It was a cultural moment in which medicine, technology, and the sciences were beacons of hope for human progress. *More than Gold in California* tells

Dr. Ritter's own story, but it also tells a story of her time, when women were increasingly entering public and professional spheres.

A DETERMINED WOMAN

Dr. Ritter's memoir is highly readable, engaging, and historically significant.[3] It shows the author's keen sense of observation, humor, and courage in the face of adversity. As Dr. Ritter recounts her eventful life, she reveals a determination to succeed, a mastery of persuasion to accomplish her goals, and a commitment to promote the welfare of those in need. She recalls in her chapter Childhood Memories a time at age five when she first displayed her strong will. Her mother had asked her to wear a hat but she refused. No amount of reasoning, persuading, or threatening would change her mind. Once she had made up her mind, she stood by her decision. Reflecting on this event, Dr. Ritter muses: "I really think that the same dogged determination which prompted the five-year-old child, regardless of spankings and being shut in a dark smoke-house, to insist, 'I don't want to wear that hat,' had something to do with the surprisingly small death list that fell to my lot."

Dr. Ritter was determined, persistent, and persuasive; she had a strong sense of indignation when she encountered injustices, whether these affected women, the poor, or the needy. She used a sliding scale to charge for her medical services and often worked without charge, but she also insisted on payment from those who had the means to do so. As she recounts in her chapter Medical Practice, when the family of a well-to-do patient complained about her fees, Dr. Ritter responded:

> To me money was never the paramount question. The poorest patient received the same devoted care as the richest ... It was the life I was battling for. But when I was asked by this patient's family for my bill, I sent one for five hundred dollars to a brother who was executor of his father's large estate. I received a partial payment check with a reference to the size of the bill. This wounded me greatly. I wrote him that if his sister's life was not worth that amount he might reduce the bill to what he considered was equitable, but that as for me, had another cipher been added to the amount it would not have been adequate

recompense for what my devotion to his sister had taken out of my life. I received an abject apology and the full amount of the bill.

This story—and many others she tells in her memoir—reflects Dr. Ritter's pragmatic approach, her commitment to social justice, and her rhetorical powers. Dr. Ritter had a way with words that could disarm even the most vociferous critics, especially critics of women determined to bring about social change. But Dr. Ritter also recognized that there could be a fine line of going too far, as she notes in her Childhood Memories chapter: "The strength of will and determination to succeed in whatever I undertook has stood me in good stead many times later in life, as well as being a characteristic I have had to learn to control."

A PIONEER IN MEDICINE

Dr. Ritter was a pioneer in the field of medicine. She was progressive, pragmatic, and feminist in orientation and would not let the "powers-that-be" deter her from pursuing her goals. She received her MD in 1886, ten years after women were first admitted to Cooper Medical College (now Stanford School of Medicine). Since Dr. Ritter did not come from a family of wealth, she had to earn the money needed to pay for a medical education. She accomplished this by working as a schoolteacher and later as a school principal (another first for a woman of her time). Once she had gained a sound financial footing and announced her plans to pursue a medical education, she encountered numerous objections. She writes in her chapter An Interlude:

> There were the usual caustic remarks about feminine unfitness for the profession of medicine, woman's lack of strength, her instability, natural timidity, and all the other hackneyed objections.
>
> Predictions of failure were universal but varied. Beside all of the above reasons for failure there came this blast: "After you have spent all your money and the best years of your life studying medicine, you will 'up and marry' and it will all be wasted." "Even if I knew I should 'up and marry' I would most assuredly study medicine," was my retort. "Surely no one needs such training more than the mother of a family."

Dr. Ritter was very aware of the double standards women in medicine faced. Reflecting on her experiences as a medical student, she recounts a time when her class observed a particularly gruesome operation. When several male students fainted, this occurrence was attributed to "poor circulation." But if a single woman student had fainted, Dr. Ritter realized, the whole female gender would have been maligned. This incident speaks powerfully to the prejudices medical women faced, but Dr. Ritter was not to be deterred.

When she graduated from Cooper Medical College, she and the only other woman in her graduating class were invited to serve as interns at the Pacific Dispensary (now Children's Hospital) in San Francisco, an institution founded by two women physicians for the express purpose of supporting women's medical education.[4] Here, Dr. Ritter learned firsthand about the power of women's professional networks. In an essay written for the Cooper Medical College alumni newsletter *Recollections*, Dr. Ritter describes how women physicians at the time collaborated and supported one another's work.

> The hospital staff [at Children's Hospital] was composed for the most part of the early women physicians who had created it largely for the purpose of affording hospital opportunities for themselves and those who came after them. Prominent among them were Dr. Charlotte Blake Brown and Dr. Lucy F. Wanzer . . .
>
> One of her [Dr. Brown's] first activities was to call together the few other women physicians and several women of wealth and lay before them a plan to establish a free clinic for poor women and children. As a result, the Pacific Dispensary was opened . . . This finally grew into a hospital and clinic combined.

Witnessing Dr. Brown's successful strategy for advocating social change—gathering professional women and women of wealth around a common cause—provided a critically important lesson for Dr. Ritter, and it became a strategy upon which she would rely many times.

Early on Dr. Ritter recognized the importance of professional networks that allowed women physicians to collaborate, support, and consult with one another and create opportunities for professional advancement. Dr. Ritter ran her own practice in Berkeley for twenty years and became part of an informal network of women physicians who practiced medicine in the San Francisco Bay area that included Dr. Mary Delano Fletcher (her classmate in medical school), Dr. C. Annette Buckel, and Dr. Sarah Shuey. These women would consult with one another when they encountered difficult medical cases and cover one another's duties during vacations, illnesses, and other absences from their practices. Of these experiences, Dr. Ritter writes in her Medical Practice chapter: "Thus we four women physicians were near enough to work together when necessary, and relieve each other when one took a vacation" [or became ill]. Such professional networking became a cornerstone in Dr. Ritter's work and life. Indeed, not only did such a network of women physicians flourish on the Pacific Coast, but it was a national phenomenon, necessitated by the relatively small, though rapidly growing, number of women physicians at the time.[5]

A WOMEN'S RIGHTS ADVOCATE

Because Dr. Ritter was one of the few women physicians in Berkeley, she became the go-to person for women students, also few in numbers at the time, who sought the medical advice and moral support of a woman doctor. In fact, with her strong-mindedness, knowledge, and compassion, Dr. Ritter greatly contributed to women's self-esteem and determination to demand change in university affairs. Reflecting on all of this in her University Interests chapter, Dr. Ritter writes:

> Again it seemed to be my lot to be a "starter," for I was the "crank" that turned over the machinery for several innovations in the lives of the women students. Although the number of women students had increased rapidly from three or four in each class in the [18]80s to as many hundreds in the classes of the mid [18]90s, they were still inconsiderable numerically, and not at all to be considered in the various activities enjoyed by the men students.
>
> For example, the men had had a gymnasium and instruction in gymnastics for years. It was assumed to be beneficial to their health

and therefore a necessity. But this argument did not apply to the girls. The idea seemed rather to be that regular gymnastic exercise would be detrimental to their well-being. I sometimes felt as if the masculine powers-that-be thought that women were made of glass and might break to pieces if they fell down. But the girls did not think that way.

When in 1891 a group of University of California women students summoned their courage to request expanded access to the gymnasium (beyond the allotted few hours on Wednesday and Friday afternoons),[6] they were told by the physical education instructor that they first needed to have a medical exam, but that there were no funds for this purpose. The women decided to approach Dr. Ritter to inquire whether she would be willing to give them free medical exams. As Dr. Ritter recounts in her University Interests chapter, she immediately volunteered to do so:

> Alas for his foxy loop-hole! He had not counted on feminine determination. When a woman wants a thing, she wants it. The girls talked matters over and a day or two later the same group called on me and told me their story, asking if I would be willing to make the medical examinations without pay. I readily consented.

At the same time, philanthropist Phoebe Hearst, the only woman serving on the board of the University of California Regents had designated money to build a campus center, Hearst Hall, as a place for dining, socializing, and entertainment.[7] When Hearst learned from Dr. Ritter about the plight of the women students—limited access to the gymnasium—she decided to designate a section of the newly constructed Hearst Hall as the "Women's Gymnasium," offering students a splendid new facility, superior to that used by the men, Harmon Hall.

The building remains standing today (expanded and rebuilt by Phoebe Hearst's son after a fire destroyed the original in the 1930s), prominently lining Bancroft Way, a major thoroughfare on campus, and a reminder of the gesture made by Hearst in support of women students more than a century ago. Dr. Ritter was delighted with this turn of events, noting in her University Interests chapter with a bit of glee:

Thus the entering wedge was made for the vast amount of fine training of many sorts which the women students have enjoyed these
later years in the beautiful Hearst Gymnasium. Until this present
year [1933] I have never passed the palatial women's building and
then old Harmon Gymnasium [used by the men] without a broad
and somewhat sardonic grin.

The strategy Dr. Ritter had learned from her mentors—collaborating
with women of power and wealth (Phoebe Hearst in this case) to advance
a social cause (women's access to physical education)—proved to be successful in her work with university women, as it would later on in her
civic, social, and medical work.

In 1903 Dr. Ritter took her advocacy on behalf of women students
to a broader audience by addressing the thirty-third annual meeting of
the California State Medical Association and publishing her research in
the *California State Journal of Medicine*. Dr. Ritter advocated strongly for
women's rights to health, safety, and higher education. She argued that
a college education *benefits* women, both mentally and physically, and
does *not* interfere with their reproductive functions or devotion as future
mothers, two factors often raised by those opposing higher education for
women.[8]

Dr. Ritter rapidly became counselor and confidante to many women,
as she recalls in her chapter University Interests: "Since I was the only
woman on the campus to whom the girls could turn for any personal advice,
such advice, perforce, spread and spread like spilled treacle. . . . Every sort
of personal problem was brought to me." Notably, many women students
faced a lack of safe, affordable, and clean housing. Dr. Ritter helped these
students to implement their idea of setting up residential self-governing
"club-houses," taking upon herself the job of convincing the university
of the importance of this enterprise. To bolster her case, she conducted a
comprehensive survey of living arrangements for women. Not taking any
chances, she surveyed *all* boardinghouses in which women students lived,
not just a sampling, visiting hundreds of women students living in Berkeley and the surrounding area. Dr. Ritter added these visits, or inspections,
to the end of her long days spent in medical practice. What she found

during her visits were unsanitary and cramped living conditions, outlandish rents, and a lack of privacy for many tenants.

Showing her hallmark thoroughness with research, she described in detail the conditions she had encountered. Once she submitted her report to the university (as well as to Hearst), the facts were undisputable, convincing the administration of the need for safe and affordable student housing. Soon thereafter, Dr. Ritter and Hearst drew up a plan to set up the first two cooperative clubhouses that would be operated, furnished, and run by women students themselves and overseen by a concierge. Writing to Phoebe Hearst on August 25, 1903, Dr. Ritter rejoices:

> I grow more and more enthusiastic over our plan. I truly believe the scheme is ideal. The Club Houses are overwhelmed with applications this year and many inquiries come to me about future possibilities.
>
> By "ideal scheme" I mean the small club houses, managed by the girls themselves, so that they can regulate their own cost of living and have the pleasure and discipline of a home for the dignity and character of which they are responsible. The supervision of a chaperone and of some University person is of course essential, and it seems to me not unreasonable that a University might build and furnish such houses for renting to the students.

Once the first two model clubhouses had been set up, Dr. Ritter continued her work with women students for more than thirty years, serving on the Club House Loan Fund Committee, which coordinated fundraising efforts for loans to buy and furnish more than three dozen clubhouses over several decades.

For their part, the University of California women students, especially those who were or are members of the Prytanean Women's Honor Society, of which Dr. Ritter was a founding member, continue to acknowledge Dr. Ritter's important contributions to women's rights in the areas of health, well-being, and housing. To this date, the Prytanean Society website describes Dr. Ritter's contributions as a founding member, and the group donated funds to name a conference room in Dr. Ritter's honor at the Tang Center, a building that houses the University Health Services at the University of California, Berkeley.

A CIVIC LEADER

Dr. Ritter became an important civic leader when she helped to establish the first sanitary guidelines for dairies in Berkeley (to improve the safety of milk for infants), lectured on social hygiene under the auspices of the State Federation of Public Health during World War I, and supported many civic and women's organizations in her later years, such as the YWCA, the National Federation of Women's Clubs, the Traveler's Aid Society, and the League of Women Voters.

Systematic research continued to be a hallmark of Dr. Ritter's work on the "Milk Committee." At this time, Dr. Ritter and several of her peers—the women physicians who collaborated with one another in the Bay area—were invited to join the "Home Club," an organization that promoted home safety and sanitation. Unclean, unpasteurized milk from local dairies was a major concern at the time, a fact that caused many of Dr. Ritter's patients to become ill or die, especially infants and young children. As she describes in her "Ply-wood" of Life chapter, Dr. Ritter decided that something had to be done:

> One of the first [Home Club] committees formed was the Milk Committee whose purpose was to investigate the milk supply in the East Bay region and to try to secure pure milk. Dr. Buckel was chairman and Dr. Shuey, Dr. Fletcher and I the committee. Dr. Shuey and I were delegated to investigate all the dairies in Alameda and Contra Costa counties supplying milk to the cities and towns around the Bay. Such conditions of mud and filth as we found are indescribable. No wonder babies were ill.

Dr. Ritter's strategy of conducting systematic research, combined with the support of professional women working together, brought about an important new public health policy. As she had with the Berkeley woman's housing problem, she completed an exhaustive survey of dairies—*all* of them in Alameda and Contra Costa Counties (not just a sampling). The survey results, presented by a group of professional women, carried great rhetorical power, enough to convince policy makers to establish regulations that provided safe, clean, and pasteurized milk to the greater Berkeley region. These examples—just a few in the life of a fascinating woman physician who practiced medicine more than a hundred years ago—illustrate Dr. Ritter's determination, persuasive powers, and networking strategies to effect social change.

AN EARLY POWER COUPLE

In 1891, Dr. Ritter married William Emerson Ritter, a professor of zoology, and they began a highly unconventional relationship. They were partners and equals, supportive of each other's work, yet remained independent spirits. Today, they might be described as a "power couple."[9] Early on they had "come to an understanding," as Dr. Ritter states in her Medical Student and Interne chapter, that before they would marry, Dr. Ritter would complete an internship and set up a medical practice, and Mr. Ritter[10] would attend Harvard University for his doctoral studies. They spent as much time apart as together, coordinating meeting points on cross-continental or transatlantic voyages. They would use extended travels as opportunities for advancing professional knowledge and extending their networks: Dr. Ritter often toured hospitals and clinics and networked with women physicians while Mr. Ritter attended scientific conferences, conducted fieldwork, and met with fellow scientists.

Humor was a glue in their relationship, as can be seen in many of the stories Dr. Ritter narrates, and in several letters they wrote to each other and family members. For instance, Mr. Ritter writes in a letter to his uncle Nelson on October 8, 1905:

> Should you be curious to know what I am doing here [in La Jolla], I should explain that I am keeping house for Mrs. Dr. Mary B. Ritter, and incidentally doing a little in the way of Natural History in the

capacity of Director of the laboratory, located here, and belonging to the San Diego Marine Biological Association.

Our University is gracious enough to give its long and faithful servants a year off now and then for studying and housekeeping away from home; hence further explanation of my presence here.

Or consider this note written by Dr. Ritter, dedicating a bathrobe to her husband:

Whereas my husband, William Emerson Ritter, having proved by his use and care of a certain blue and gray lounging-robe during the period covering several months when said robe was loaned to him that he has the necessary qualifications to put said robe to its proper use, I hereby give the above mentioned robe to him for his use and pleasure.

Just as important as humor seems to have been in their relationship, there is evidence of true, deep, and abiding appreciation and respect for each other's intellect, work, vision, and accomplishments. Their letters to each other are tender, thoughtful, intellectually rich, and supportive. In an invitation sent to friends and family on November 19, 1931, on the occasion of Mr. Ritter's seventy-fifth birthday, Dr. Ritter writes:

For besides the desire to give my husband a pleasant evening, and to enrich his later years with happy memories, there was the hope that before the close of the evening each one of you might know him, *the whole man,* a little better; might see a little more clearly, the relatedness of his various activities and interests . . . So it is that this modern naturalist [Mr. Ritter] has striven all his life to help demonstrate not only the "Organism as a Whole" but the "complete reality" of Nature, that thereby human welfare might be enhanced. (emphasis in original).

Clearly, Dr. and Mr. Ritter provide an early model of what a relationship of deep mutual respect, support, and affection can look like.

A Founding Contributor to the Scripps Institution of Oceanography

In 1905 Dr. Ritter faced one of the most difficult decisions of her life: giving up her medical work. It became clear that her husband would be required to move to La Jolla on a full-time basis to oversee the establishment of the Marine Biological Station, now the world-renowned Scripps Institution of Oceanography of the University of California, San Diego. Dr. Ritter's own health was failing at the time, as it was on and off during her entire life (described below), so that the decision to give up her praxis (in 1909) and resign her work at the University of California, Berkeley, (in 1905) was perhaps made a little easier as she already had asked colleagues to cover her duties. But Dr. Ritter's lifework as a physician had shaped her identity, her values, and her vision. Her medical work enabled her to speak confidently, publicly, and persuasively. It formed the core of her activism and civic leadership. In letters to her friends, she comments about missing her medical work. In February 1905, she writes to Phoebe Hearst:

> I miss my work very much. One cannot lightly give up a work into which much of one's life has gone, nor is it easy to readjust one's life to the trivial round of duties that fall to woman's lot. Perhaps they are not trivial, and the outside demands upon my time keep me more than busy in various forms of philanthropic work.

And on September 9, 1910, she writes to her friend Mrs. Kofoid:

> Another element in the pleasurable week was getting back into the old harness [attending to a patient]. It was like a taste of blood to an old caged lion. I am more convinced by experience than I was formerly by observation, that it is a serious thing to deprive one of a long accustomed occupation.

Once the Ritters moved to La Jolla on a full-time basis, Dr. Ritter, true to her pioneer spirit, rolled up her sleeves and managed the day-to-day affairs of the newly established "colony," the Marine Biological Station. She became a critically important contributor to the development of the new campus, supervising the construction of the first buildings as well as the early landscaping of the Scripps Institution of Oceanography. In a letter to Hearst on December 29, 1909, she writes,

> [Mr. Ritter] is in the East again this Winter—has quite contracted the habit, it seems to me, of being away at Christmas time.
>
> I am kept occupied by foresting a hundred and seventy acres of land with some twenty-thousand trees, and superintending the numerous contracts necessary for the completion of the new laboratory and Station.

Situated on a piece of land about six miles by dirt road from downtown La Jolla and eighteen miles from San Diego, the colony became its own settlement. That meant providing housing and meals for staff and students who came to work and live there, hosting visitors from near and far, and entertaining San Diego's civic and business leaders, on whose financial support the success of the Marine Biological Station would depend. In her chapter The Half Decade—1913–1918, Dr. Ritter remarks, tongue-in-cheek:

> Once established in our residence, I often said that all we needed to do was to put out a sign, "RITTER INN—Entertainment Free." Officials from the University—president, comptroller, surveyor—as well as scientists from all over the world, were our house guests, to say nothing of the friends and acquaintances who kindly dropped in, in the course of their tours.

Furthermore, Dr. Ritter was an active editor and reviewer of her husband's manuscripts (e.g., typing and proofreading reports, articles, and book manuscripts) and supported his laboratory work (e.g., preserving specimens).[11] The combination of opportunity, necessity, and duty compelled Dr. Ritter to become an active collaborator with her husband as they, together with many San Diego businessmen and philanthropists, undertook the founding of what would become the Scripps Institution of Oceanography.

WORLD TRAVEL

Dr. Ritter traveled quite extensively, especially in later years, often accompanying Mr. Ritter to scientific meetings and conferences. They took extended voyages to Japan, Australia, the South Sea Isles,[12] and several trips to Europe. On occasion, Dr. Ritter would invite family members to accompany them on these trips. She took great delight in getting to know her nieces and nephews and their children. One time, she invited two of her grandnieces and one of their friends to come along on a trip to Europe, where they shared many adventures while touring England, France, and Italy. When the young women returned home, Dr. Ritter traveled to Geneva to the seventh annual convention of The League of Nations in order to attend lectures offered by the International Institute of Education—the reason she had decided to travel to Europe even when Mr. Ritter was unable to accompany her. On another occasion, she invited her grandnephew immediately after his high school graduation to come to Washington, D.C. for six months to see the inauguration of President Calvin Coolidge and assist her as companion and driver because she was ill at the time and did not want to be housebound. Thus, the young man toured the East Coast extensively and discovered his love of travel and adventure, later exploring South America and Europe on his own. As the quote (on the dedication page) from her niece, Ruth Bennett Cody, suggests, Dr. Ritter inspired several generations of nieces and nephews with her brave, courageous, and unconventional life.

HEALTH CHALLENGES IN DR. RITTER'S OWN LIFE

Dr. Ritter's determination, accomplishments, and success are perhaps all the more remarkable when one learns about her own lifelong health challenges. At age twelve, she was diagnosed with typhoid fever. She was vulnerable to contracting influenza and the common cold. At age thirty-five, she was diagnosed with an enlarged heart. She suffered a number of serious physical breakdowns, spending weeks, months, even years confined to her bed, a wheelchair, or a sanatorium. In 1889, while Mr. Ritter was traveling to the East, her mentor, Dr. Charlotte Brown, urged her to undergo a serious operation for intestinal ulcerations.[13] When her prognosis did not look good, and her caretakers, believing she would not survive, wrote a letter to Mr. Ritter, urging him to return home, she took matters into her own hands. As she tells in her chapter First Years in Berkeley, she sent a telegram to Mr. Ritter that read, "Do not believe letter. Am not going to die. Do not come home."

Dr. Ritter also suffered several life-threatening accidents: a near-drowning in the Pacific Ocean during her youth, driving off a cliff with her horse and buggy, and, many years later, plunging down a canyon with an automobile. In the latter two accidents, she was lucky to survive with only severe bruises and broken ribs. Finally and devastatingly, she lost her eyesight at age seventy-three, just after the publication of *More than Gold in California*. Undeterred, she learned to read Braille as she describes in the pages appended to the second printing of the memoir in 1939, "After Five Years," included here as Afterword.

A WORK OF ENDURING IMPORTANCE

More than Gold in California is a lost classic of women's memoir. It is inspiring, engaging, and filled with adventure. It speaks to readers today, addressing contemporary issues, such as overcoming gender stereotypes, working toward equality, engaging in civic leadership, and promoting a greater common good. Readers of memoir and autobiography will appreciate the vivid details, sense of adventure, and narrative style of Dr. Ritter. This memoir will be of interest to scholars and students of women's studies, medical history, and California history who want to learn more about the life of an early woman physician, women's rights activist, and civic leader. While there are other works that narrate the lives of early women physicians, few speak so eloquently to how an early woman physician combined her medical training, persuasive powers, and lifelong commitment to women's rights to promote social change. Deborah A. Day, former archivist at the Scripps Institution of Oceanography, recognized Dr. Ritter's legacy early on and made her materials widely available to interested scholars and readers. She describes Dr. Ritter in correspondence with the editor as "one of the most important forgotten women in the history of sciences, especially here in the west, and her life and its obstacles are both instructive and inspiring."

This book illuminates recent work in the history of women in medicine. There are a number of books that examine the obstacles women have faced in their quest for a medical education;[14] their roles in the medical field as nurses, midwives, and physicians;[15] and their contributions to medical research, medical writing, and medical reform.[16] Dr. Ritter's memoir adds another dimension to this ongoing scholarship by providing an in-depth look at one woman physician and the collective of professional peers she assembled at the turn of the twentieth century.

This work enriches scholarship in women's studies and illustrates how one physician used her medical education, network of peers, and rhetorical powers to bring about social change, thus contributing to our understanding of women's activism. In recent years, scholars have begun to uncover the writing of many women, both famous and ordinary, who have made major contributions to civic and social life.[17] Having access to Dr. Ritter's autobiography, readers will be able to interpret her legacy in a contemporary context while gaining firsthand knowledge of her lived experiences, accomplishments, and insights. Importantly, this project contributes to the literature and history of California. Dr. Ritter's life illustrates how a determined young woman could become a medical doctor, civic leader, women's rights activist, and major contributor to the development of two universities—University of California, Berkeley, and University of California, San Diego—long before women had the right to vote.

Dr. Ritter's many contributions to public life, medicine, and women's history have never been fully recognized. She was awarded an honorary doctorate from the University of California, Berkeley, in 1937 to recognize her role as the first unofficial Dean of Women at the university, and she had a women's residence hall named in her honor (the Mary Bennett Ritter Hall, a building sold to a fraternity in the 1960s), but no full account of her life exists. With the republication of *More than Gold in California*, Dr. Ritter's many contributions to public life—her pioneering role in the field of medicine, her work as a woman's advocate, and her major contributions to public life—will be rightfully restored, and an important piece of missing American history recovered.

NOTES

1   Deborah A. Day, longtime archivist at the Scripps Institution of Oceanography, first introduced me to Dr. Ritter's remarkable life and suggested I read *More than Gold in California*. I have narrated several of my archival adventures in researching Dr. Ritter's life in a book chapter, "Being on Location: Serendipity, Place, and Archival Research."

2   Ellen S. More, Elizabeth Fee, and Manon Parry, three medical historians, write "the creation of all-women's and coeducational schools, regular and sectarian, became the engine behind a noticeable increase in the number of women medical graduates in the United States by the end of the nineteenth century, with their numbers increasing from a few hundred in 1860 to approximately three thousand five hundred by 1900" (2).

3   This memoir is particularly accurate because Dr. Ritter reviewed—and cites—many sources she consulted as she drafted the manuscript: personal diaries, letters, university reports, medical reports, visitor logs, her husband's notes, papers, and correspondence, thereby verifying exact dates, times, places, visitor names, travel itineraries, and more.

4   See "A Century of Service;" "The Story of Children's Hospital;" Eliassen.

5   One place where this phenomenon becomes visible is in the *Woman's Medical Journal* (1893–1952), a national publication that served both as a scholarly journal reporting the latest medical research and as a networking tool through which women physicians stayed in contact, shared knowledge and resources, and published their research. See also Ellen S. More, *Restoring the Balance: Women Physicians and the Profession of Medicine, 1850–1995*, and Carolyn Skinner, *Women Physicians and Professional Ethos in Nineteenth-Century America*.

6   Roberta J. Park notes that in 1891, the University of California registrar listed one course in physical education available to women on Wednesday and Friday afternoons.

7   For more details about Phoebe Hearst's contributions to the University of California, see J.R.K. Kantor, "Cora, Jane, and Phoebe: Fin-De-Siecle Philanthropy," an article about the three most important women philanthropists at the university at the turn of the twentieth century. For additional information about prominent early Berkeley women, see the online exhibit, Women at Cal: When California Passed the Woman Suffrage Amendment, 1910–1915; http://vm136.lib.berkeley.edu/BANC/Exhibits/womenatcal/index.html.

8   e.g., Smith-Rosenberg and Rosenberg.

9   The urban dictionary defines a power couple as follows: "A relationship between two people . . . Neither one depends on the other for their feelings of self worth—they know in their heart that they are just as valuable to the world as the other." This definition captures a distinct part of the Ritters' relationship. http://www.urbandictionary.com/define.php?term=power+couple.

10   I use "Dr. Ritter" to refer to the writer of this memoir, Dr. Mary Bennett Ritter. I use "Mr. Ritter" to refer to her husband, in keeping with Dr. Ritter's usage throughout the book and to avoid confusion; Mr. William Emerson Ritter held a PhD in zoology from Harvard University.

11   In a letter to Mrs. Kofoid on November 16, 1905, Dr. Ritter writes, "I have worked hard . . . Preserving specimens is harder than the ordinary task of 'preserving,' inasmuch as each jar must be classified, labeled, and arranged systematically. It does not show for all the work that has been put into it, but yet makes a very respectable showing."

12   Readers might find a few of Dr. Ritter's descriptions or comments about citizens of the countries she visited derogatory when viewed through a twenty-first-century lens, but they would have been considered fairly progressive for her times, when she followed the intellectual trajectory of her husband, Mr. Ritter, who was interested and wrote about human history, culture, and evolution, trying to answer the question his longtime friend and collaborator, Mr. E. W. Scripps, had posed: "What kind of animal is the human?"

13   Dr. Jim Ollhoff, a historian at Saint Mary's University of Minnesota, who has an abiding interest in Mr. Ritter's work and life, in 2004 asked a group of health care practitioners at a highly

respected teaching hospital and clinic to make a diagnosis based on the numerous symptoms Dr. Ritter describes throughout her memoir. This team ventured the following diagnosis—speculative at best—yet informative nonetheless, according to Dr. Ollhoff:

> The medical staff . . . talked through about a dozen different possibilities of what ailed Mary Bennett Ritter. There is one diagnosis that seems to cover most of the symptomology . . . Crohn's disease. This is an inflammation of parts of the intestines. Those who suffer from it tend to have loose and frequently bloody bowel movements. This might explain why she spoke so ambiguously about her health (i.e., saying she was "not well" or that her health was "delicate"). As was the custom of the time, she wouldn't have wanted to be specific about such an intimate matter.
>
> Her major operation in 1889 that revealed, in her words, "abseses walled off by adhesions among the intestines" would be very consistent with Crohn's disease. Crohn's disease creates ulcerations that burrow through the intestinal wall, which is, perhaps what they found when Dr. Brown did the surgery. In fact, the doctors described her condition as "intestinal tuberculosis," which was an early name for Crohn's disease. Crohn's disease would explain her constant fatigue. Further, intestinal ulcerations frequently get infected, which explain her jaundiced color, her low hemoglobin, and high white [cell blood] count. It also explains her "susceptibility to influenza" and could even explain her heart problems.
>
> Crohn's disease wasn't identified as a specific pathology until 1931 . . . Even today, with steroids and antibiotics, Crohn's disease is a very nasty, painful syndrome. With no anti-inflammatory medication or antibiotics, and a prescription of complete bed rest (which would make the problem worse), it must have been torturous.

14 e.g., Abram; Bonner; Chin; Morantz-Sanchez; More; More, Fee, and Perry.
15 e.g., Ehrenreich and English; Furst; Robinson.
16 e.g., Hayden; Skinner; Theriot; Wells.
17 e.g., Enoch; Gere; Johnson; Kates; Logan; Mattingly; McHenry; Royster.

BIBLIOGRAPHY

Abram, Ruth. *"Send Us a Lady Physician": Women Doctors in America, 1835–1920.* New York: Norton, 1985.

A Century of Service: Children's Hospital of San Francisco, 1875–1975 Centennial Year. A publication issued by Children's Hospital of San Francisco, 1975.

Bonner, Thomas Neville. *To the Ends of the Earth: Women's Search for Education in Medicine.* Cambridge, MA: Harvard University Press, 1992.

Chin, Eliza Lo, ed. *This Side of Doctoring: Reflections from Women in Medicine.* Thousand Oaks, CA: Sage Publications, 2002.

Day, Deborah A. "MB Ritter." Email correspondence. February 16, 2016.

Ehrenreich, Barbara, and Deidre English. *Witches, Midwives, and Nurses: A History of Women Healers.* Second Edition. New York: The Feminist Press at City University of New York, 2010.

Eliassen, Meredith. "The San Francisco Experiment: Female Medical Practitioners Caring for Women and Children, 1875–1935." *Gender Forum: An Internet Journal for Gender Studies.* Vol. 25 (2009). Accessed January 13, 2014. http://www.genderforum .org/fileadmin/archiv/genderforum/.

Enoch, Jessica. *Refiguring Rhetorical Education: Women Teaching African American, Native American, and Chicano/a Students, 1865–1911.* Carbondale: Southern Illinois University Press, 2008.

Furst, Lilian R., ed. *Women Healers and Physicians: Climbing a Long Hill.* Lexington: University Press of Kentucky, 1997.

Gere, Anne Ruggles. *Intimate Practices: Literacy and Cultural Work in U.S. Women's Clubs, 1880–1920.* Urbana: University of Illinois Press, 1997.

Hayden, Wendy. *Evolutionary Rhetorics: Sex, Science, and Free Love in Nineteenth-Century Feminism.* Carbondale: Southern Illinois University Press, 2014.

Johnson, Nan. *Gender and Rhetorical Space in American Life: 1866–1910.* Carbondale: Southern Illinois University Press, 2002.

Kantor, J.R.K. "Cora, Jane, and Phoebe: Fin-De-Siecle Philanthropy." *Chronicle of the University of California: A Journal of University History.* Special Issue: Ladies Blue and Gold. 1.2 (Fall 1998): 1–8.

Kates, Susan. *Activist Rhetorics and American Higher Education, 1885–1937.* Carbondale: Southern Illinois University Press, 2001.

Kirsch, Gesa E. "Being on Location: Serendipity, Place, and Archival Research." *Beyond the Archives: Research as a Lived Process.* Eds. Gesa E. Kirsch and Liz Rohan. Carbondale: Southern Illinois University Press, 2008, 20–27.

Logan, Shirley Wilson. *We Are Coming: The Persuasive Discourse of Nineteenth-Century Black Women.* Carbondale: Southern Illinois University Press, 1999.

_____. *Liberating Language: Sites of Rhetorical Education in Nineteenth-Century Black America*. Carbondale: Southern Illinois University Press, 2008.

Mattingly, Carol. *Appropriate(ing) Dress: Women's Rhetorical Style in Nineteenth-Century America*. Carbondale: Southern Illinois University Press, 2002.

McHenry, Elizabeth. *Forgotten Readers: Recovering the Lost Histories of African American Literary Societies*. Durham, NC: Duke University Press, 2002.

Morantz-Sanchez, Regina. *Sympathy and Science: Women Physicians in American Medicine*. New York: Oxford University Press, 1985, 2000.

More, Ellen S. *Restoring the Balance: Women Physicians and the Profession of Medicine, 1850–1995*. Cambridge, MA: Harvard University Press, 1999.

More, Ellen S., Elizabeth Fee, and Manon Perry, ed. *Women Physicians and the Cultures of Medicine*. Baltimore, MD: Johns Hopkins University Press, 2009.

Nerad, Merasi. "The Situation of Women at Berkeley between 1870 and 1915." *Feminist Issues* 7 (Spring 1987): 67–80.

Ollhoff, Jim. "Re: Mary's health." Email correspondence. September 23, 2004.

Park, Roberta J. "A Gym of Their Own: Women, Sports, and Physical Culture at the Berkeley Campus, 1876–1976." *Chronicle of the University of California: A Journal of University History*. Special Issue: Ladies Blue and Gold. 1.2 (Fall 1998): 21–48.

Prytanean Women's Honor Society, University of California, Berkeley. Accessed on March 13, 2014. https://sites.google.com/site/prytaneanmembership/.

Ritter, Mary Bennett. *More than Gold in California, 1849–1933*. Berkeley, CA: The Professional Press, 1933.

_____. "Medical Student and Interne." *Recollections of Cooper Medical College, 1883–1905*. Published by Stanford Medical School, May 1964.

_____. "A Study of the Health of University Girls; The Relation of the Physician to Preventative Medicine." *California State Journal of Medicine* 1 (1902–1903): 259–64.

_____. Letter to Phoebe Hearst. August 25, 1903. William E. Ritter Collection. MSS 71/3c box 24. Correspondence and papers of Mary Bennett Ritter. The Bancroft Library, University of California, Berkeley.

_____. Letter to Phoebe Hearst. February, 1905. William E. Ritter Papers. MSS 71/3c Box 24. Correspondence and papers of Mary Bennett Ritter. The Bancroft Library, University of California, Berkeley.

_____. Letter to Phoebe Hearst. December 29, 1909. William E. Ritter Papers. MSS 71/3c Box 24. Correspondence and papers of Mary Bennett Ritter. The Bancroft Library, University of California, Berkeley.

_____. Letter to Mrs. Kofoid. November 16, 1905. Kofoid Papers, 2007-01, Box 6, Special Collections and Archives, University of California, San Diego Library.

_____. Letter to Mrs. Kofoid. September 9, 1910. Kofoid Papers, 2007-01, Box 6, Special Collections and Archives, University of California San Diego Library.

_____. Note from Mary Bennett Ritter dedicating a bathrobe to her husband on Hotel Claremont letterhead. No date. William E. Ritter Papers. MSS 71/3c Box 18. The Bancroft Library, University of California, Berkeley.

———. Letter to "Dear Friends," an invitation to celebrate William E. Ritter's 75th birthday. November 19, 1931. William E. Ritter Papers. MSS 71/3c Box 18. The Bancroft Library, University of California, Berkeley.

Ritter, William Emerson. Letter to Uncle Nelson. October 8, 1905. William E. Ritter Papers. MSS 71/3c Box 24. The Bancroft Library, University of California, Berkeley.

Robinson, Elizabeth Ann. *The Soul of a Nurse.* Santa Barbara, CA: SpannRobinson, 2012.

Royster, Jacqueline Jones. *Traces of a Stream: Literacy and Social Change Among African-American Women.* Pittsburgh: University of Pittsburgh Press, 2000.

Ruyle, Janet. "The Early Prytaneans." *Chronicle of the University of California: A Journal of University History.* Special Issue: Ladies Blue and Gold. Vol. 1.2 (Fall 1998): 49–56.

Skinner, Carolyn. *Women Physicians and Professional Ethos in Nineteenth-Century America.* Studies in Rhetorics and Feminisms series. Carbondale: Southern Illinois University Press, 2014.

Smith-Rosenberg, Carroll, and Charles Rosenberg. "The Female Animal: Medical and Biological Views of Woman and Her Role in Nineteenth-Century America." *The Journal of American History* 60.2 (1973): 332–56.

The Story of Children's Hospital. A publication issued by Children's Hospital of San Francisco, 1975.

Theriot, Nancy. "Women's Voices in 19th Century Medical Discourse: A Step toward Deconstructing Science." *Signs: Journal of Women in Culture and Society* 19 (1993): 1–31.

Wells, Susan. *Out of the Dead House: Nineteenth-Century Women Physicians and the Writing of Medicine.* Madison: University of Wisconsin Press, 2001.

PART I:
HIGH LIGHTS AND LOW

CHAPTER I

Childhood Memories
1862–1870

MY EARLIEST RECOLLECTION WAS CAUSED BY AN ACT OF DISOBEDI-
ence which made such an indelible impression upon me that the physical
scar still remains on my forehead. Although I was only about two years of
age the memory-pictures of two factors in the incident are as vivid as any
memory of later years, and as no one else recalls these trivial factors, the
pictures I so clearly visualize must have been photographed on my retina
and on some hidden brain cells.

I had followed my father and eldest sister out to the barn to gather
the eggs and while they searched for the nests in the hay-loft I played
outside. Father had warned me not to climb into the high ox-cart standing near. It was tilted at a sharp angle resting on its heavy shafts. I proceeded to climb up the sloping shafts and succeeded in getting into the
body of the cart, but in trying to mount the sloping seat I slipped and
catapulted earthward head first. But I did not reach the earth. A pointed
piece of iron on one shaft stopped my downward flight by piercing my
scalp at the edge of my hair, driving it an inch or more into my forehead
between skull and scalp. Father was just coming out of the barn and was
only a few steps away, so I was instantly lifted off the cruel rack.

Though most of the memory of this incident is hear-say memory, I
think the falling at least is actual remembrance.

But the two factors of the event which no one else recalls and which
remain so vivid in my mind, were surprisingly trivial. As my father carried

me to the house, instead of going through a gate into the dooryard, he went over a little flight of steps nearly as high as the fence, a kind of farmyard gate that prevented cows, horses and pigs from passing from the barnyard to the household garden through a left-open gate.

Doubtless I climbed up and down those steps hundreds of times during the year my family lived on that farm, but my only recollection of the exterior of the place or of the arrangement of the house and barn is the picture of myself in father's arms with the blood streaming down my face while he went over the stile.

The memory of mother's fright and of the washing and bandaging of the wound are hazy, but an after picture is as clear as any of adult years. With bandaged head I was lying on pillows in a large rocking chair tilted backward to make a safe resting-place in the sitting room facing the dining-room door. Mother was serving the noonday dinner. Father and the farm-hands were seated at the table when mother came through the kitchen door bringing a dish piled high with fleecy mashed potatoes. Though no one else remembers this, that picture is as distinct in my memory as a great picture of Washington crossing Delaware, which made a deep impression on my mind twenty years later in college days.

My next distinct memory was of moving from that farm some months later into the village of Old Gilroy, a few miles away. The labor and turmoil of the occasion made no impression upon me. I only remember sitting on the high seat of our old-fashioned lumber wagon and swinging my feet. It seemed an infringement of my privileges that someone held onto me. The sense of freedom, of exhilaration away up there in the air was akin to that of a youthful aviator making his first ascent, leaving the ground beneath him.

My exact age at this time can be determined only by the fact that my brother, three years younger than I, was born after we moved into the village. Here we lived half of my first decade but the memories of it are mostly indistinct. The adobe house of the neighbor across the street where my particular playmate lived I recall clearly, as well as a hayloft in which we sometimes played. This memory lasts because of a disagreeable experience.

3

One of my earliest recollections of this village life was an incident that occurred one day on the broad stoop of this old adobe house as I sat alone on the porch playing in a corner with a little doll-house and some dishes. I was so intent that I heard no tip-toed steps nor other sound until a mysterious growling seemed right over my head and a hand was laid on my shoulder. I looked up to see three terrible forms bending over me, miles high seemingly, clad in sheets and pie-dough masks with great holes for eyes and mouth. My scream of terror rent the air and I fell over senseless. The terror was now transferred to my innocent but cruel tormentors, my older sister and two other girls older than she. Frightened at the result of their fun they tore off their masks and tried to restore me to consciousness by rubbing and shaking me, telling me who they were and that they wouldn't hurt me.

The cruelty of youthful fun! Can the life-long tendency to be startled by something coming up behind me be traced to the agony and horror of this memory-picture? If a stile and a dish of mashed potatoes can make an indelible impression on the mind of a child of two, what might not the terror of seeing such ogres do to the soft gray matter of the brain of a child three or four years old? At any rate I have ever since disliked having anyone steal up behind me, and now, sixty years later, I can feel the terror of my early experience.

When I was three years old my brother, William Joseph was born. I have no recollection of this event.

At three and a half years of age I started to school because the teacher who boarded with us was fond of me and took me with her. I did not study but somehow learned to read and spell, and at four recited Wordsworth's poem, "We are Seven," on the last day of school. After my baby lips had lispingly recited:

> I met a little cottage girl
> Who was eight years old she said,
> Her hair was thick with many a curl
> That clustered 'round her head.

4

and the fifteen subsequent stanzas, Miss Fisher humiliated me beyond expression by grabbing me up in her arms on the platform before all the assembled pupils and parents, kissing me enthusiastically and exclaiming, "You blessed baby!" She never guessed the shame and chagrin I experienced. But the next year she retrieved herself by making me as proud as before I had been shamed.

One day as I was nearing the age of five, the youngest member of this ungraded village school, Miss Fisher became exasperated when every one of the third reader class failed to spell the word "umbrella."

The class varying in ages from eight to sixteen years, standing in front of the teacher's desk, reached across the room. According to the progressive method a pupil failing to spell a word went to the foot of the line. At the head on this day stood Sinferano Fallon, a tall lanky youth of sixteen, half Spanish and half Scotch, while a few places below him stood his brother, Pedro. These two are the only members of the class of eighteen or twenty whom I remember, but the incident of this day and the subsequent tragic end of these two brothers make them living pictures in my mind.

Sinferano was not very bright and was at the head of the line only because, following the progressive method, the pupils failing to spell a word went to the foot of the line. The word "umbrella" fell to Sinferano. He failed to spell it—likewise the girl next to him and then Pedro. When Miss Fisher's impulsive temperament was displayed, panic struck the class and that poor word was torn and twisted into every conceivable combination of letters except the right one. As the last pupil stumbled over it, Miss Fisher, almost in a rage, told them how stupid they were, exclaiming, "I believe little Mary Bennett could spell that." She called me to the foot of the class and I spelled it in the simplest manner, whereupon she exclaimed, "There, I told you so! Mary, go to the head, and from now on you are in the third reader class." I shall never forget my pigmy size as I stood beside that nearly six-foot youth.

Why do I remember Sinferano and Pedro and almost no others in the school? Because a few years later Sinferano became a bandit and Pedro was killed when a base-ball struck him in the temple. At this time California was terrorized by bandits headed by a young Spaniard named Vasquez. This horde of marauders would descend from the mountain fastnesses upon a lonely cattle farm or a village store and drive off the cattle or rifle the store of provisions, clothing, ammunition or whatever they desired. No house was safe. Everyone was in terror, for they were excellent marksmen with a liking for human targets. Many a county sheriff with his volunteer posse felt the sting of whizzing bullets. The name Vasquez became a household terror to most of us, but to certain youths it fired the imagination with love of adventure, and more than one not-bad boy was tempted to follow in the lead of this daring desperado who seemed to lead a charmed life and who for years evaded every trap or ambush of county officers. Poor simple Sinferano was one of these, yielding to the excitable temperament inherited from his Spanish mother. A price was put upon his head and he was finally killed in a raid. Pedro was killed in a baseball game at a Catholic school near San Jose some years later.

My cousin Alice tells me that her father, George Bennett, was assistant sheriff of Santa Clara County at the time of the capture of Vasquez in which he aided. The bandit was confined in the county jail at San Jose. He was a likable young fellow and he and Uncle George became quite friendly. Before his execution Vasquez gave Uncle George a small beaded bag for his little girl as a souvenir, of his robberies I suppose. Alice treasured this purse during all her girlhood.

Another personal incident connected with this public terror was related to me by Julia Canfield, later one of my friends. Mr. Canfield's farm was about three miles south of San Juan. One evening about dusk two Spaniards rode up to the house and asked for supper and a place to sleep. Mr. Canfield told them he had no extra bed but if they wished they might take their blankets into the living room and make a bed on the floor by the fireplace. They accepted the offer and asked particularly that their horses be put in the stable among Mr. Canfield's horses. This aroused Mr. Canfield's suspicions but caused him to be only more polite to his guests. The men were especially kindly to the children. They were off the next morning by daybreak. A few hours later a sheriff's posse arrived in search of Vasquez and a pal who were supposed to have escaped in this direction. Their description of the men and horses exactly fitted the genial guests of the night before.

Another clear memory links up with our University and introduces another of the fine families that early found their way to the Pacific Coast. Old Gilroy was favored in having for its minister John Edwards, a Princeton man, descendant of two Princeton presidents. He had come to California seeking a mild climate for his delicate wife. They had two children, George and Clara, about thirteen and nine years of age. George had a mischievous twinkle in his eyes that remained through his more than four score years. As a boy he was noted for his ingenuity in perpetrating jokes on both old and young.

The little church stood on the bank of a typical dry stream-bed lined with sycamores around whose roots the swirling waters of winter washed deep holes, leaving pools in springtime.

One day when mother was calling on the minister's wife, Laura and Clara disappeared to play, leaving me behind as too young for them. I wandered out to the creek with my doll. Then this picture appears. Beside one of the pools at the foot of a large sycamore tree stood a small girl of three or four years weeping and stretching her arms helplessly upward. Astride a branch of the tree was a thirteen-year-old boy grinning gleefully and tantalizingly holding the small girl's doll by the foot over the pool. The anguish of the moment made an indelible impression though the sequel is forgotten save that the doll was not drowned and later reposed safely in my arms.

What freaks memory plays and how little elders can tell what incidents are making lifelong impressions on a child's mind!

Another memory-picture of George Edwards is one on a warm drowsy Sunday in church. Near the pulpit were some side seats facing each other. On one of these sat an old man and directly opposite an old woman. Gradually as they succumbed to slumber, first one nodded and then the other as if exchanging greetings from dreamland. It was too much for humorous George and he burst out laughing, much to the scandal of the congregation and his own sorrow later.

Why do I remember these trifling incidents when all other memories of the church and nearly everything pertaining to the community have faded? Doubtless intimate contact with the Edwards family in later years made their personalities living images.

Other freakish yet vivid pictures stand out here and there. A Spanish wedding party witnessed one day on the way to school; an unjust punishment by my doting teacher, Miss Fisher, being made to stand in the corner for something of which I was innocent, at least in intent; some habits indulged in by older girls which I now know were vicious, and even then disgusted me. I could not tell my mother of these things because of a lack of that intimate confidence which must be established by mothers. Children cannot establish it.

During the first few years of my life the Civil War was fought. Not a glimmer of memory of it have I. The assassination of President Lincoln made not the least impression upon me.

After the close of the war another detached memory-picture clings to my mind. There was a picnic somewhere, I do not know where, but there were trees under which were long tables made of boards laid on wooden horses. These were laden with good things from all the neighborhood hampers and baskets.

Evidently a local company of soldiers had returned, for men in blue uniforms with funny little caps marched around while a brass band played stirring music. Then there was some speech-making, I suppose, for the people sat down before a raised platform where the men in blue where seated. Then they all began to sing campaign songs. Some were familiar, but there was one new to me, the only one I remember, "Babylon has Fallen." Babylon and the Bible were connected in some way in my mind and I wondered what Babylon was and how far it had fallen. Then the picture faded, but this much of the aftermath of the war remained clear in memory's album.

My last memory of our life in Old Gilroy is of our whole family having the measles at once. One by one we three children came down with it. Mother cared for us until she too was stricken. Then came the discomforts entailed by having to depend upon the kindly but intermittent attention of neighbors. There were no trained nor even practical nurses to be employed in those days.

My sister tells me we lived in New Gilroy for a short time before father purchased the farm one mile northeast of Gilroy, where we lived as long as our family circle remained unbroken.

Memory of only one corporal punishment lingers in my mind. Mother attempted once to "break my will," but after the contest she decided it was better to avoid open strife and use more diplomatic measures to gain her point.

The scene of action was the back yard under the oak trees. It was a hot summer day. I was five or six years old. As I was going out to play mother put on my hat. I took it off and threw it on the ground. She replaced it … I again tore it off saying, "I don't want to wear that hat!" "You must! It is too hot to play bareheaded." "I don't want to wear that hat!" At each repeated assertion I threw the hat on the ground. With each command of mother's, and the explanation of her reason for doing so, the hat was replaced on my head.

This altercation was repeated several times until finally the dictum was pronounced: "If you do that again I shall spank you!" Again the hat was thrown on the ground with what seemed to me the entirely logical statement, "I don't want to wear that hat!"

The spanking began. At first there were a few tearful reiterations of the same statement. The spanking continued. Then, strategy, "Mother, look at those dogs!" Some dogs had come in sight frolicking as dogs do. Mother's soft heart relented but she must not give up the battle. What to do next?

A short distance away stood the smoke-house used annually at hog-killing time for curing hams. It had no windows and when the door was closed was totally dark except for the light coming through the key-hole. Mother put me in this dark solitary building and closed the door, though like Mary's loving lamb she lingered near, doubtless suffering more than I did, for anger still ruled me. With eye glued to the key-hole, I continued to vociferate "I don't want to wear that hat!" At last mother took me out and resorted to the diplomacy which would have been better at the outset. She said, "You are getting tired and overheated. I will put you in bed to rest until you can be a happy, obedient little girl again." So we both lost the battle, and yet won it.

Mother told me in later years of one other tussle against my determination when I was a creeping babe. Naturally I do not remember it, but that, too, was a battle of wills. She never again resorted to corporal punishment but as in the dish-washing episode related elsewhere, used a form of punishment that brought out my sense of shame and justice instead of my combativeness. The strength of will and determination to succeed in whatever I undertook has stood me in good stead many times in later life, as well as being a characteristic I have had to learn to control.

When I was about seven years old, a second brother was born, the fifth and last child in our family. On Christmas Eve we all, except mother, went to the Christmas tree festivities at the church. I have no idea why mother did not go and was grieved to start off without her, but the excitement soon chased my sorrow away. It was a boisterous stormy night. The rain fell in torrents and the wind blew so hard that we children were put in the bottom of the carriage with a blanket over our heads to prevent us being drenched with the rain which drove through the curtains. The trees, the lights, Santa Claus and his gifts are but hazy memories.

But three days later we were sent into town to spend the day at Aunt Jane Clifton's. Father came for us in the evening and after an animated conversation with Aunt Jane, told us that we had a little brother . . . that the doctor had brought a baby to our house.

I accepted this story unquestioningly, and also accepted with joy the acquisition to the family. But would not the whole situation have been sweeter, holier, if I had been lovingly instructed beforehand about the great expectation? I am sure it would have been not only better for me but would have given me a different attitude toward my mother—that our relations would have been closer, more sacred.

Poor, dear, sweet mother, an orphan from infancy, married in early girlhood, she could never overcome her timidity and natural shyness regarding sex subjects. Then, too, the ethics of that day would have been outraged by such revelations of Nature. Children's minds must be kept clean and pure. The barrier between my mother and me was never broken down, and what I learned regarding adolescence, I learned later from my sister and other girls.

This baby brother was destined for only a few months of life. In less than two years baby Frank and Abby, Uncle George's infant daughter and also the last child in the Clifton family, were victims of an epidemic of pernicious dysentery, which nearly took the lives of Aunt Eunice and my sister Laura as well.

* * * * * * *

The extension of the railroad from San Jose southward as far as Gilroy—at least the dedication of the great acquisition to that portion of Santa Clara County—was one of the great occasions of my childhood. A huge barbecue picnic was held in the railroad yards. The new freight buildings were filled with temporary tables and benches for the use of the assembled crowd. Seemingly everyone living in the southern part of the county was present.

There were speeches and band-playing and there were the usual vendors of all sorts of articles to tempt the gullible public. The big pink popcorn balls and pink lemonade rivaled those of the circus. Added to these delectables there was to me a new allurement, little rubber balloons, the first I had ever seen. Father bought me one. Such rapture was mine! But not for long. As the balloon bobbed about it evidently annoyed a big gruff ogre who struck it and pulled the string out of my hand. Aghast, I watched it soar until it rested in the tip of the gable of that great barn-like freight building. Would that that cruel man could have known something of the grief he inflicted on a little child, turning supreme happiness into sorrow, the poignancy of which still stands out sharply after sixty years. Were it not for my personal grief I should not have remembered this historical event.

Sometime later our Sunday school used this new acquisition to give the children (and grown-ups) a great thrill as well as an educational experience. For the annual May Day picnic an excursion to Woodward's Gardens in San Francisco was planned. This was the first railroad ride for many of us, the first sight of a large city, and our introduction to a zoological garden. My recollections are principally of the animals, especially the bears, and of a lake with a boat that went 'round and 'round.

I wish here to pay tribute to Mr. Woodward who established those gardens in early San Francisco. To this day I hear gray-haired people refer to those gardens as one of the greatest joys and inspirations of their childhood. The memory of the founder is blessed by many.

The railroad journey to and from San Francisco on that May Day figures but dimly. The early morning start, the impatience to reach our destination, and on the way home the impatience of an elderly woman passenger over the ill-mannered children, as she dubbed the excited, restless picnickers. That remark clouded the happy memories of a wonderful day in a child's life.

Living too far from school to walk, we were either driven there and back by father, or road horseback. Just when I learned to ride I do not know. It seems to me that I had always ridden. Father held the theory that one did not die until his time came so perhaps he took unusual risks in allowing us to ride none-too-tame horses. For some time I rode astride behind my sister's side-saddle. One beautiful horse we rode had a fondness for running away, and we took more than one thrilling ride, when I seemed to flop in the wind holding tightly to my sister's waist.

Uncle George lived on a farm a couple of miles farther out of town. Nearby was a hill where wild flowers grew in profusion, and gathering them was a favorite pastime. The hill was a veritable great Persian carpet of cream cups, baby blue eyes, yellow buttercups, pink gilias and very delicate little white lilies. I can still smell the fragrance of those flowers.

One Saturday some children from town came to visit us and we all decided to go wild flower gathering. Father was away with the family carriage and there were no saddle horses available. The only quasi horse was an old mule, gentle as a lamb but very determined as to where he wanted to go and the gait he wished to travel. Seven of us children piled on his bare back, astride, reaching from neck to tail. As usual, being the youngest, I brought up the rear clinging desperately to the boy in front of me from my perilously sloping seat on the mule's haunches. It was a slow and hard-worked passage as seven pairs of legs left no place to ply the whip, and our heels were not very effective speed promoters.

Another horseback escapade occurred one day after we had all been to the circus and were filled with a desire to emulate the standing-up stunt riders. Our cousins Ed and Will came over on a pet horse, cream-colored, very gentle with a broad back. The horse had been trained to herd cattle by vaqueros, and to obey the slightest touch of the Spanish bridle then in common use.

The boys succeeded in riding barefooted standing up behind the saddle ridden by the one who guided the horse. My turn came, and in stocking feet I mounted behind cousin Ed. When the horse had struck an easy, steady lope I raised my hands from Ed's shoulders and with arms wide-spread fancied I was a trick rider. As a joke Ed thought he would disturb my balance a little by slowing the horse's pace a bit. He pulled gently on the bridle and the vaquero horse true to his training stopped dead still. I did not! I flew over the heads of boy and horse and came down with a thump in the deep dust of the farm road, sitting upright. The dust fortunately softened the fall and I was not hurt.

The great earthquake of 1868 occurred when I was about eight years old. Again an indelible memory is due to an act of disobedience which to my mind brought in its wake a disciplinary act of God.

There had been a birthday in the family and as usual a birthday cake, frosted white and decorated with tiny pink peppermint candies and the name of the honored child in pink granulated sugar across the top. Some of these trimmings had been left over and mother had carefully put them away on the top shelf of the dish cupboard. One day when I had been helping wipe the noon dinner dishes, I climbed up on a high chair to put them back on the proper shelf. The left-over candy was temptingly near and I was just helping myself to a bit of it when the whole house began to shake. The dish-cupboard swayed from the wall; my high-chair pedestal toppled and I was thrown to the floor, thoroughly convinced God had been watching me and had shaken me down to save the candy and to punish me for my wickedness. Mother was too distressed upon finding the pantry floor and shelves swimming in milk and cream from the rocking milk-pans to take any notice of my share in causing this seismic catastrophe.

CHAPTER 2

Youthful Days

FOR THE MOST PART MY GIRLHOOD WAS A HAPPY ONE. SCHOOL DAYS were always joyous to me. Most unfortunately at the age of twelve, I had a severe illness diagnosed as typhoid fever. I have always doubted the diagnosis as it left me with internal adhesions and a focus of infection from which I have always suffered and which later necessitated a serious surgical operation. But suffering or not, I never stopped so long as I could keep going, and doubtless increased the trouble by intemperate sports, such as excessive horseback riding and dancing. And, yes, by excessive work in my medical career. The demands of that profession take no account of the physical condition of the doctor. Many times, day and night, I have attended patients less ill than myself.

Adjoining Uncle George's farm to the west, lived the Turner family, one of whom, Eva Turner was my girlhood chum. There were no girl cousins of my age and much as I loved the boy cousins and enjoyed playing with them, even Ed could not take the place of a girl confidante with whom to have prodigious secrets as we learned the mysteries of life. Going home from school with this chum to spend the night, or having her come with us, were memorable events of the first half of my second decade. It was with this friend that I first left home to begin independent life and to be inducted into the experiences of a mountain "school-ma'am."

Doubtless to modern youth our sports would seem tame but not so to us. Our games at school and various contests in athletics were just as exciting and our prowess equal to that of football teams in the grammar grades now-a-days.

To be sure there were no movies to entice us as children. There were no automobiles, no railroads even in our earlier years, no telephones, no radios nor any electrical devices nor conveniences, save the telegraph. And the telegram was so sacredly reserved for business or the announcement of death or dire disaster that I doubt not the receipt of one would have alarmed our parents.

Not knowing of present day methods of amusement, we did not miss them. Our parties were just as gay and perhaps more so than the present day formal. Buggy-riding was as entertaining as the automobile, possibly less thrilling because less speedy, but it was also less destructive of life and possibly of morals as well. While the auto has a great advantage in getting somewhere speedily, driving a spanking team or riding a prancing steed can give as great thrills as driving an automobile sixty miles an hour on paved roads.

Horseback riding was my chief joy but dancing and dramatics followed a close second. At sixteen I thought the one thing I should demand in a husband would be that he must be a perfect waltzer. To float through space to the strains of Strauss' "Blue Danube Waltz" seemed unalloyed joy to me.

Next to our relations, the family of Uncle Albert Willson were our most intimate friends. Visits to their dairy ranch occupied a week or two of nearly every vacation. The trip of twelve or more miles to their ranch near San Felipe beyond Tule Lake was always a great adventure. Aunt Eliza Willson was the personification of hospitality, and having no daughters she seemed to have a special fondness for Laura and me. Anyway we were often invited to pay visits.

There were three Willson boys but only two, Carlon and Fred, were old enough to be companionable with us. As little tots we would play housekeeping among the then seemingly huge boulders on the hillside in a pasture across the road from the house and dairy. Huge those boulders were to an eight- or ten-year-old child. Yet that child drove by there fifty years later and could see only medium-sized rocks on that hilly slope— Uncle George's experience with the home farm over again.

Laura married when I was thirteen and named her first child Albert for our beloved Uncle Albert Willson.

In my middle 'teens I sometimes took a girl friend with me on these visits. One such visit stands out vividly in my mind because of a memorable adventure. We two girls went up into this same pasture for a walk and also to read. I recall that the book was Owen Meredith's *Lucile*. We sat down on some rocks under an old sycamore tree by the side of one of California's innumerable dry creeks.

We were engrossed in Lucile's harrowing love affairs when a bellow brought us rudely back from fancy to stern reality. We knew we were in the pasture of the dairy cattle but supposed them all to be harmless milch cows. But alas! There was the lord of the herd, and apparently not in a friendly mood, for he was bellowing and pawing the dust, though he was still a considerable distance from us.

I knew this to be a sign of danger. We jumped up to run. This attracted his attention and he started toward us with lowered head and angry mien. We realized that we could not reach the fence. What should we do? The sycamore tree! We were not tree-climbers and the long full skirts of those days were not aids to agility. By good fortune there was a great limb of the sycamore stretching out over the dry creek. We could easily straddle that and work our way out on the almost horizontal limb to a point over the middle of the creek bed where our dangling legs were out of reach of the angry beast, which had by this time reached the tree.

Great was his disgust at losing his prey and he demonstrated his wrath by circling the tree trunk, bellowing and pawing for what seemed an eternity. The afternoon waned and dusk approached. There we sat astride that life-saving branch of the tree, one part of its huge divided trunk. Below was the angry bull. Occasionally he would go off some distance, causing our spirits to rise, but soon he would return as if just waiting for us to come down. Needless to say, we did not gratify his expectations.

Finally when we did not appear for supper, Fred Willson started out on horseback to find us. When his horse hove in sight, loud were our shouts for help. He drove the now somewhat calmed-down terror across the field and then returned and herded us safely to the fence which we climbed with alacrity.

Despite numerous such near fatalities I have lived to round out my three score years and ten, and as I recall the first two decades of my life, one of the richest experiences of my later 'teens was the friendship with Carlon Willson. It was one of those fine normal friendships which sensible boys and girls can have. Next to Cousin Edmond he was my closest companion in all of the parties, picnics and other gaieties of our high school days. Although other young gallants began to figure on my horizon, our friendship never flagged until I became a school teacher in San Juan and he went to Oakland to a Military Academy. After that our pathways drifted apart.

This was one of those boy and girl friendships which one can recall in old age with genuine pleasure and without any blush of shame or regret for youthful familiarities. We had royally good times horseback-riding and buggy-riding but in those buggy-rides there was never a thought of "petting parties." Such things were not unknown in those days any more than now, though the automobile and darkened movies have doubtless increased the opportunities. But human nature has not changed. It was the same then as now.

* * * * * * *

Almost every summer our family went camping below Monterey where Pacific Grove now thrives. Sometimes we went farther to Carmel, Point Lobos, or up the Carmel Valley into the hills. Always the trip meant an all-day trek across the San Juan or Gavilan Mountains and the Salinas Valley. Until very recently the San Juan grade has been unloved by autoists, but the old grade now supplanted at a lower level by a wide highway was a mere bagatelle compared to the old-time wagon-road which went over the top of the range. So steep was the ascent that everyone able to do so walked to lighten the load. As a child I often guided the reins of the horses which climbed as far as they wished to and then stopped to blow.

Many are the pleasurable memories of the rocky coast, the coves, the shells which we carried home by the sackfull. Light House Point, Moss Beach and the white sand-dunes could tell many tales of our childhood escapades. Rolling down the sand-dunes was one exhilarating sport. But alas for the present-day children, the dunes have largely been hauled away by carloads to make fine glass.

The old Carmel Mission was a favorite playground. "Hide and Seek" could be successfully played in the roofless old church with its corner staircases, belfrys, and other nooks and crannies. Mother was always worried lest the crumbling walls should fall and bury us. Beautiful old ruin!

To add to its beauty, mystery and charm, there lived or existed near by an old woman said to be a hundred and fifteen years old, who had carried mortar to help the builders of the Mission. A living skeleton was she, lying on a skin rug in the corner of an ancient adobe. The Mission was built in 1777, and we saw this woman in the early 1870s. She was said to have been about fifteen or sixteen when the church was erected. We also met her grandson, who was over eighty years old.

Years later Mrs. Stanford had the old church restored, but not to its pristine beauty—its typical Spanish architecture. Instead of the low tile roof a steep shingled roof was substituted.

Soon after the restoration of the Mission I took a friend to see it. We drove over the famous Seventeen-Mile Drive and finally came in sight of the Mission. As I saw the tall gabled roof I gasped, turned the horses' heads and drove away. I could not endure this desecration of my childhood idol.

* * * * * * *

At sixteen I finished the Gilroy school in a class of which I was the youngest member. Several of the older pupils were going to San Jose to take the State examinations to secure teachers' certificates. The principal urged me to go as he wished to test my ability. I went, and secured a second grade certificate which entitled me to teach in grammar grades.

My chum, Eva Turner, obtained a school in Bitter Water, a country district in Monterey County. She learned there was another school twenty miles farther south in a sparsely settled district named Peachtree. To me this name suggested large orchards of the luscious fruit. Later I was told that once a lone peach tree had sprouted in this treeless region but had long ago succumbed to the arid soil. Probably John Clifton's version of the origin of the name was more nearly correct.

Eva urged me to apply for this school and go with her. I was eager to do so but mother objected because of my youth and delicate health. Our family physician advised her to let me go as it was only for the Spring term and he thought the change would be beneficial.

So one day Eva and I set forth anticipating thrilling experiences as school teachers. We took a train to Hollister whence a stage made bi-weekly trips down into the country for which we were destined. It had been raining for two weeks. All the streams were swollen and rampant and the rough mountain roads were ground into mud almost axle-deep.

Late one Thursday afternoon we reached the hotel in Hollister where we were to spend the night and where the stage driver made his head-quarters. In the evening we sought out the driver who had arrived late. We found a gruff middle-aged man who utterly refused to take us as he had not been able to bring the usual stage-coach and had barely got through the mud and swollen streams with an open spring wagon. He could not take any extra load nor assume any risk for our lives.

We argued and implored. Our schools would open on Monday. We must be there. We would take our own risks. He was adamant. So were we. We insisted we would go if we had to hang on behind the wagon. Finally our determination broke down further resistance and he said, "Well, you can't take any trunks." "All right!" He would have to start very early in the morning as the roads were so bad. Again, "All right! We'll be ready." The bargain was sealed.

At five next morning we were ready. With only a handbag, we made our start at about six o'clock, seated with the driver on the one and only seat of the open vehicle. A cold wind was blowing, but fortunately the rain held off. Chilled to the marrow, our teeth almost chattered during the first hour or two. The road wound up a canyon through which a moun-tain stream tore its way. Usually an easily forded stream, it was now filled to the brink. Never a bridge was there and the stream had to be crossed twenty times or more. The river bed was virtually the road for many miles. Soon we realized why the driver had been so loath to take us. Many times the horses had to swim the turbulent stream.

Eva reached her destination in the late afternoon but more hours of travel confronted me. By now the adventure did not seem so delightful as I had anticipated. About dusk I found myself an unexpected guest in the only house within three miles of the school. The clerk of the school district who had engaged me as teacher and had supposedly made arrangements for my board had neglected to negotiate with the people with whom he had told me I was to live. Fortunately we settled the matter satisfactorily and I had a pleasant home in a family with three grown daughters who provided companionship of my own age.

The school-house was situated on the top of a hill about a half-mile distant. It was a one-room, roughboard, unpainted structure. Fortunately the rear end was well anchored in the sloping hill-side or it would have blown away in some of the late winter storms. The front entrance rested on stilts or light timbers four or five feet high with flimsy steps leading up to an equally flimsy porch. To my surprise I found myself janitor as well as teacher, but I accepted it as "all in the day's work."

On Monday nineteen pupils, ranging in age from the stupid five-year-old son of the Clerk of the Board to an equally stupid young fellow of twenty-two presented themselves. The rest of the pupils were of average age and intelligence. I have forgotten all of them except these two, the youngest and the oldest. Nearly all of the primary and grammar grades were represented in the school.

Life was humdrum enough after the first excitement had settled into a routine. Out of about one hundred and twenty days spent in the arid, treeless region ironically called Peachtree, two days only stand out—days in which something exciting occurred. Is not that true of life? The incidents one remembers are the few outstanding ones, the days that are different from the ordinary routine?

During the four months school term the usual day meant climbing that half-mile hill path rain or shine, before half past eight, sweeping the school-room—a room about eighteen by twenty-four feet—starting the fire and having things both physical and intellectual, in readiness for the straggling pupils and the nine o'clock call to order. I could usually inveigle some of the boys into chopping kindling and bringing in wood for the next day, so I escaped that irksome task.

Day after day for four months, there were the same recitations and explanations of "readin', 'ritin' and 'rithmetic," plus "gography." Two Saturdays during this time I remember vividly, because they included my favorite sports of horseback-riding twice, and dancing thereafter, once. One of those rides might easily have been my last.

Of all my horseback experiences the riding of a locoed horse was the most hair-raising. I had determined to vary the monotony of my life by hiring a saddle horse to ride after school. The horse was represented as being well-broken but the information that he had been pasturing on loco-weed and was therefore virtually insane, was not forthcoming. The fact that he had to be blind-folded and led up parallel with the garden gate in order that I could mount through the opening, out of the way of his heels, was explained by the statement that he was nervous owing to having been out at pasture for several months, but would soon be all right.

I had misgivings about entrusting myself to an animal of such vicious behavior, but priding myself on being a good sport I was vaulted into the saddle by one man while another held the horse.

No sooner was the blind lifted and the bridle loosed than he bounded off on a dead run across the rough country, regardless of roads. The men seeing my danger followed, but could not overtake this wild steed.

The great peril came when a gulch, a deep crack in the earth's crust yawned before us. It was about six feet wide at this point and probably ten or twelve feet deep. With all my strength I sawed on the bit and tried to turn the horse's course but on he flew. Loco-weed is said to affect an animal's vision causing shortsightedness, but this time the frantic steed measured his distance fairly or else my good angel intervened. The horse leaped into the air and came down on the other side of the gulch. I had visioned a sad mix-up of horse and rider at the bottom of the gorge.

On he flew. The next obstruction was a fence. A farm road led to the gate. This he followed and sailed into the air to hurdle the gate which fortunately was a pair of bars. This time he misjudged the distance or the hurdle was too high, as only his fore legs scaled the bars. My rescuers were close behind and before the horse could recover his balance, they grabbed the bridle and one man held him while the other let down the bars.

Ignominiously my horse was led home, and I alighted unharmed, through the gateway where I had mounted the maddened beast.

The following day a vaquero tried the animal, certain that he could conquer anything in horseflesh. The next we heard was of a dismounted rider limping along, and scraps of a saddle strewn for miles down the valley. The horse was never heard of again so far as I know. I anticipated a bill from the owner for one lost horse but neither the owner nor the bill ever appeared. I decided to do without a saddle-horse the rest of the term.

One more memorable ride I had in Peachtree. This time it was an antic rather than a frantic one. It was May Day, the holiday picnic of the whole country-side. There was to be an all-day picnic about fifteen miles away where there was a stream with some trees. This was to be followed by an all-night dance in the school-house. People came from such distances and the roads were so bad that they could not go home until daylight.

Near Bitter Water lived the family of Mr. E. Tully, noted in John Clifton's diary. Mr. Tully was a brother of Judge Tully of Gilroy. He had three sons, whom I had met when they visited their cousins, my schoolmates. Occasionally one of these young men had ridden over on a Saturday leading an extra horse for me and we would take a horseback ride.

On this May Day they all came, bringing Eva Turner with them. They also brought me their finest vaquero horse. Such a beauty! But so excitable! He had never been ridden by a woman and the unusual side-saddle plus the long-skirted riding habit of those days excited the mettlesome steed still more.

There was a whole troop of riders and this horse must be in the lead. Reining him in only made him chafe at the bit all the more. If the distance was fifteen miles, I am sure I rode thirty additional ones on that prancing steed. Frolicking and playing games filled the day. A repetition of the forty-five mile ride (as I estimated my horse's prancing) and dancing all night on a rough floor with country youths, was an experience of rural festivities sufficient for a lifetime!

CHAPTER 3

Undercurrents

AFTER MY FIRST EXPERIENCE IN TEACHING I ENTERED A PRIVATE school preparatory for college, but another opportunity to teach lured me away. One evening a gentleman called and introduced himself as the principal of the San Juan School. He said one of their teachers was ill and I had been recommended by the County Superintendent to replace her. They wanted someone at once. I accepted and rode to San Juan with him that evening and found myself installed as teacher of the intermediate grades. There were three teachers, the principal, the primary grades teacher and myself with the lower grammar grades. I remained there two years, from the time I was seventeen until I was nineteen, two eventful years of my life.

Great was my joy the second term to have Clara Edwards installed as the primary teacher, the same Clara Edwards with whom I was not permitted to play when a four-year-old. Her father was now minister of the San Juan church. Once when I was about fifteen I had visited the church, and Clara, who was then a Mills College student, entered and walked up to the organ. She was dressed in a bottle-green riding habit with a black silk-felt hat, a miniature "stovepipe hat" as the men's dress-up hats were dubbed. As she began to play my heart bowed in silent adoration of the superb creature. Now, several years later she was to be my fellow teacher. The association was one of the happiest of my life and ripened into a lifelong friendship.

One of the attractions in San Juan was a group of fine people into whose circle I was admitted. Among them were the Flints and Bixbys of old-time fame in California history, both civic and political; the Canfields, also old-time settlers; and other fine families, more recent comers. They formed the Harmony Club to enliven the winter and to go camping in the summer-time. All ages were represented in these camping parties from Dr. Flint, for many years State Senator, down to the Bixby children. There were also several San Francisco members. I especially remember the Searles brothers and Lily Shipman. A regular caravan we formed as we started over the same old San Juan grade, and a village of tents soon arose on the camping ground, now the site of Pacific Grove.

For two summers it was my privilege to join this merry group. The second summer came near ending my career, for as far as consciousness is concerned I was drowned. Dr. Flint restored me after I was rescued, but the full experience of drowning was mine.

It was Sunday. Someone proposed going swimming. I hesitated for I had had the commandment, "Remember the Sabbath day to keep it holy," thoroughly instilled into my mind and principles. It still clings. Clara Edwards and I discussed the question as to whether we should join the majority of the party or stay in camp. Finally Clara ended the discussion of our conscientious scruples by saying, "Cleanliness is next to godliness. If we cannot be godly, let's be clean. Come on, let's go!" We went though my conscience still troubled me.

Russ Canfield was teaching me to swim. The surf was heavy and a huge wave washed us out far beyond my depth. He lost hold of me and I became frightened and sank. I went to the bottom, about twenty feet I should judge. It is said a drowning person reviews his whole lifetime. I did not do that but I thought of my mother, of my failure to do all a daughter should do for her and of her grief at my death. My mind was so filled with fear, that death seemed certain. Then I rose to the surface. One man swimming to my rescue was at hand, and with the traditional instinct of a drowning person I grabbed his throat in such a way that he had to shake me loose.

Before I sank the second time I saw Jim Searles, the champion swimmer of the camp, dive from a point of rocks and I knew he was coming to save me. But as I lay on the bottom for what seemed to me an endless time, my fear departed and was replaced by a sort of ecstacy. As consciousness left me my last thought was, "I hope they will not find me; this is so beautiful." Glorious coloring, wonderful beauty and peace formed my semi-conscious experience.

Unaware of anything I again rose to the surface. Jim Searles was not quite near enough to reach me but as I sank the third time he dived and caught hold of my pleated bathing-suit skirt. Thus he towed me ashore. The next I knew I was being rolled on the beach to get the water out of my lungs.

In passing let me speak a word in favor of the full bathing-suits, now a subject of humorous caricature for modern beach-fans. Pray tell me what my rescuer could have caught hold of had I been clad in a modern, skin-tight, postage-stamp bathing-suit? Anyway I am thankful for the wide knee-length skirt which enabled James Searles to save my life. Also my gratitude includes Dr. Flint for his services in restoring me to consciousness.

As I indicated, my experience verified the tradition that drowning is one of the pleasantest of deaths. This is a way of departing this life from which those who fail to reach the other side of the River Styx, may return to relate their sensations. But no one to my knowledge has related the sensations of being restored. That to me was most painful. Such a headache for twenty-four hours I have rarely suffered. And the respiratory tract also resented its internal bath of salt water. I recovered without further evil effects.

Another narrow escape from drowning occurred during my two years in San Juan, an occurrence somewhat similar to the Salinas River flood; though this time the danger was needless.

Another almost dry river, the San Benito, lay between San Juan and Gilroy. Like most California rivers rising in the mountains and crossing the narrow state toward the sea, it had a wide sandy bed with but a narrow fordable stream in summer, but became a tempestuous torrent carrying everything before it, after heavy and protracted rainstorms.

On one such occasion I wanted to go home one week-end for an important party. Friends tried to dissuade me but I decided to drive down to the river and see how it looked. As noted in the childhood hat episode it is very difficult for me to give up an idea once my mind is set on it.

The river was nearly bank full, a surging, muddy torrent. The stage came along just as I reached the river. The driver said he was going to cross and would wave to me as to whether or not I should try it. He knew the "ford" well so could keep his four horses on the narrow strip of rocky roadway. He signaled me not to cross. I mistook his signal and plunged in.

My horse was a large bay loaned me by Uncle Albert Willson for my week-end trips home. In a moment the water was well up on the horse's sides and coming into the buggy. He lost the only solid footing, the regular ford, and was soon forced to swim for his life and mine. The buggy swirled around down stream with the force of the current. The horse was swimming valiantly. I plied the whip to urge him on. Well I remember thinking, when in the middle of the stream, "What will Uncle Albert say if his horse drowns?"

The river seemed miles wide. The stage-driver was yelling directions which I could not hear because of the roar of the water. The women passengers were screaming and the men passengers were shouting, "Do this!" "Do that!" I could only ply the whip and shout encouragingly to the horse. How that splendid animal did swim!

At last, after what seemed eons, he touched bottom. And how that stage driver did scold me. I am alive to tell the tale, and I went to the party. This occurred in my eighteenth year.

* * * * * * *

The next incident is too painful to tell merely as a story. I would omit it but for the fact that it influenced my whole after life and was indirectly the cause of my choosing the profession of medicine.

This sad experience changed me from a thoughtless girl interested chiefly in good times. It caused me to think much more seriously on the meaning of life, and I thought hazily of becoming a missionary or doing something for the world that would make my life worth while. How it was to come about I did not know but one thing I decided on. As soon as I could save enough money I would go east to my grandmother's, to learn something of the eastern culture which Aunt Mary and Aunt Ruth had held out as a lure for one born and raised in the Wild West.

October of that year brought the hard experience which not only made an indelible impression, but told heavily on my emotional nature and my health.

I have said nothing of beaus or love affairs. Of the latter there had been no real ones. During the two years since escorts had been permitted I had not been interested in any one but liked them all and accepted the invitations of various young men. This, I thought, was the more honorable course—showing no partiality. As soon as one became sentimental I would avoid him. But I was quite a favorite and had difficulty in keeping several of them on friendly terms.

The principal of the San Juan school was a young Tennesseean, morose in temperament and not at all attractive to me. In fact I disliked him at first, but had to keep on friendly terms with him. He was fond of horseback riding and so was I, hence a few times I accepted his invitation for a gallop over the hills.

On one of these occasions he told me his life story. His father had become insane before his, the son's, birth. When he was but a few days old an insane act of his father's had cost his mother's life. He was orphaned early for his father had to be confined and soon died. The nurse in whose care he was placed was evidently unwise and embittered his mind with the tragedy, which he could not have remembered. He had dwelt on this all his life and anticipated his father's fate, but said he would never live to endure it.

This explained what Clara Edwards and I had considered his moroseness, and thereafter I tried to be kinder, but at the same time avoided buggy-rides or close proximity to him.

One evening he called to tell me he had been asked by Julia Canfield to bring me to a "bee" of some sort at her home. As Julia had written me to the same effect, I could not refuse. Mr. H. smiled and said, "This time you will have to go buggy-riding with me." During this call he assumed more of a lover-like attitude than he had ever displayed before, but I pretended not to notice it.

The evening of the party came. The Canfield ranch was about three miles from town. Mr. H. drove up with a spanking span of grays, known to be the most temperamental team in the livery stable. The buggy was an open one. We started. I was nervous about both the team and the driver, though I tried to be lively and nonchalant.

When about half way to the ranch, he suddenly turned some nonsense into a dramatic proposal, stopped the horses and dropped on one knee while holding that unreliable span of horses. Later he told me he was glad I did not love him for it would mean sorrow to me and that he must never marry anyone, but that he had loved me ever since he had known me. This was the third semester of our association as teachers and I had never guessed his state of mind.

My pleasure for the evening was spoiled and I wondered how I could go on teaching with him.

Finally the evening ended and we started homeward. The team was cold and weary of standing. Scarcely were we seated than off they went and were soon beyond his control. Mr. H. managed to keep them on the road. The mettlesome horses wanted to get home more speedily than was safe and resented any effort to stop them or guide them. Fortunately the road was straight so we ultimately dashed into the livery stable unharmed. Needless to say I insisted we should walk to my boarding place.

This happened on Thursday evening. Friday evening Mr. H. went to Watsonville to visit his old nurse as he often did over week-ends. He had just been conducting a lively candidacy for the office of County Superintendent of Schools and had been defeated by a small margin the week before.

Doubtless the excitement and pre-election strain had upset his mental poise and were partly responsible for the tragedy which followed. He had spoken of it to me, saying life held only defeat and disappointment for him.

The following Monday afternoon he came into my school-room and asked if he could call that evening. I pleaded a mythical engagement. Then the next evening? I was going home with Clara Edwards, though I had not thought of it before. Wednesday evening? Again a lame excuse. Thursday evening? My inventive ingenuity was exhausted so I reluctantly said yes.

When Thursday afternoon came I felt I could not spend an evening with him, but had no excuse to offer. However, I was troubled. As I started home I passed the stairway to the upper floor where he taught the higher grades. Scarcely knowing that I did it, I flew up the stairs and walking up to his desk said, "Mr. H., I am sorry but I cannot see you this evening." He replied, "You mean you will not." "No, I cannot. Please excuse me." He turned very pale and said, "I have something important to tell you." I could not relent. So, seeing my misery, he added, "I see how it is. Goodbye."

Two or three pupils were still in the room. One of the older girls whom I knew well was among the number. She chanced to be the last one to leave the room. As she reached the street, possibly five minutes later, she heard a shot. So did the janitor, who found Mr. H. lying on the platform behind his desk mortally wounded. On the blackboard was written, "To Mary: The problem is solved. Remember my virtues; forget my vices." On his desk lay a book of poems with a pencil in it. Heavily underscored were the words, "It is better to have loved and lost than never to have loved at all." He died two or three days later. Clara and I went to see him the second day. He recognized us and tried to smile, but no word ever explained his act.

The effect of this tragedy upon me was a great nervous shock, but I had to keep up a brave face as no one except Clara Edwards knew that I was in any way involved. Though not blaming myself this tragic episode made such a deep impression on me that I resolved never to allow myself to be placed in the position of refusing another man. I concluded that I was hard-hearted and could not love anyone, or that my ideas of love were too exalted to be realized.

While the incidents related thus far may give the impression of a thoughtless, head strong girl (which was partly true), these characteristics were somewhat in the common ratio of ordinary life, of exciting days to steady, plodding work-days. Persistence, faithfulness, devotion to duty, made up the deep pool of character under the ripples, or at times, high waves of gaiety on the surface. But waves may be blown in wrong directions by strong winds and so do great damage. Emotions such as faithfulness and devotion to duty, good in themselves, may cause one to be tempest-tossed and landed on dangerous rocks or shoals.

The emotional storm caused by the San Juan tragedy, innocent of it though I was, landed me on an island reef from which it required considerable time and effort to rescue me and set me upon terra firma again. After the shock I was left with two conflicting convictions: The deep, still waters asserted, "You must make yourself worth something to the world"; and the restless surface dashed against the stony shore with, "You must never hurt another man through thoughtlessness, as you evidently did hurt this man with whom you were associated as principal and teacher."

Thus tempest-tossed, I struggled on to the end of the school year, meanwhile planning to go East for a year and thus try to escape from myself and at the same time see something of the world, with the hope that some worthwhile and congenial avenue of self-expression would present itself. Unfortunately the disturbed surface was the first to again feel the force of life's currents.

In Gilroy a young man of apparently admirable character and one especially pleasing to mother had been paying me attention for a year or more. I was away teaching most of the time but he was always on hand during week-ends and vacations. A few years earlier he had come to Gilroy to accept a position of responsibility. Although most "proper" in every way, he was not my ideal, but I respected him and mother preferred him to the town boys. It was convenient to have someone to rely on, so things had drifted during the two years I taught in San Juan.

The summer of 1878 found me busy getting ready for my first transcontinental trip, the first of so many that I cannot remember them all. The great adventure of going three thousand miles from home was thrilling. I was to accompany a friend who was returning to Wellesley College after the summer vacation.

Just before the time to start the attentive young man avowed his love for me and his great need of me in his life. I was stricken dumb. The horror of the San Juan tragedy came back to me. What could I do? The thought of the trip East seemed a loophole. Perhaps while I was away he would forget. So I replied, "Give me time to think."

After he had gone I went out into the rear garden and under the stars fought out the question with myself. Which was to be sacrificed, this fine young man or myself? I decided that I should be the one and determined that I could make myself love him, and would do so. So I told him that if he would be satisfied with a Platonic engagement and an arms-length friendship, I would consent. Anyway I was going away the next week and would write to him. Thus I tried to quiet the surging waves.

The change to my grandmother's home in New Preston, Connecticut, was a decided one. As I indicated in the opening chapter, grandmother was a delight. To me she was a beautiful picture, and her stories of her youth, and her songs were bewitching for a time. But she was nearly eighty years old and confined to a wheel-chair. Aunt Ruth, Aunt Mary and Uncle Hiram made up the family. I realize now that these maiden aunts and bachelor uncle were not antediluvian even though aged somewhere between thirty-five and forty-five, but as the weeks dragged on the difference in our years seemed to increase.

Soon Aunt Louise Beeman, the oldest daughter of the Bennett family, invited me to make her a visit. Her home was about three miles away. It was a large square house on a hilltop overlooking the beautiful Lake Waramaug. Uncle Ed Beeman was a jolly soul with a fondness for young people. And they had four of them—a daughter Loraine of my own age, who was away at boarding school; a second daughter, Helen, fifteen; and two boys, Will and Edwin Jr., aged ten and eight years. Here was the environment I wanted. Such fun I had with the children and such wonderful rides along the lakeshore to New Preston, either for pleasure or marketing. After one of these rides Helen came home with a severe headache and sore throat. It proved to be diphtheria. Quarantine must be established.

Thus entered into my life one of its finest friendships. A cousin of the Bennetts, hence my second cousin, happened to come in that day. He lived in Texas and was home for a visit. Having been a captain in the Civil War he had remained in the South.

Aunt Louise suggested to this cousin, Captain John Whittlesey, that he take me to his sister's home in Washington Green, eight miles beyond New Preston that I might be under the watchful eye of her husband, Dr. Orlando Brown, and where I could be with young people. The Browns had two daughters and a son near my age. I cannot dwell on these kind friends, but "Cousin John" became one of the greatest influences of my life. Although older than my aunts and uncle in the New Preston home, he was thoroughly congenial and a hero in my eyes.

The long, cold buggy-ride a week later to Helen's funeral provided opportunity for him to probe into the deep waters of my soul. This heart-breaking occasion, Helen's untimely death, brought my most serious self to the surface. John Whittlesey knew the real me by the time that long sad day was over, and he proved to be the one friend to help me years later carry out my heart's deepest desire although neither of us dreamed at that time what it would prove to be.

Soon Cousin John returned to Texas for the winter. Before going he warned the serious-minded girl he knew, that "Your devotion to duty will be the death of you if you are not careful."

During the holiday season Loraine came home, and soon after her newly-acquired fiancé, Edward Hayes, followed to make a visit and meet Loraine's parents. Jolly times ensued as there were plenty of young people around for sleigh-rides, skating and what to me were novel winter sports.

At this same time a distant cousin who was associated in business with John Whittlesey came from Houston, Texas. Cousin John had asked him to help me have a good time. He did. Never will I forget one sleigh-ride! Four of us, Loraine and Mr. Hayes, Mr. Cogswell and I started out with a spanking black team for a moonlight ride. The night was clear and cold—oh so cold! But ample robes and hot stones at our feet left only the cheeks to feel the stinging wind.

We were singing, joking and laughing when suddenly I noticed the black horses were white. Such a freak of Jack Frost was unknown to me, and my amazement caused great merriment. The point of this story is that John Whittlesey later wrote me: "Cogswell has returned and remarked, 'My! what a jolly girl our California cousin is!' It had never occurred to me that you were jolly. I found you a very serious girl." The deep waters had been stirred by one man—the ripples by the other.

So the winter passed, but before I leave the subject I must tell my young Californians of some other surprises Jack Frost, or "King Cold" had for me. It was bad enough to find the water in the pitcher frozen solid in my room in the mornings, but when I tried to make a cake and the solid eggs would not break, and the milk was a cake of ice, I was puzzled. Again, a steak was a board-like hardness. But when Aunt Louise asked me to go to the pantry and bring her a pan of squash prepared for pies and I found that frozen also, I decided that anything that stood still would freeze in a New England winter. Therefore I kept on the move.

In the Spring, Aunt Mary and I made a trip to New York and Washington—my introduction to the country's metropolis and capital. Little did I dream as I visited the interesting points in Washington, particularly the United States Senate and Supreme Court, how many months I later would sit on those hard benches, an attentive listener to these highest law-making bodies of our nation.

Visits in Boston, Hartford, New Haven, Bridgeport and other places filled in the early summer. Then Cousin John Whittlesey returned for his annual summer with his parents. Before I was to leave for home, he planned a trip to the White Mountains with friends. Of course we went to the top of Mount Washington where we had the unique experience of being above the clouds and coming down through them on the little funicular railroad.

October 1879 found me home again. The wrench in leaving New England was caused by the parting from my lovely grandmother whom I never expected to see again. The others I saw repeatedly in my many trips across the continent in later years.

My fiancé had visited me in Connecticut. It had been quite a feather in my cap to have a lover come all the way from California. On the other hand it was a relief that his visit was very short, about a week. Upon my return he met me in San Jose and I again undertook the self-education of making myself love him. No thrills resulted, but I honestly and sincerely respected and trusted him. I thought of him as a paragon, superior in honor and ideals to most young men.

Therefore when a few months later, without the least warning something occurred which caused him to tell me he was not worthy of me and that he could not marry me although he loved me, and me only, my faith in mankind received another severe shock. The blow was a heavy one for I had trusted him implicitly.

How well I remember dear Cousin Ed coming to the rescue and taking me the next evening for a long buggy-ride during which we discussed life's problems most solemnly. Already I had reacted to the "intervention of Providence" theory, and had decided that this meant that I was to devote myself to some vocation that would be of service to the world. What it was to be I had no clear idea. The vague vision of a missionary in Madagascar again presented itself, but did not satisfy me. I ended it by telling Edmond that I would go to Professor Norton for advice. I felt sure he would be the Moses to lead me out of the wilderness.

Professor Norton was a teacher of the Natural Sciences in the San Jose Normal School. He was also a minister of the Gospel and the most Christ-like man I ever knew. There had been a schism in the Presbyterian church in Gilroy a few years previously, and a Congregational Society had been formed by the more liberal members, largely New England Congregationalists. They held services in a small hall and Professor Norton became the minister. He came down from San Jose on Saturdays and remained over Sunday, entertained by the various families of the congregation. Thus we came to know him intimately. To him I turned in this great crisis of my life.

I told him my story and said that I wanted to find some work that would make my life worth something to the world. Innately I felt that I had been entrusted with life and it was my duty to use it in some way that would make the world a little better for my having lived in it. "Teaching does not satisfy me," I said, "and I fear being a missionary is not quite to my liking." After questioning me closely but kindly, he said, "There is a form of missionary work that the world sadly needs, and as yet the number of workers is woefully inadequate. It means endless hard work, necessitates the sacrifice of ordinary pleasures, but I know of nothing that yields such rich rewards." Then he proceeded to delineate the opportunities for service for a woman physician and illustrated by telling me of the work of my future preceptress, Dr. Euthanasia S. Meade of San Jose.

I listened enraptured. My heart had never known such satisfaction as came from the picture he drew. When he had finished I sprang up from the sofa on which I sat opposite him and with hands tightly clasped, exclaimed, "Oh, Professor Norton, that is what I have always wanted but I had never known about it!"

"Think it over carefully," he cautioned. "It is a very serious undertaking." "I don't need to," I replied, "I know now."

Never for a moment did I waver in that resolution although it took years to accomplish it. I flew home on wings of air and announced explosively, "Mother, I'm going to be a physician." She looked surprised, but knowing the excitement under which I was laboring, said quietly, "Well, we'll see." "No, it is settled now for all time!" It was. The ways and means had yet to be earned and educational preparation was necessary. Mother relied on the effect of time and obstacles. My goal was far off.

CHAPTER 4

An Interlude

DURING THE SUMMER MONTHS MOTHER DECIDED SHE WANTED TO visit her sister in Sonora. She had never returned to Sonora, and had not seen her sister since she left there a young wife and mother nearly twenty-five years before. So with my brother as driver we three set forth to combine a camping trip with a visit to an unknown aunt.

Amelia Noble, mother's younger sister, had married Charles Tupper, an editor in Sonora, a man much older than herself. She had had a large family and had had a hard life. Mr. Tupper was a brilliant man but addicted to the cup that cheers, and in consequence had neglected his business, causing suffering to his family.

The oldest son, named for his father, had inherited his flair for writing. Besides attending school he had worked in the printing office and written poems and articles for the paper. Two or three years before our visit he had had a fall which injured his hip-joint. "Hip disease" or tuberculosis of the bone had developed and for more than a year he had been confined to the bed, lying flat on his back with a heavy weight for extension attached to his leg.

There he lay as we entered, pale as a ghost, with large, blue eyes shining out of his pallid, delicately-carved face. A shock of blond hair crowned his head. He looked like a poet and he was a poet at heart. His first reaction toward us was one of resentment—anger at the fates which had chained him to that bed up there in the mountains, while my brother and I, his cousins, were free to go whither we pleased.

As the week of our visit passed his mood changed and we two found ourselves kindred spirits, restless spirits, yearning for something beyond our reach. Educational opportunity was what he longed for. He could never have it there. A mission opened before me. Here was a patient, needing a doctor's care. To be sure I wasn't a physician but I felt sure I could help this boy to get well.

One day when our conversation led up to it, I blurted out, "Charlie, would you be willing to risk dying on the way if I would attempt to move you to Gilroy?"

"Indeed I would, gladly," Charles answered.

"All right," I said, "I'll ask mother's permission, but I know she will consent. But first you must get better. You cannot be moved until that abscess in your hip is healed. If you will grit your teeth and determine to improve, I'm positive you can get well enough to stand the journey, and once there you will recover, I'm sure."

My prophecy came true. In a few months Charlie Tupper was in our Gilroy home, having been carried there on a bed. I had promised mother that I would assume the extra care. With hope and courage renewed, with extra feeding, fresh air and tonics he gained miraculously. We spent the winter studying hard. One phase of our studies has brought great pleasure to me all my life, especially when in foreign lands. It was learning the constellations. When conditions were favorable, with map and a small lantern (there were no flashlights) we would go out in the garden and study the constellations visible during the first half of the night. Another time we would set the alarm clock for the wee small hours and study the skies until dawn.

By varying these studies during the seasons, at the end of the year we were acquainted with all the constellations in the northern hemisphere and they have greeted me as familiar friends in many strange countries. Often out on an ocean or in the Orient I have felt like saying, "Hello Orion, old friend, you here too?" Only in the South Seas did these old friends fail to greet me.

When I left home in the spring for my next school Charlie was walking on crutches; later one crutch was discarded and a cane substituted. In the course of two years he could walk easily with only a cane though one leg was permanently shortened. He secured a position on the Gilroy newspaper as type-setter, reporter and writer of special articles.

Years after, Charlie moved to San Jose and finally became an editor of a small paper. After his father's death his mother, with her large family, moved to San Jose and three generations of the Tupper descendants still live there. One is at present in the State Legislature. Charlie married and left two half-grown children when influenza carried him off.

Gradually the barriers to my ambition were cleared away. The cost of a medical education had been the greatest obstacle. To teach long enough to earn all the money necessary would take several years. In addition to mother's opposition she could not undertake the expense. All my friends save one objected to my plan, so there was none to whom I could turn for encouragement, nor from whom I could borrow money on the precarious security I could offer.

Here let me pay tribute to the one friend who understood and encouraged me from the first. She was my Sunday-school teacher, Mrs. Ball, a quiet Quaker woman. Her own life was largely devoted to a semi-invalid husband. She counseled with me and gave me courage. She said that each one had the right to choose his or her life-work; that ofttimes home life was as exacting as any outside career. She urged me to persevere in my purpose if I was sufficiently in earnest. Friendly advice however was the only help she could give me, but that was beyond price. The memory of that woman's kindly encouragement still warms my heart.

One other friend came to my aid. The summer following my return from Connecticut, John Whittlesey came to visit his California cousins, or at least one of them. My decision to study medicine had been made before his visit, though when I had known him in the East, a domestic life had apparently been settled upon. The upheaval in my plans for the future had been a major cause of his journey to the Pacific coast. He wanted to discuss the situation with me face to face.

Naturally he did not approve of my aspirations either concretely or abstractly. The general proposition did not appeal to him. He was not particularly attracted to professional women, nor did he feel any enthusiasm in my individual case. All the arguments he could muster were brought forth but to no avail. I was determined. After a month of discussion he said to me just before his departure, "Are you unalterably set on this plan?"

"Unalterably!" I exclaimed. "I shall study medicine if it takes half my life-time to prepare."

"Very well," he said, "then I will make a bargain with you. You teach school for two years and save up every dollar that you can. If at the end of that time you are still determined upon this course I will lend you whatever you need over and above your savings." The offer was accepted. My course was clear.

The unforeseen episode of my efforts in the restoration of my cousin Charles Tupper's health and my teaching extended my probationary period to three years.

By the time I was free to leave home after six months' care of my cousin, it was too late to secure a town school. In the early Spring a San Juan friend offered me a school at Firebaugh, one of the headquarters of the great Miller and Lux cattle ranges which stretched the length of the state. It was a common saying that Miller and Lux cattle could be driven from the Mexican to the Oregon border and rest every night on their own land. Their holdings were enormous.

Firebaugh is about thirty-five miles northwest of Fresno. Again the trip from Hollister must be made by stage. This time I went alone. The trip was uneventful save for the stop-over at night. The half-way house which the stage reached at nightfall was another Miller and Lux station, but a very dreary one. It was a barn-like hotel on a sheep range. As the driver stopped at the watering trough, another man was watering his team. I recognized him as one Jack, an Englishman, who had worked a few years before for my father. He recognized me also and asked, "What are you doing here?" "Going to Firebaugh to teach school."

"I'm sorry you are here tonight. I'm afraid there'll be a high old time. Sheep-shearing is just over and the men, mostly Mexicans, are coming in for their money and will be drinking and gambling. They won't molest you, but don't worry if you hear a little shooting." Then he added, "I don't usually mix with these men but I'll stay up tonight until they quiet down so you can know you have someone looking out for you."

This news was disquieting enough, but I had no alternative but to spend the night there, so tried not to worry. But when I went to the hotel door and was greeted by the proprietress, I thought I should faint. Of all women in the world, this one!

In Gilroy, years before, there had lived across the street from the school grounds, a queer woman whom we children were warned to avoid as she was known as a very bad woman. "Never go near that fence," we were told. Of just what her badness consisted, we did not comprehend, but we knew she was sometimes drunk and beat her children. She had disappeared years ago. As I entered that ramshackle hostelry this woman greeted me. The only woman within many miles! Had it not been for Jack's proximity I think I should have succumbed.

Swallowing, or endeavoring to swallow a hasty supper, I hastened to my room before the sheep-shearers appeared. My room! A small, one-windowed, carpetless box with no lock on the door. It was directly over the barroom. Through cracks and knot-holes in the floor I could see the bar and the men moving about. As a barrier I moved the light pine bureau against the door, and then my bed against the bureau. The window I locked with a nail in a hole for that purpose, and proceeded to suffocate, air-loving creature that I am.

Had sleep not been impossible because of fear, the noisy men would have prevented it. As they gambled and drank, drank and gambled, there alternated tense silence and noisy quarrels. Finally the quarreling became serious and a pistol shot rang out. Another and another. Quaking in my bed I wondered if the mattress would stop the stray bullets.

The fighters were dragged apart, the row quelled, and finally the gamblers one by one sought their beds to sleep off their drunkenness.

The wee sma' hours were getting large before nature's sweet restorative came to me. No "ten nights in a barroom" for me! One over a barroom was enough.

Arriving at Firebaugh, I was greeted by my San Juan friends now living there. Firebaugh was the main headquarters of the Miller and Lux holdings of that portion of the San Joaquin Valley. It was relatively quite a village although there were no residences, but the hotel, store, blacksmith shop, barns and other essentials for the vast ranches were commodious and well administered.

The hotel-keeper, Sam Wollenberg, was the former husband of an old family friend. His family consisted of two small boys, Roy and Russell, my pupils, and a housekeeper Amelia Spangler, all of whom were acquaintances, so I felt quite at home. Amelia was a good housekeeper and a famous cook. Everything was neat and clean and I was thoroughly comfortable. In this case, the inevitable barroom was not in evidence.

Scattered on the many ranches within a radius of fifteen miles, were families whose children made up the pupils of the school. Several nationalities were represented, among them a good sprinkling of Mexicans. The name of one of these made an indelible impression on me. All the other names have faded from my mind but "Jesus Christo" is a living memory. I was relieved to learn that the first name was pronounced, "He-soos," accent on the second syllable, which made it seem less a sacrilege.

To my dismay I found only six desks for about twenty pupils. Around the room were high benches on which the others were to sit. For two or three weeks I endured seeing those poor children sit hunched over on those benches, too high for their feet to touch the floor. The weariness of the little folk! The curved spines and bent legs were too much for me. I went to the school trustees, Mr. Wollenberg and the foreman of this region for Miller and Lux. My request for more desks was met with the reply, "There is no money." My most eloquent pleadings were of no avail. A few warped children apparently did not count in a ranch expense account. The same number of abused calves or lambs might have been a different matter. That would have been remedied at once.

I was indignant and determined that those children should have decent seats if it were the last thing I ever did. My announcement to this effect was met by incredulous smiles. Amelia and I put our heads together. She was an indefatigable worker and not much my senior in years. We decided to earn the money. We would give an entertainment followed by a dance. Thus everyone would contribute to the enterprise. But where should it be held? There was no town hall. The schoolroom was a mere box of a place with a rough floor. That would never do.

There was a fine large barn with a spacious loft, the floor of which was planed and would be fit for dancing when waxed. We appealed to the foreman, a kindly young man and a special friend of Amelia's. Yes, we could have the loft of the barn but it was still about a third full of last year's hay. Could that be taken out? "Well, yes, the hay could be put down below but there is no one to do it." We reconnoitered. The baled hay was piled high across the front end of the barn. On the floor near the rear was a large trapdoor through which the bales were dropped as needed.

Amelia and I were on our mettle. If the men were so mean that they wouldn't help us we would move the hay ourselves. We experimented and found that by pushing the top bale off it would bound along the floor some distance, and by keeping it rolling we could guide it to the trapdoor and down it would go—we didn't care where. This required agility rather than sheer muscle although we expended our full supply of both. The men were not really mean, but they considered our idea hare-brained and took this way of deterring us.

Finding their ruse did not work, after a few days they came to the rescue. Amelia and I had done our "daily dozen" after school, rolling off the higher bales. But to move the lower tiers was a different matter. That required sheer muscular power. We asked no quarter but soon helpers strayed in and the hay-rolling became quite a "bee." Likewise the cleaning of the barn, the building of a rude platform and the arrangements for seats. The school house benches, the hotel chairs and even the stock-chairs in the store, light rawhide bottomed chairs, were spirited to the barn for the audience. On the great evening, after the performance they were quickly ranged around the walls to make room for the dancers.

But the performance! What about that? Amelia and I were the main actors in what my nephew, Bert Warner, in a letter received last week, kindly called a "pageant." I cannot recall the whole program but it contained a one-act playlet, songs and recitations by the two stars. "Stars" is literal, for in the only song which I remember, Amelia was the morning star and I the evening star. "Star of the morning, beautiful star." Do you know the old song? We were clad in appropriate costumes made of five cent cotton material, the morning star in azure blue, the evening star in the deep grey of twilight. Huge gold stars on paper crowns adorned our heads. Can anyone deny our claim to stardom?

For the playlet we inveigled to our aid an Englishwoman and her daughter, recently from San Francisco, now living on a Miller and Lux ranch. I trained the whole school in a song or two, not so much because of their melodious voices as to enlist their interest. This was an advertising dodge, part of the plan by which to induce the parents to attend and contribute their fifty-cent entrance fee.

One preliminary to the success of the evening was a trip to Fresno one week-end, to procure the materials for our stage curtain and the various costumes. Everything had to be properly costumed. Amelia and I induced the foreman to provide us with a nondescript span of horses and a two-seated carry-all. It was my purpose to bring my sister, Laura Warner, and her three children back with me to see the pageant. My sister had offered to make my costumes while I taught and trained the children and other performers.

We started from Fresno Sunday morning with our passengers and purchases, for our thirty-five mile drive to Firebaugh. It was one of the coldest, rawest days that Fresno County can be guilty of. I remember the biting wind but Bert Warner speaks of the "cold, foggy day." Anyway it was bitterly cold. The road was simply rough wagon-tracks over thirty-five miles of uninhabited hog-wallows, as the peculiar knolls of sand are called. There was not a house on the way except one at White's Bridge, ten miles from Firebaugh. This was a toll-bridge across the San Joaquin River.

When miles from houses, water or aid of any kind, one horse began to lag. He appeared to be ill. Amelia and I got out to see what was the matter. The horse's tongue hung out of his mouth, dry and parched. What could we do? The only water within reach was that in a bottle for the children. But how could we make a horse drink out of a bottle? "Necessity is the mother of invention." We soaked our handkerchiefs and squeezed the water on the horse's tongue. He seemed to like it. One of us pushed his head up while the other trickled the water on his tongue until the bottle was empty.

The situation was really serious. To have the horses give out meant the stranding of three children and three women out in those plains on that bitterly cold day. The road was seldom traveled. The nearest help was at White's Bridge, five miles or more distant. By walking the horses and letting them rest occasionally, we finally reached Mr. White's. There we got another horse, and after resting both the team and ourselves and getting thoroughly warmed, we completed our journey.

Needless to say, the entertainment was a financial success. The hall, or barn, was crowded. The fiddlers and the dancers made merry after the program was ended. After expenses were paid we had one hundred and twenty dollars for the school. This provided the needed desks and some other necessities. It was worth the effort.

I remained at Firebaugh only during the spring term, as I secured a position in the Fresno schools. Before leaving the story of Firebaugh, I will record one event which has recently become historic.

The sheep-men and cattle-men from all over the San Joaquin Valley came occasionally to Firebaugh to lay in stores. Beside what they purchased they usually laid in store several of Amelia's good home-cooked meals. One of the occasional visitors was an old man who looked and lived like a hermit. He had taken up a large claim of sheep-grazing land through which the San Joaquin River ran. He lived alone in a cabin and tended his sheep. He surely approved of Amelia's cooking and I used to tease her about him much to her disgust, for she was devoted to the genial foreman.

Before I left she said to me, "If C—(the foreman) does not marry me I'll do something desperate." I tried to laugh it off and parried, "What? Commit suicide or marry old H. (the sheepman)?" She would not answer, but she did marry the old man. After some years he died leaving her with two daughters and the sheep ranch.

Many years later, the Southern Electric Company developed a great water and power supply for Southern California by damming the head waters of the San Joaquin River and creating Huntington Lake and its power plants. This was claimed to lessen the flow of water through the above-mentioned sheep-lands. The ensuing great battle of riparian rights in California was fought out in the courts. The early day enactment to protect placer-miners was held to be the law of the state, and a verdict of a million dollars was awarded to Amelia H. and her daughters.

* * * * * * *

My last school was in Fresno, where I taught for two years, by which time I felt that my savings warranted beginning my medical training. Mother had followed Laura to Fresno and built a house which chanced to be within three blocks of the school grounds. Here I was established with my mother and brother, living a normal life both socially and in my schoolwork. My sister's family lived only a few blocks away and the little folk were always a great joy to me. I was soon surrounded by a group of congenial friends and for the first year my existence was relatively placid.

Fresno prided itself on its one schoolhouse, a large white building of eight rooms, if I remember correctly, although I can recall the names of only four teachers. The principal was a Mr. Underwood, a man over six feet tall. Mr. C., the vice-principal was another tall man. Miss Mary Ellis, a life-long friend, taught the next grade, and I had the primary grade with between eighty and ninety pupils.

The school had the reputation of being unruly. Several principals had had serious times with the bigger boys. One had been put out of a window, and similar experiences had been the fate of others. Annoying the principal to the limit of endurance had become a tradition. There were rumors of trouble in the school at this time. It was reported that both men were liable to be struck with rotten eggs if they ventured in a conveniently dark place of an evening. The women teachers had never been disturbed as their pupils were younger.

All went well in my primary department although handling so many youngsters was an arduous task. My nephew, Bert Warner, was one of my beginners. Several good friends of today, notably the Helm girls, began their education under my tutelage. One little chap, not remarkable for anything so far as I could see, twenty years later became a great champion base-ball player, Frank Chance.

In the second year, Mr. Underwood came to me one day and said he had to go to San Francisco on business. He asked me if I would be willing to take his place during his absence, which he hoped would be for only a few days. He would procure a substitute for me. I felt greatly flattered by his request and said I should like to oblige him but felt inadequate to handle those boys. Why not get a man teacher? He replied, "I think the boys will be chivalrous with you, but I fear a man would have a hard time of it." So it was arranged and the following Monday I assumed the duties of acting-principal.

I had no trouble with the boys who were not vicious, but whose tradition it was not to be controlled by any teacher. The few days stretched into two weeks before Mr. Underwood returned, but the boys lived up to his expectations of chivalry to a young woman who was only substituting for a few days. We parted the best of friends on the Friday afternoon of the principal's return.

It was soon learned that the purpose of Mr. Underwood's trip to San Francisco had been to secure the position of Wharfinger, and that he was returning to begin that work at once.

On Friday evening he tendered his resignation to the school-board. They expostulated at his leaving them thus in the lurch. Where could they find a principal? There wasn't a man in the county who could manage those boys. "No," replied Mr. Underwood, "there isn't a man, so far as I know, but there is a woman. Miss Bennett has handled those boys splendidly during my absence. If you will let the school go on as it is now, all will be well." Alas! he should have given the credit for the peaceful two weeks to the boys, to whom it belonged.

I knew nothing of all this until Saturday morning. As I was going down town I met Judge Sayles, the chairman of the School Board. He greeted me more warmly than usual, stopping and holding out his hand, saying, "I was just coming to tell you that Mr. Underwood has resigned and you have been elected to fill his place. You are to begin as principal of the school on Monday." I was nearly bowled over. Could I do it? Dared I risk it? He repeated what Mr. Underwood had said and expressed his own confidence in me, adding, "The boys will probably make you some trouble but the Board will stand behind you." Thus encouraged, backed by the thought of the fifty per cent increase in salary, I accepted the position. As I walked on down town my head whirled while I somewhat fearfully considered the difficult undertaking, but I could not back out now.

Monday and Tuesday came and went. There was considerable flurry in the school. The vice-principal's verdict was, "A pretty situation! No head to the school!" Other teachers criticized. Only Mary Ellis championed my cause. Knots of children, especially my little ones, excitedly discussed the change. The big boys were restless but not disobedient. By Wednesday morning things had apparently settled down and I was greatly relieved. But it was the calm before the storm.

At recess there was great excitement among the boys. A sound of pounding was heard. I went to a rear window to investigate. There was no sewage system in Fresno then. Two large octagonal outhouses were built in the two school yards, one for the boys and one for the girls. The noise of pounding came from the boys' outhouse. It sounded like chopping. All the boys of the school were gathered around and greatly excited. I asked Miss Ellis to ring the bell while I watched to see who came out of that building. Five of the large boys filed out.

When the pupils were seated I appointed a monitor and went down stairs to inspect the building. The entire center had been chopped out. Returning to the room, I told the five boys to go into the library. I asked them who had done the chopping but got no satisfaction. Then I said, "Boys, you have destroyed school property. Your fathers will have to pay the bill, but if you will tell me why you did it, perhaps we can come to an understanding." No answer, or a surly, "Don't know anything about it."

I stepped out and said to Miss Ellis, "I am going to be forced to punish those boys. I don't know whether I shall come out alive or not. Listen and if I need help, call for it." "Oh, don't attempt it," she urged. "I have to," was my reply. This was my Thermopylae. The boys had thrown down the gauntlet. Moral suasion would not do. A small boy had told me they had said I would not dare to touch five of them.

Returning to the library I picked up a rattan and said, "Boys, you have done this to defy me. I am sorry. I like you, but I must control this school. I will give you another chance." And turning to the leader, I said, "Sidney, will you tell me what happened?" "I don't know anything about it." To the next boy I put the same question and received the same answer, and so on to the last one, the tallest in the lot. "Alfred, what have you to say?" Somehow I pinned my hopes on Alfred. He flushed and blurted out, "Well, I'm not going to lie about it. Of course I know; we all do, but we swore we wouldn't tell, so I can't."

Turning back to the stubborn heavy-set leader, I said, "Take off your coat, Sidney." "I won't." "Take off your coat, Sidney Shannon," I repeated more sternly. "I won't do it." We stood and glared into each other's eyes. It was a battle of wills. I weighed only one hundred and three pounds. Every boy was heavier, and some taller, than I. Putting all my "do or die" determination into my voice and holding his eyes steadily, I commanded, "Take off your coat or I will." His eyes dropped, his face flushed, and slowly he began to tug at one sleeve. Finally the coat dropped to the floor. I grasped his arm tightly and delivered slashes with the rattan across his shirted back. He winced decidedly. It hurt. Then the next boy. He yielded a little more readily and received the same treatment. The third coat came off with less effort and also the fourth. By this time my arm had nearly given out as every lash had had to be given upward, the boys being so tall. Alfred's coat was off before I got to him. "I'm sorry, Alfred," I said. "But since you shared in the defiance of school rules, you must share in the punishment." But he did not suffer much from his whipping. My arm was too tired.

When it was over I said, "Now boys, you have carried out the tradition of the school; let us go back to our work and be friends. I like all of you, but I must have order in the school." We all went into the school-room together, and as I entered the door I heard another one of the big boys say, "Gee, ain't she got some spunk!"

At noontime, utterly exhausted, I went home to lunch and to lie down until one o'clock. Returning, I entered my schoolroom by a side door. There sat Sidney Shannon, his face flushed, his arm inside his desk. I had to pass him to go to my desk and I had visions of being struck with a club as I passed. I was terror-stricken! Should I retreat and go around the hallway to another door near my desk where I could enter facing him? No, he had seen me and would know that I was afraid of him. With trembling knees and pounding heart, I walked up the aisle. As I expected, when I reached his desk he sprang up. My heart stopped. Out of his desk came—not a club—but a huge bouquet! With the single word, "Here!" he thrust it at me and bounded down the stairs. The battle was won. Henceforth those boys were my champions. I had no more disciplinary trouble.

The fathers of the boys paid the carpenter's bill without a murmur, so far as I know, and the incident was never reported officially to the school board.

Years afterward when I was practicing medicine in Berkeley, I heard this story which Sidney Shannon had laughingly related to his family physician. He was then living in Alameda with his wife and children, and the physician was my chum in medical college, Dr. Mary Delano Fletcher. My nephew Bert Warner writes me that Mr. Shannon is now living in Fresno and is United States Marshal of the Federal Court. I should like to meet him after this half century.

Since writing the above, another echo of this episode has come to me. The story was told by the mother of the boy to Dr. Fletcher's sister and herself a few days after it occurred. The mother said, "When John came home from school at noontime the other day I noticed something wrong with him and said, 'What is the matter, John?' 'Nothing,' he replied. 'Oh yes there is. Now tell me what it is.' 'Well, I've just been thrashed by a woman, and a little one at that!'"

The contest was not one of will only. On my part it necessitated success then; otherwise I could expect nothing but failure to control the school. On the boys' part, they were carrying out a tradition. They had not anticipated the issue of having to yield to a young woman smaller than any of them, or use brute force on her. As Sidney Shannon and I faced each other he realized that he had a chivalrous issue before him. His better nature conquered and he submitted to the whipping. The bouquet was an acknowledgment of fair play and friendly good will. Alfred B. was actuated by a sense of honor. He had given his word to the gang and could not break it. So he too accepted the consequences. These boys I respected at the time and have always remembered; the other three merely followed their leader and I do not remember them.

After completing the year as principal of the Fresno school, I resigned to begin my preparation for medicine. This determination on my part brought out afresh all the family opposition as well as that of my friends. There were the usual caustic remarks about feminine unfitness for the profession of medicine, woman's lack of strength, her instability, natural timidity, and all the other hackneyed objections.

Predictions of failure were universal but varied. Beside all of the above reasons for failure there came this blast: "After you have spent all your money and the best years of your life studying medicine, you will 'up and marry' and it will all be wasted." "Even if I knew I should 'up and marry' I would most assuredly study medicine," was my retort. "Surely no one needs such training more than the mother of a family."

Then a financial blast! "Here you are giving up a fine salary in a profession in which you have succeeded so far, and you will run yourself heavily in debt to undertake an uncertain livelihood." As to this prediction I can only say that in the first month of my practice I earned as much as the principal's salary in the Fresno school, and after that an increasing amount until my income soon equalled that of the highest paid university professor of that time. Regarding running in debt, that was true. I used up all my own money and drew on Cousin John Whittlesey to the extent of two thousand dollars. This amount, plus six percent interest, was repaid in a few years.

So all the bug-bears proved to be harmless bugs, not destructive bears.

CHAPTER 5

Medical Student and Interne

PRELIMINARY TO ENTERING MEDICAL COLLEGE I SPENT A YEAR IN San Jose under the tutelage of Dr. Meade and Professor Norton in premedical work. There were no pre-medical courses offered then. I lived with Dr. Meade in order to see as much of her actual work as I could. Meanwhile I was "reading medicine" most persistently and also studying chemistry under Professor Norton.

Dr. Meade felt that my health decidedly needed building up, so she kept me out of doors as much as possible. One of my great privileges was driving her span of spirited black horses.

This was an important year in my formative life. The spirit of the profession at its best was imbued in me by this indomitable, high-minded woman. Professor Norton was an occasional visitor at the house, and it was a great privilege to listen to those two noble souls discuss world problems.

Naturally it was only among Dr. Meade's poorer patients that I could watch her work. It was usually among the foreign population that I accompanied her in maternity cases and helped in the preliminary work of general cleaning up of the bed and premises to make conditions relatively sanitary.

One amusing incident I must relate—a huge joke on myself. I was walking along the main street of San Jose one day on my way to the livery stable for the team, when I saw a countrified group that amused me greatly. A tall man with a straggling, unkempt beard and clothes which gave him an appearance of middle age, lurched along. Hanging to his arm was a woman with a wide skirt sweeping the sidewalk, and such a funny hat! Clinging to her skirt were two or three equally quaint, peculiarly dressed children. I tried to control my risibles but confess to staring at them impolitely. Possibly my gaze fastened on them, caused the man to notice me particularly. At any rate he returned my stare, stopped, smiled, thrust out his hand, and said, "Wife, this is my old school-teacher." Ye Gods! Old school-teacher to that patriarch? I was then twenty-three. But sure enough, it was my eldest pupil in Peachtree! He had given his age as twenty-one when he entered the school seven years before. Old as he now appeared, he could be no more than twenty-eight. Moral: Girls, do not begin teaching at sixteen if you don't want to be an "old-school-teacher" at twenty-three!

During that year mother was suddenly stricken with a fatal illness, living only about a week. I hastened to her bedside. Finding her desperately ill, I telegraphed for Dr. Meade who came at once and remained two or three days. As noted before, this experience with a woman physician caused mother to withdraw her objections to my studying medicine. Her opposition had been based solely upon two factors: Her own experience as a friendly nurse to her neighbors which had given her a keen appreciation of the hardships of such a career, and her knowledge that notwithstanding my determination and strenuous activities, my health was far from good.

That she could approve of my choice of life-work in those last three days of her life, and give me her blessing, has always been a great consolation to me. Mother died December 12th, 1883, and her body was carried back to Gilroy to lie in the tri-family plot.

The following spring I matriculated in the Cooper Medical College of San Francisco, now the Medical Department of Stanford University. Few incidents stand out during those years except hard work. There should have been thirty hours in the day in which to accomplish all the work laid out by the various professors, to say nothing of hospital work and clinics.

The women students were relatively few, less than ten in all three classes. Only one other woman student, Mary Delano Fletcher, was in the class of 1886. She has proved to be one of my closest friends from the day we entered as freshmen to the day of this writing, 1933—fifty years. The men students were for the most part friendly. Some left us severely alone but all save one were gentlemanly. He, although a scion of a wealthy San Francisco family, was not a gentleman in any sense of the word. He was simply vulgar; gloried in obscene stories, and so could make us very uncomfortable, especially in the dissecting room. But some of the men students squelched the vulgarity, which, with the utter indifference on our part, put an end to his petty persecutions. Splendid friendships were formed with some of those fine men in "Cooper."

The dissecting room was naturally the hardest break for us, but not more so than for some of the men. It was not a pleasurable procedure, but to my surprise I received a prize for my dissecting. I was not working for the prize—in fact did not know there was one offered, but my natural desire to do the best I possibly could resulted in the preparation of one "upper" (shoulder and arm) which was pronounced the best work done that year. The feature that made my work unusual was this: After removing the skin and adipose tissue, I carefully separated all the muscles, blood-vessels and lymphatics without severing any of them. The arteries I painted red, the veins blue, nerves yellow, and lymphatics white. The muscles I varnished. Thus all the parts were *in situ*. The professor of anatomy took it for demonstration in his lectures and I was enriched by twenty-five dollars. With this I purchased an old-fashioned mahogany writing-desk and book-case combined. This souvenir of medical college has been in constant use ever since.

In dissecting, five students work on one "subject," which is divided into two uppers, two lowers, and the head. Our work in this course began shortly before the Fourth of July. Being alone in San Francisco, I decided to make use of the holiday to get farther ahead with my assignment. I therefore appeared at the Medical College door about nine o'clock in the morning. The janitor let me in but was not at all enthusiastic about my plan, protesting that he wanted the holiday, and the building must be locked. After some persuasion he consented to lock me in but would leave a latch so that I could get out.

I mounted the five flights of stairs to the dissecting hall, a large room occupying almost the entire floor. As I reached the door and opened it, I will confess I had to swallow hard. The few times before when I had entered the room I had been in the company of the class, and the "subjects" had been all in readiness, prepared by the janitor. Besides, there had been a good deal of talking and some merriment among the students. Now, all alone, locked in a great building, I opened the door to see twenty or more "stiffs" as the boys called the bodies, covered with sheets. The sight was gruesome and the odor sickening. I hesitated and would have retreated but that monitor, Duty, said scornfully: "A pretty way for a physician to act!" Gritting my teeth, I entered, put on my dissecting apron, opened all the windows, removed the sheet from my subject, and started work.

I had unfortunately been allotted a share in a fat, liquor-soaked body. The adipose tissue made the dissecting more difficult, and the odor nauseating. Anatomical drawings in light frames lined the walls. The strong sea-breeze through the open windows rattled them spookily. Every few minutes a sheet would be blown off, revealing a grinning, partially-dissected head or a seemingly moving foot. How many times did I replace those sheets? The nerve-tension was tremendous but I stuck to it. When a cat, somewhere in the building, set up a dismal "meow, meow," it capped the climax. The cold sweat ran down my back but I stuck to it until luncheon time. Somehow I did not feel like working that afternoon, and I never celebrated another holiday in a dissecting room.

Surgical operations came next in testing one's self-control. This work was carried on at the City and County Hospital, at that time a group of old buildings, long since replaced by the present plant. The trip across the city to the hospital was a long one requiring three changes of cars and a walk of about three-quarters of a mile down a road with no sidewalks or paving. It was muddy in winter and covered with deep dust in summer. Various mud-holes were alluring to the geese and goats that paraded back and forth. While I do not consider myself an arrant coward that old gander was my *bete noir*. He delighted in putting me to flight. Dr. Fletcher still laughs over the way she would ward him off with the point of her umbrella when I was terrorized by him.

Although we made weekly trips out there, but two vivid memories come at my call. One was a bedside case at which we were quizzed as the professor made his examination of the patient. The professor of internal medicine was a Hebrew with a caustic tongue. Absolute accuracy in the use of medical terms was required. One day I ventured to use the term

"Rheumatism" in reply to a question. I can still see him draw himself up to his full height, as with flushed face and pursed lips he turned on me and scathingly hissed: "Will you kindly tell me what you *mean* by rheumatism?" How "mean" I thought he was! Then followed a lecture on the indefiniteness of that term—which did not signify any specific disease. I was a sadly withered sprig when he finished his dissertation.

The other memory is of an operation—the most sickening one in my clinical experience. It was a case of cancer of the face. The result was a foregone conclusion, but the patient insisted on the attempt at relief. A facial operation of such magnitude is far more repellant than one on any other part of the body. As it proceeded, a student fainted. Soon another; and then a third. The three men were stretched out on the floor and no further attention was paid to them. As the gruesome operation proceeded I gritted my teeth, clenched my hands, and held on. Next to me stood a senior woman student. I watched her turn a greenish white and sway a little. Contrary to the ethics of an operating room, where silence is the rule, I hissed in her ear, "Don't you dare faint." She jumped, and flushing with anger, turned on me. In turn I flushed with embarrassment. But the return of blood to our heads by blushing saved the situation. The two women students did not faint and thus disgrace the sex. That three men did faint was merely due to a passing circulatory disturbance of no significance; but had the two women medical students fainted, it would have been incontrovertible evidence of the unfitness of the entire sex for the medical profession.

The student days passed happily and for the most part uneventfully. During most of the time I lived with the family of Mr. Emmet Rixford on the corner of Sutter and Webster Streets, only four blocks from the college building at Sacramento and Webster. It was a charming family with two delightful little children. Mr. Rixford was an attorney and the uncle of the now famous surgeon who was his namesake and was, at that time, a student in the University of California. The house was managed by Mrs. Rixford's sister, Miss Halsey. Three men students also boarded there and we grew to be staunch friends, often studying together, especially at examination periods.

During our senior year we were given practical experience in obstetrics by being assigned cases to attend. Anyone desiring student care in a confinement case could apply to the college. Two students were usually allotted to a case. If anything went wrong the professor of obstetrics was summoned. Owing to my experience with Dr. Meade such work was not new to me, although the responsibility placed upon me was. My memory of this angle of our preparation lies chiefly in our prowling around dark streets in the middle of the night searching for the number of the house, usually a tenement. Naturally this was in the poorer parts of the city where there were few street cars or street lights. Since we went in pairs, we felt relatively safe, and apparently were as nothing untoward happened.

One experience I had with morphine may be worth relating for its moral. When our final examinations began I was suffering one of the attacks of pain which I had had occasionally ever since that indefinite illness at twelve years of age. I studied until late, then went to bed and tried to sleep. But the pain made sleep impossible. Feeling that I must have some rest before facing three final examinations on the morrow, I arose and searched for relief. Finding a sample bottle of morphine tablets, I took one—a very small dose. It relieved the pain but instead of inducing sleep, it stimulated my brain which simply raced along until morning.

Physically weary, I dragged up the hill and the two or three flights of stairs to the examination room. Resting my heavy head on my left hand, I started to write. Heavy though my head was, my brain was still racing as never before. It seemed as if the pages of my text-book were photographed on my retina, so clearly could I see them. It was difficult to write rapidly enough. Suffice it to say, both morning examinations were marked one hundred per cent. But I realized that a drug which could have such a profound effect upon a brain was something to be left severely alone. I have never repeated the experiment. Doubtless I experienced a bit of the exhilaration felt by the narcotic addict without the consequent stupor of repeated dosage. But that experience has caused me to realize how easily one could become an addict.

Finals over, there came the graduation exercises and the banquet. Dr. Fletcher and I were of course in line with our class to receive our diplomas as Doctors of Medicine, and proud we were of our titles. But when it came to the graduation banquet—that was another matter. We were not urged to attend. In fact our classmate friends strongly advised us not to go as there would be much drinking and lewd story-telling. We were told that some members of both class and faculty would be under the table before the dinner was over. We later learned that this had indeed occurred. That, it seems was the established custom in 1886. Imagine a class banquet of the University of California or Stanford now, where the women members would be outlawed because of either drunkenness or obscenity on the part of the men. During all my years in Berkeley, women students have been a recognized, if not an honored part of most university functions.

During the vacation periods I returned to Dr. Meade with whom I could be constantly acquiring experience, as well as getting plenty of fresh air while driving her lively team. She also needed me as she was not well.

One week-end we drove up to Alum Rock Springs that she might have a little rest and profit by the hot sulphur baths. Alas! many week-ends passed—more than three months—before she could return to her home. Desperately ill as she was, she directed her own case, with me as all-round helper. At her command I summoned her favorite nurse, and we two undertook a life-and-death battle. For three weeks we scarcely undressed except to bathe and change our clothes. When either one slept she was ready for immediate call. For two weeks at least, neither of us went regularly to bed. It was one of the severest physical and emotional strains which I have ever undergone.

Our patient recovered and lived another decade or more, when she met an untimely and unusual death. Walking on the street she slipped on a banana-peel and fell heavily on her back. She lived only a few days. The autopsy showed that her spleen had been ruptured by the force of the fall. Many of the poor and the rich of San Jose felt that they had lost their best friend when Dr. Euthanasia Sherman Meade died. Her girlhood, her marriage, motherhood, and her professional career had been as dramatic, as unusual and as tragic as was the termination of her life.

But this end did not come until I had been well established in medical practice in Berkeley for several years, and settled in my own home as well, for I had been married in the meantime. To whom?

As Christmas 1885 approached—the end of my junior year in college—my sister urged that I should visit her during that last vacation. I had not returned to Fresno since the death of our mother two years before, having spent all my spare time with Dr. Meade. As an inducement, my sister advanced the information that my cousin Alice and my brother Will would be there also, and we could have a family reunion.

The morning before Christmas I left Dr. Meade's, and after the regulation weary wait at Tracy for a south-bound train, I arrived in Fresno on Christmas Eve. To my distress I found myself invited to a Christmas dinner party in my own former home, the house in which my mother had died. I felt I could not go there, and made every possible excuse, especially my duty to my sister.

On Christmas morning the host came to intercede with my sister, saying he had a strange young man as his house-guest, an old-time schoolmate, one of those bookish fellows, and he wanted me to be the dinner partner of this stranger. My sister agreed that I should go as she had postponed her Christmas dinner because Alice and Will were going to the same party. I was forced to yield much against my will, but evidently Fate was driving me to meet my future husband, William Emerson Ritter.

Being emotionally upset by having to go into that house so full of memories, it was to be either a case of tears or unnatural gaiety. I chose the latter. Our host was a young bachelor who was taking advantage of his sister-in-law's absence on a visit to the East. The dinner party was composed of some twenty young people.

The day was warm and sunny. We adjourned from the table to out-of-door sports and soon many of our childhood games were on the tapis—anti-over, marbles, and so forth. My table-partner challenged me to a game of mumble-peg and produced a most appropriate knife with open blade. I accepted the challenge. He won the game. Later he challenged me to add the duties of wife to those of physician. Again I accepted the challenge, and again he won. But that is a long story as we were not married for over five years.

Mr. Ritter had been drawn to California by a text-book on geology by Professor Joseph Le Conte which he had studied in the Wisconsin Normal School. The desire to study under this famous author had determined him to choose the University of California as his alma mater. But he also had to earn the money for college by teaching. At that time he had secured a school in Fresno County.

Before entering the University he came to Cooper Medical College to take a course in practical anatomy, dissecting, and laboratory work. One day he and I were working on a human brain—trying to trace those elusive structures, the hippocampi, major and minor. His Fresno friend and host was standing near. When Mr. Ritter finally discovered the hidden structure, I exclaimed, "Fine! You are a man after my own heart!" "Most evidently so!" somewhat cryptically remarked the visitor, much to my discomfiture.

Before my graduation in November, 1886, we two had "come to an understanding," but that understanding included a university course in Berkeley for him, and then two years residence at Harvard to obtain his higher degree. On my part it meant a year of hospital interneship, and then ample time to settle somewhere and demonstrate that I could succeed in my chosen field. This we carried out faithfully, but to my own surprise I found myself located in Berkeley instead of going back to Dr. Meade or to Madagascar or to some other end of the world.

After graduation both my classmate chum, Mary Delano Fletcher, and I were invited to serve as internes in the Children's Hospital. At that time the hospital was located in the old building on Thirteenth Street near Folsom. A new building was in process of erection on the present site at California and Maple Streets.

The last day of January, 1887, was the day set for moving the patients to their new and more capacious hospital. The patients were both women and children. This proved to be a rare California day, but not "A rare day in June." The rare January day brought one of those infrequent snowstorms of this vicinity, and a real snowstorm it was!

The new hospital buildings were some blocks beyond the residence district, and only a straggling horse-car spanned the distance beyond the end of the California Street cable-car line. The electric line on Sacramento Street came years later. Opposite the hospital were two cemeteries. The horse-car line ran too infrequently to suit our purpose and automobiles had not yet been invented. Ambulances and carriages conveyed the patients, but in the numerous round trips incident to moving, we internes and the nurses had ample opportunity to witness the fun for boys, large and small, old and young, incident to a snowstorm. We also experienced its disagreeable side as we waded through several inches of drifted snow, and later in the day, through mud and slush.

The hospital staff was composed for the most part of the early women physicians who had created it largely for the purpose of affording hospital opportunities for themselves and those who came after them. Prominent among them were Dr. Charlotte Blake Brown and Dr. Lucy F. Wanzer. Association with these noble women brought another rich friendship into my life. Charlotte Blake Brown was one of the most notable women I ever met, and as beautiful as she was talented. The daughter of an army chaplain she early married Henry Adams Brown. After bearing three children she could not resist the family trend toward the profession of medicine. Her older brother, Dr. Charles E. Blake, was a prominent physician in San Francisco, always a friend of women and an ardent assistant to his sister in her later charitable work.

Dr. Charlotte Brown went to the Women's Medical College in Philadelphia for her training, at that time almost the only place a woman could study medicine. While not one of the earliest pioneers in medicine, she was a pioneer in that profession in California and did much to make the pathway of the medical women who came after her a smoother road to travel.

One of her first activities was to call together the few other women physicians and several women of wealth, and lay before them a plan to establish a free clinic for poor women and children. As the result the Pacific Dispensary was opened on Post Street near Dupont, now Grant Avenue. This finally grew into a hospital and clinic combined, which at the time we entered was located on Thirteenth Street near Folsom.

In connection with the hospital came the first training school for nurses in San Francisco. At Thirteenth Street only eight nurses could be accommodated. Immediately upon occupying its more commodious quarters, the number of student nurses was increased to seventeen. One of the first graduates was Kitty Estep now living at the Crocker Home in San Francisco. Those early day nurses were unusually fine as they were all women with a mission in life, and were most carefully selected.

The removal of the hospital to the inaccessible location out on the sand-dunes necessitated finding a location near the old site for the clinic and dispensary. This in turn necessitated two internes instead of one and it was to Dr. Brown that Dr. Fletcher and I owed our appointments.

It was arranged that we should alternate as interne and externe, the latter having charge of the out-patients in the clinic and dispensary and occasionally in their homes. I was the first to assume the outside work, while Dr. Fletcher served her term as interne. The work of the internes was alternated between the various wards, the surgical and medical for children, the maternity ward and the private rooms for women. We were on call both night and day, and the night calls came quite frequently.

Our days off were occasional, not regular. One such I recall. I went with my fiancé to Mill Valley for an outing and rest. We took a book along—Wordsworth's poems, as Mr. Ritter was an ardent admirer of that poet. Having been up most of the preceding night I was extremely weary. After we reached a wooded spot for our picnic luncheon, I settled myself under a tree while Mr. Ritter read aloud. Soon I was sound asleep and slept all the afternoon. Such a holiday was a fair, but not an exciting introduction to life with a woman physician.

Another unromantic incident for the same young man occurred at the clinic. Dr. Brown, who was the leading surgeon among the women physicians, was preparing to remove a patient's kidney. Preparatory to this she secured a dog from the pound where it was destined to be killed, and took it to the clinic where a room was fixed up for it. Under the most sanitary conditions possible the dog was anaesthetized as a patient would have been, and the doctor removed one kidney and then assigned the canine patient to my care, in the room prepared for it. The difficulty was to keep the patient quiet, as it was not seriously ill. The wound healed rapidly and in a few days the dog was as frisky as ever. For a few weeks it lived a charmed life being bounteously fed and meticulously cared for. Then one day my zoological friend was invited over from Berkeley to demonstrate the results of the operation. Quietly chloroformed, the dog slept the sleep that knows no waking, and Mr. Ritter performed as careful an autopsy as he would have made on a human being. The purpose was to see what nature does when one-half of an eliminative system is suddenly removed.

Dr. Brown witnessed the autopsy and found a healthy kidney considerably enlarged to perform its double function. Thus reinforced in her conviction, she saved the life of her otherwise doomed patient by performing this—at that time, unusual—operation. Charlotte Blake Brown was the peer of any man in the profession, and to me was a life-saving friend because of her surgical skill.

During my hospital days she had watched me medically, and in one of my repeated attacks of suffering tried a minor operation. This giving no relief she was convinced that a more serious cause underlay my condition. Three years later she saved my life by as serious surgical means as the case referred to above, but in the meantime I had finished my hospital experience and practiced medicine for two years.

It had been Dr. Meade's wish that I should return to San Jose and enter into practice with her. The wisdom of this course was questioned by me and some of my friends. Anyway I decided on the year of interneship and awaited my future destiny.

Before my year of interneship was over, Dr. Brown told me that Dr. Sarah I. Shuey of Berkeley was planning to remove to Sierra Madre, above Pasadena, where she intended to build a private hospital and run it with the aid of her friend, May Treat, now Mrs. Alexander Morrison. Dr. Shuey wished to dispose of her practice and Dr. Brown considered me the most suitable person to succeed her. Satisfactory arrangements were made. To my regret this necessitated my leaving the hospital before my year of interneship expired, but the opportunity was too good to be lost.

Sarah Shuey and May Treat had been classmates in the University of California in the class of 1876 and formed a deep and lasting friendship. After graduation in Toland Medical College, now the Medical Department of the University of California, Dr. Shuey established herself as the first woman physician in Berkeley. She was remarkably successful and soon built up an enviable reputation and practice.

Unfortunately the hospital venture was not a financial success. After two or three years, Dr. Shuey returned, having lost all of her invested capital and with a heavy indebtedness which burdened her remaining years. She settled in Oakland with Dr. C. Annette Buckel and soon established another good practice. Fittingly, she died in the harness, expiring suddenly when on duty at a maternity case.

Dr. Shuey and Dr. Buckel were my most intimate friends and advisers in the East Bay region, while Dr. Brown in San Francisco was a frequent consultant and always like a mother to me.

Dr. C. Annette Buckel was the real pioneer among our group of women physicians. She had been graduated from the Women's Medical College in Philadelphia before I was born and later had hospital training in Boston.

About the time of her graduation the Civil War began. When she had completed two years of hospital interneship, the gloom in the North was at its deepest. She offered her services to General Grant. The medical staff of the army would not recognize a woman as physician, but they offered her the position of head nurse with General Grant's army. She accepted and was on duty with Grant for many weary months, including the siege of Vicksburg and the previous battles down the Mississippi.

Dr. Buckel seldom mentioned this subject, as the experiences were too heart-breaking to be spoken of lightly. I simply know that after conflicts she went onto the battlefield with the stretcher-bearers to succor the dying and give relief to as many as possible. This was in addition to her duties as chief of nurses in the tent hospitals, where often the work required unremitting duty days and nights on end.

For her service General Grant brevetted her as Major Buckel and commissioned her to establish as many hospitals as possible near the fields of operations. This service she continued until the end of the war. I am not certain whether the number of hospitals which she established was seven or nine.

During part of this period, Dr. Meade was with her and their friendship continued through life. Dr. Buckel hearing of Dr. Meade's illness at Alum Rock, came to her aid, and remained several days. She was the only physician we saw during those long, trying weeks. As with Dr. Buckel, Dr. Meade seldom mentioned her war work.

Dr. Meade was the first to break this circle of pioneer women physicians in California. Dr. Charlotte Brown was the next, and Dr. Shuey third.

Dr. Buckel outlived the others by several years though she was the oldest in the group. After nearly forty years of practice in Oakland, she spent her declining years in the beautiful Piedmont home of a friend and patient, Miss Charlotte Playter. Though declining in physical vigor, her mentality was alert to the end.

At a dinner given to celebrate her eightieth birthday, she was persuaded to display, for the first time in public, the documents given her by General Grant, brevetting her as Major and commissioning her to establish hospitals.

These four women physicians were living monuments of the kind of highly trained "missionary" work which Professor Norton had idealized to me. Likewise their skill in the art of healing, whether medical or surgical, ennobled the profession and added prestige to the cause of women in medicine.

CHAPTER 6

First Years in Berkeley

ON JULY 7TH, 1887, AGED TWENTY-SEVEN YEARS, I CAME TO BERKE-ley to begin what I considered to be my serious life-work. It was serious beyond cavil. I was soon established in Dr. Shuey's office as well as in her living quarters. Both were in the residence of Mrs. J. R. Little, 2223 Durant Avenue. Here I lived until my marriage four years later.

Berkeley when I first knew it was a straggling village clustered around the University, the site of which had been chosen by men who could envision the glory of the prospective campus. The college had been moved from Oakland in 1868, and received its charter as the State University. Three farm houses were then its nearest neighbors, but the town, Berkeley, named by the same group of men, soon sprang up.

Dwight Way Station was the center of the village. There were no public buildings, no paved streets, no sidewalks except rattling boards. Strawberry Creek meandered across Shattuck Avenue where Allston Way and the Hotel White-cotton now are. It was spanned by a bridge on Shattuck Avenue. Great oaks lined the banks of the stream, a few standing on the avenue. Southern Pacific trains made up of a decrepit engine and old red cars made hourly trips from the San Francisco Ferry to North Berkeley Station. A wheezing little engine of ancient vintage drawing a rattling old street car frightened the horses as it tooted its way out Telegraph Avenue to near the University entrance, which is now adorned by Sather Gate.

The University consisted of old North and South Halls and the square brick building occupied by the Engineering Departments. These recitation halls and laboratories were grouped around the Bacon Library and

Art Gallery, another red brick structure with a clock tower crowning an elongated reading-room, above which was the art gallery. In the rear was a semi-circular stack-room for books.

Located on Strawberry Creek, Harmon Gymnasium was at that time a single "ink-bottle" as it was dubbed because of its shape. Octagonal, with a small tower for neck and cork, it certainly looked like a mammoth ink-bottle. Shortly after, to enlarge it, another building of the same size and ridiculous architecture was built along-side of it and joined by removing three of the octagonal segments and building straight connecting walls. Offices and locker-rooms were built in the rear adding to the monstrosity. That old structure has been used for the men's gymnasium until this year, likewise serving as an auditorium for the entire University. When I first ridiculed this unique building, little did I think how intimately I should be associated with it later.

Dr. E. S. Holden, the astronomer, was then president of the University. At this time the student body numbered about seven hundred men, and the graduating class in 1888 consisted of eighty-one men and three women students.

Small though the college was it had several outstanding men on its faculty—men of world renown. Notable among these were the two Le Contes, John, professor of physics, and Joseph, professor of natural sciences; Eugene Hilgard in agriculture; George Howison in philosophy; and Bernard Moses, professor of "History and Political Science."

It was often jokingly said that Doctor Joseph Le Conte did not occupy a "chair" in the university, but a "settee." Later, as the student body increased, this settee was divided into four chairs—geology, botany, zoology, and paleontology. Dr. Le Conte retained the chair of geology until his death in Yosemite in the summer of 1901. No instructor was ever more beloved, nor did anyone leave a deeper imprint upon his students than did Joseph Le Conte.

When I came to Berkeley, William Ritter, my future husband, was a special student in the University. During his first year he lived and tutored students at the Boone Academy. In his second year, finding himself taxed for time, he gave up tutoring and came to partake of Mrs. Little's bounteous table although he roomed elsewhere.

Entering the University in 1886, he was graduated with the class of 1888, having completed the required work in two years. After the finals I well recall his having to take entrance examinations on some required subjects which he had completed before coming to the University. Dread of these "exams," on subjects long out of his mind, was greater than for the finals. He survived the ordeal and was granted the degree of Bachelor of Science. He continued graduate study for another year, meantime serving as an assistant in Chemistry.

Being awarded the scholarship of the San Francisco Harvard Club he went to Harvard University in 1889, enrolling in the graduate department of zoology. Living in Memorial Hall with other graduate students for the required two years of residence, he received his Master's Degree in June, 1891. He was also sufficiently advanced toward the highest degree awarded, that of Doctor of Philosophy, to enable him to return to Berkeley to prepare his thesis.

During his student days in Berkeley, another special student at the Little residence was John Campbell Merriam. He, as well as Mr. Ritter, was a devoted follower of "Dr. Joe" Le Conte, and likewise succeeded to one of the "chairs" into which Dr. Joe's "settee" was divided—that of paleontology. A romance developed under our eyes, and John Merriam married Ada Little, the daughter of the household.

In middle life Dr. Merriam was elected president of the Carnegie Institution of Washington, one of the most important positions in the scientific world in this country. A close friendship has existed ever since those student days.

* * * * * * *

The traditional fate of the young medico entering practice did not fall to my lot—that of hanging out a "shingle" with his name on it, and then watching for weeks, and perhaps almost starving while waiting for someone to ask for his services. Instead of this doleful experience I fortunately stepped into Dr. Shuey's capacious "shoes"—the clientele which she had built up. To be sure those shoes were too large for me although I found work waiting for me on the first day of my occupancy of her office. While not all of her patients accepted the new fledgeling, a sufficient number patronized me to keep me busy and give me a comfortable means of support. As remarked before, my income the first month more than equaled my salary as principal of the Fresno school, and gradually increased.

One of the first accessories requisite for active practice was a horse and buggy. Automobiles had not been invented at that time. It was not until my first visit to Europe eight years later that I saw the first "horseless wagon" that appeared on the streets of Paris. It was indeed merely a horseless wagon—a typical two-seated spring-wagon in form with the usual carriage wheels and the tiny hard-rubber tires which were a luxury on a few buggies in those days. The running-gear was somewhere under the body of the wagon. There was nothing in front of the dashboard, so the term horseless-wagon used by the Parisians was most appropriate.

To the close of my years of medical practice, horses were my means of transport. The choice of a suitable horse had its comic side. All sorts of equine quadrupeds were brought for my inspection. Finally a large, spirited dark-bay was brought, a glorious creature which took my fancy at once. After trying him out on a short drive, he was soon mine and served me faithfully until I went to Europe nearly a decade later. He well earned his name, "Prince."

Prince and I started out each morning after breakfast on days when a routine could be carried out, but the life of a physician is anything but a matter of routine. When emergencies did not interfere, Prince and I traveled the streets of Berkeley, Oakland, and sometimes Alameda, that I might make bedside visits to my patients. Home for luncheon when possible, the afternoons until four o'clock were devoted to office work. After four Prince and I again set out to make our rounds.

Fortunate we were when our work ended with the close of day, but for a physician, going to bed was by no means indicative of staying there until morning. Scarcely a week went by without a call which routed both Prince and me out of our respective beds to roam about the unlit streets in search of an ofttimes unknown house. If the distance was short and the destination known, I did not interrupt Prince's slumbers, but prowled the dark streets alone. Even flashlights had not been invented then, and street lights were few and clustered about the business center only. These were either kerosene lamps, or later, gas-jets, both of which had to be lighted singly by a man who went from post to post. No pressing of electric buttons for anything, inside or outside in those days, forty-five years ago.

As a rule, Prince, though spirited, was a safe and reliable assistant in my peregrinations. Once his ambition to lead the van came near producing serious results.

One Saturday, about six months after I began practice, I was called before midnight to Alameda on a maternity case. Prince gallantly took me over, and in return for the favor I put him in a livery stable while I worked all night. The patient was Dr. Fletcher's sister, hence a friend of mine. It was a first baby, therefore the case was liable to be prolonged, and she had sent for me early as I had so far to go. The night dragged wearily on. We both had catnaps between the preliminary paroxysms. By morning, to my disgust, she felt decidedly better, but matters had progressed too far for me to dare to go beyond call. The idea of another night did not attract me. Having heard that driving would often expedite a "lazy" case, at mid-day I proposed that we take a drive. My patient agreed and we drove off somewhere across the Alameda marshes where there was a dyked road, from four to six feet high and wide enough for two-way travel, but not wide enough for much frisking or a runaway.

It was Sunday, a glorious day, and seemingly everyone was out driving. We drove across the dyke toward Mills College then turned to go back. Prince was in gay spirits and the congestion on the dyke excited him. He simply wanted to pass everything regardless of whether there was room or not. I wanted to drive carefully because of my patient. He resented being curbed and the contest resulted in my arms having to pull the entire weight of the buggy. I realized that I could not hold him all the way home.

Two youths were walking along the dyke. I managed to rein Prince in sufficiently to ask one boy to jump in quickly and help me, and the other to get on behind. There was no argument. They obeyed instantly—and none too soon. Prince was off to make up for lost time. The boy had to sit on my lap as there was no vacant space, and together we managed to keep the horse under control and reach the house safely. Suffice it to say I never tried that method of stimulating retarded uterine contractions again.

However, it was successful, and ere night a cheery baby girl entered the world, sucking her thumb before fully making her entry. As a postlude, let me add that about twenty-two years later this same girl was married in our laboratory-home in La Jolla, where she was living with us. A beautiful wedding it was.

Beside being usually so valuable an adjunct to my work, Prince was likewise a valuable aid to courtship. Many a restful, refreshing drive did Prince give me and my chosen life-escort after the day's work was done and the setting sun cast a radiance over the world, extrinsic and intrinsic, as we drove "in the gloaming."

Night-work had some compensations. The starlight was often glorious, the moonlight on bay and hills a thing of beauty, and the glory of the dawn repaid for the broken rest, once or twice, but not for scores of times each year. Alas, it was not on such nights that calls most often came. There is definite relation between stormy nights and a patient's or the family's need for the reassurance of a doctor's visit. In the majority of instances it is only reassurance that is needed, not a newly arisen emergency. To be sure the vital resources are at their lowest ebb in the post-midnight hours and crises are apt to occur at those hours. In such circumstances any physician is glad to answer the call of distress and to work valiantly to relieve the crisis or save a patient's life.

Maternity cases too are apt to occur at night or run into the night. These are all accepted without a murmur as a part of the physician's life, but there is a psychology about sending for the doctor in the middle of the night which makes the family doctor's life much harder than it need be. With any trifling illness there is apt to be restlessness at night, the patient cannot sleep, the pain is more severe, and the mother's nerves are taut, then frayed, and the doctor is summoned. In my earliest days, or nights, of practice, the father or big brother had to be routed out and sent for the doctor. With this envoy on his way and the expectation that help would soon come, the nervous tension lessens, the mother is less uneasy, the patient relaxes and usually goes to sleep before the doctor arrives. How many times after dragging myself out of a warm bed after only two or three hours of sleep, have I wearily entered a sick-room to be received with a whispered warning, "please do not make a noise, he has gone to sleep and seems better. I don't think we really need you now doctor, but I was frightened."

May I skip over a decade and illustrate this by relating my experience on a greatly-needed vacation? A doctor is a doctor wherever he or she may be, and being away from home is no guarantee of freedom from work.

In June, 1898, Mr. Ritter and I, with Professor and Mrs. Stratton and Maude Wilkinson (now Mrs. L. J. Richardson), went on a two weeks' camping trip to Yosemite. I was weary beyond all powers of description and every member of the party was pledged not to reveal the fact that I was a physician.

On the way to the Valley we stopped over at Wawona to visit the big trees. Here, to my later undoing, I was recognized by a Berkeley woman. As we were not acquainted I thought little of it, but alas! she came to Yosemite later and immediately asked the warden about me, and reported that I was a physician.

In the Valley we sought a camping place near Mirror Lake, then remote from Yosemite Village and the usual campers. A week of unalloyed pleasure passed. I was free from care, with jolly and congenial friends, the glorious scenery and ample time to rest. What bliss!

In the second week Mr. Ritter went with Joe Le Conte Jr. and Clarence Cory, veteran mountaineers, to climb Mount Lyell, one of the highest peaks in the Sierras. They left early in the morning, scaling the Yosemite Falls trail to get out of the Valley. Although a little uneasy on account of Mr. Ritter's lack of experience in climbing dangerous mountain peaks and glaciers, I was sleeping the sleep of the just, when about three o'clock in the morning a strange noise awoke us all. Was it a hoot-owl or a coyote? As we all roused more fully we recognized a human voice and words—words fatal to me and my vacation. "Dr. Ritter, Dr. Ritter," rang out through the air in the dark forest. My first thought was of an accident to Mr. Ritter, but not so; it was the warden of the Valley searching for me.

His little child had been taken sick in the night and he wanted me to see her. After questioning him, I decided it was one of those frequent midnight scare cases. I tried to beg off, but no, I must come. Even my friends joined with the warden. Maude W. was sure the baby would die. Mrs. Stratton thought his story sounded alarming. I was positive the child had only eaten something that had not digested and that simple means which the mother could carry out would be sufficient. No, I must go. Again that evil spirit "Duty" which always hounded me, drove me out into the cold, dark night. And oh, how cold it was at that elevation at three o'clock in the morning.

In an open buckboard we rattled slowly over the three miles of rough wagon tracks through the woods. I nearly froze. At last the house. I was so cold and tired I could scarcely walk. I was met by the usual, "Sh— the baby is asleep. Don't make a noise!" Sure enough my diagnosis had been correct; the baby had vomited some raw carrots and was then all right. But I was not. I sat there waiting for the dawn in a cheerless room with but a poor excuse for a fire, rather than repeat that freezing night ride back to the camp. But my spirit was not serene!

The following night at about the same hour came the same hoot, the same unwelcome "animal" had returned. This time it was a man in one of the camps who was sick. "How long has he been sick?" "Two or three days." Again I diagnosed the ailment as indigestion, and refused to go, but dictated means of relief, saying I would see him in the morning, which I did, and found him none the worse because I had not gone at three a.m. But not a wink of sleep had that wretched "Duty" let me have after my heartless refusal to repeat the experience of the previous night. Perhaps the man might be seriously ill and I was neglecting my duty.

Believe it or not, but it is a fact that the third night, the same call was repeated. This time it was for a case of appendicitis away off in the mountains. I was not a surgeon and had no instruments. Mariposa was as near to the patient as Yosemite Valley, so I told the warden they must get a doctor from there, and read him the riot act about ruining my vacation; saying I had come there to rest not to practice medicine, and did not want to be disturbed again.

Alas, about ten o'clock the next day he came apologetically but excitedly, saying the stage had had a runaway and had met with an accident on the grade near Inspiration Point, and all the passengers were injured. Of course I went with him, bound up the wounds as best I could, and to make a long story short, had about a dozen patients to care for during the rest of the stay, which was not a vacation for me.

The length of my vacation was shortened that I might be home in time for a certain maternity case which I had promised to attend. Sufficient margin had been allowed and I agreed to be home in time. Weary and worn as I was with my so-called holiday, I came back on schedule time only to find that the baby had been born as I was en route home, two weeks earlier than he was due.

This story may sound exaggerated but it is true, and typical of a doctor's life. There is no relief from the call of duty; no regularity in one's supposed routine; no opportunity to take much-needed rest nor to consider one's self as of first importance, if one is able to work at all. Yet many people seem to think it smart, or witty, to say, "Physician, heal thyself," or, "A doctor should be able to take care of himself," or some other vapid, inane wise-crack. A physician is the last person who can either spare or care for himself, and many times responds to a patient's call when he himself should be in bed, "healing himself." Therefore such inanity or assininity is not a welcome pleasantry to a worn and weary physician. Perhaps I am unusually sensitive on this point, for I have always had to work with a handicap of poor health.

Scarcely had I reached home when I was called to the deathbed of my sister's husband, Henry Warner, in Fresno. Thus are birth, life and death constantly intermingled.

* * * * * * *

Returning to my first years in Berkeley, I struggled on with my practice without a vacation for more than two years, though my physical condition was growing constantly worse. In October, 1889, Mr. Ritter left for Harvard to be away at least two years. Then Dr. Brown "put the screws on me." She had insisted ever since my hospital days that I was suffering from septicemia and that the focus of infection must be found and eradicated.

After Mr. Ritter's departure I made arrangements for my absence and went over to Dr. Brown's private hospital in late December, hoping to have the cause of my constant suffering and anemia removed. My pallor was greenish; the haemoglobin dangerously low; the white blood count high; and microscopical examinations revealed so severe an anemia that scarcely a normal red corpuscle was to be found.

An exploratory incision revealed ample cause for these results of infection. Evidently a perforation of the intestinal wall had occurred in the obscure typhoid which I had had when twelve years old; obscure because the erratic fever continued far beyond the usual cycle of typhoid. An abscess had become walled off by adhesions among the intestines and all these years I had been carrying this focus of infection, absorbing a septic poison which produced the extreme anemia and repeated illnesses which permanently weakened the heart muscles.

The immediate diagnosis was that it was a tubercular infection, but this proved to be wrong. The prognosis was for non-recovery and all of the physicians who saw the interior of my abdomen wondered how I had ever walked, much less worked as I had.

Dr. Brown, according to promise, wrote Mr. Ritter this diagnosis and prognosis, and advised that he come home. Fortunately, severe storms delayed the mails for two or three days.

For a week I hovered over the River Styx, but by that time my mind was active enough to wonder what word had been sent to Mr. Ritter. Getting no satisfactory answers to my questions and guessing by the actions of my nurses and doctors that I was not expected to recover, I insisted that my day-nurse, my dear friend "Badge" of hospital days, should send him the following telegram: "Do not believe letter. Am not going to die. Do not come home." It was just in time. The letter had reached him that morning and he was endeavoring desperately to pack his trunk and make arrangements to take a trans-continental train that evening.

"There is no great loss without some small gain." Every seemingly great ill has some compensations. I had some. The winter of 1889 and '90 ranks as one of California's wet years. It was said at the time that it rained every day and night for forty days. Anyway, as I lay there all through the holiday season and the following January, listening to the rainfall, I was compensated in large measure by the thought that I did not have to get up and wade around Berkeley streets those stormy nights.

After about six weeks, Dr. Brown permitted me to go to my sister in Fresno for a prolonged rest. Alas, my restless nature and my sense of duty would not permit that, and I thereby made a vital mistake with life-long consequences. I was too thoroughly anemic to recuperate rapidly and should have given nature time to overcome the effects of more than seventeen years of infection. Instead, I was so eager to get back to my work that finally, when I was able to walk around the house, Dr. Brown relented and wrote, "You will find your practice so scattered after your three months' absence that you will perhaps be able to rest as well in Berkeley as in Fresno. So if you are so restless, you may go back, but take things easily."

Alas, when I reached Mrs. Little's, two patients sat in the office awaiting me. Instead of going right to bed as planned, I attended to their needs. That night I was called out and within a week found myself in a life and death struggle with one case of pneumonia and another of typhoid. Night after night I was called out. In all my years of practice there were never more night calls in any single month than in that first one when I was supposed to be resting and recuperating. It was a fatal mistake. The strain on the weakened, anemic heart muscle was too great. It took me many years to overcome the anemia and the heart never fully recovered its muscular tone. Of this more, too much more, anon.

Gradually I regained sufficient strength to go on working but always with a "chain and ball" on my ankle, on both ankles. The cause of the suffering had been removed but I have never known a really well day. My determination to make my life worth while has carried me over many mountain tops and many seas both literally and figuratively. At this epoch I plodded on for nearly a year and a half before an event occurred that determined the permanency of my residence in Berkeley.

In the spring of 1891, a new department was to be formed in the University of California—the Department of Zoology. There were naturally many applications for the post. Finally all but two of the applicants were eliminated—Mr. Ritter and a more experienced man in the East. The influence of Professor Edmund O'Neil, with whom Mr. Ritter had worked as assistant in chemistry, doubtless carried much weight. Added to this was Professor Le Conte's acquaintance with Mr. Ritter's personality and ability. The scales tipped in his favor and the decision was made. Professor Le Conte said later that he had never had occasion to regret his choice. The appointment made in May, 1891, brought to an end months of intense anxiety for both Mr. Ritter and myself.

Upon receiving the appointment, Mr. Ritter arranged to return immediately upon the close of the semester at Harvard. He reached Berkeley about eleven o'clock on the morning of June twenty-third, 1891, and that evening we were married quietly at the residence of my dear friend and patient, Mrs. T. R. Bacon. Her husband, the Reverend Thomas Rutherford Bacon made us man and wife. My sister and her husband, my classmate, Dr. Mary D. Fletcher, and my beloved Doctor Charlotte Brown and her son and daughter, now the prominent San Francisco physicians, Dr. Philip King Brown and Dr. Adelaide Brown, comprised the wedding party.

A brief getting-better-acquainted trip took us to Coronado opposite San Diego, a focal point decided upon because the young husband could thus combine pleasure and work. In this case the lure was some blind "Goby" fish, a rare species living under the rocks below Point Loma. These foolish creatures have had their heads so long buried under the rocks that Dame Nature decided that since they did not use their eyes they should not have any, and proceeded to grow skin over their now sightless eyes.

Mr. Ritter had chosen these retrograde eyes as the topic for his Doctor's thesis. Therefore a week from the day we were married we made an excursion out to the Point to secure some of these strange creatures. Hiring a sail-boat plus its skipper, we had a fine sail across San Diego Bay and secured a good "catch" of specimens. The homeward trip was dramatic to say the least. Mr. Ritter insisted on trying his skill at sailing. The afternoon breeze was lashing the usually calm water into whitecaps, and the tide was running in strongly. These two forces made it difficult to steer the boat on a straight course.

A large dredge was anchored inside our route. The dredge was tugging hard at its anchor-rope so that the rope lay but a little way under the water. We should have kept well clear of it but the amateur helmsman could not control our course. The boat yielding to wind and tide swerved toward the dredge. Our rudder caught the anchor-rope of the dredge and over we went. Fortunately the rope held our capsized boat or we should have been sucked under the dredge, as had happened once before to others. We clung to the boat until the excited men on the dredge rescued us. Mr. Frederick C. Turner, a Berkeley civil engineer was in charge. It was he who had effected our rescue and now afforded us all the comfort possible.

While the bedraggled bride tried to dry herself somewhat by the cook stove, the enthusiastic scientist was happily engaged in sifting out amphioxus, another interesting but lowly creature, from the water and sand which the dredge was pumping up from the bottom of the bay. This important find may have helped to decide the location of the Biological Research Station of the University of California twenty years later. At any rate it brought such delight to the wet groom that what "might have been" was eliminated from consideration.

Another great find on Point Loma and in San Diego was that of two of our most valued friends of a lifetime, the Doctors Fred and Charlotte Baker. To Dr. Fred's interest in science and his enthusiasm over San Diego is largely due the fact that a score of years later our paths were turned in that direction, and more than two decades were spent in that locality.

But this is hurdling over a quarter century.

CHAPTER 7

The "Ply-wood" of Life

RETURNING FROM OUR WEDDING TRIP, MR. RITTER AND I BEGAN our life together in one-half of a double house directly across the street from Mrs. Little's, where we could still partake of her table-board. The other half of the house was occupied by the owner and her grandson, Billy Waste, as he was called by his college classmates. He is now formally addressed as the Honorable William H. Waste, Chief Justice of the Supreme Court of California. I doubt if anyone could foresee a career of future greatness in the callow youth at that time, though he was considered a good student.

Mrs. Townsend, a character of early Berkeley days, took care of our house. When the railroad was laid on Shattuck Avenue a lot owned by her was condemned against her will. She vowed no train should run over that lot except across her body. When that great event, the approach of the first train occurred, she sat down in the middle of the track, on her lot. The train was forced to stop, but Berkeley's burly policeman with adequate assistance, succeeded in carrying off the kicking, scratching woman whose property rights she considered had been unjustly usurped. This incident was a classic of early Berkeley history. Later the same fiery little woman served me faithfully and cheerfully in various capacities for many years. Whenever I needed extra help I could rely upon Mrs. Townsend.

A year or two passed, but living in one house and eating in another was not home. How to manage housekeeping I could not see. But problems solve themselves.

One of my university girl patients who was now teaching in the Los Angeles High School had been breaking for years under the strain of her work. We exchanged letters about it, but she finally phoned me that she could not continue teaching. I replied, "Come and keep house for me." Agnes Crary was one of the most brilliant and competent women I ever knew. She often laughed at my giving her housework as a rest cure. But before that there were weeks in a private hospital. I forbade teaching for a year and a leave of absence was granted her. So with Mrs. Townsend's help Agnes started me in housekeeping.

The building bee was in my bonnet, but first a permanent house-keeper must be found. One day a north-of-Ireland woman came and asked for the position. I knew of her and of her ability and was greatly surprised, but she insisted that she wanted to make me a home and look after me. She came and fulfilled her promise to the letter as long as we remained in Berkeley. Thus Josephine Clifford became a valued member of our family.

How can one picture one's life? A straight continuous story cannot be told since life is so complex. One might as well try to describe a patch-work quilt. Life, or at least my life, has consisted of layers, not like those of an evanescent chocolate cake but more like "ply-wood" made up of crisscross layers for greater flexibility and endurance of strain. Anyway my interests were many and I am sure the strain of medical practice was made more endurable by the addition of outside interests which formed my four- or six-ply life-board.

First and foremost came my practice. Everything had to give way to that as does the Wednesday and Saturday afternoon golf-game of many modern physicians. I had no regular time off as is now the custom, but one cannot work at the same thing all the time. Recreation may be diversity of work as well as games.

My second great interest was social welfare work of various sorts. I was connected with several organizations, the work of which finally led to my occupations in after years. Church and clubs were given their due. I united with the Congregational Church soon after coming to Berkeley. This was the first church built in Berkeley, with Clinton Day as its architect.

When the call came for a group of women to meet with Mrs. Bunnell at her home on Dwight Way to form a club, I was one of the thirty invited and hence became a charter member of the Town and Gown Club of Berkeley.

A National Young Women's Christian Association was formed in San Francisco, and I was appointed a member of the Pacific Coast Branch and served on it as long as it existed—about thirty years. My function on this Board was always along the line of different phases of betterment work. It seems to me that I have always functioned as a "starter" and then let the "magneto" take over the job of keeping the machine going.

Later, for many years I was a board member of the State Federation of Women's Clubs. My office was usually that of chairman of the committee in the line of social work in which I was most interested at the time. Thus it was I could be "starter" and steer the wheel of the machinery which carried on the work in all parts of the state. As an illustration, I was made chairman of a committee by the National Young Women's Christian Association Board to organize Traveler's Aid work in San Francisco. While I was nominally the leader, Mrs. John F. Merrill, one of San Francisco's most philanthropic women was my team-mate and a stronger "wheel-horse" no team ever had.

In the course of our investigation Mrs. Merrill and I interviewed the railroad and steamship presidents, men to whom she had access because of her social position. These men would talk freely to Mrs. Merrill and we thus learned that the "white-slave" traffic was being carried on as systematically in this state as it was in New York and Chicago, where thousands of girls disappeared every year, a large proportion of them from railroad trains. While the traffic in California was numerically small, the system was well organized and persistent, and the railroads were largely the means of such exploitation. These railroad officials were glad to abet our work although they would not openly aid us. We learned that procurers, mostly men, were going throughout the length and breadth of the state in search of young girls, promising good positions of various sorts in San Francisco, their fares paid and even their trunks checked to the given address. Arriving at the depot or Ferry Building, these girls were met by someone in a carriage and that, as a rule, was the last heard of the poor victims.

This sort of information I carried to the State Federation Board and was made chairman of a Traveler's Aid Committee for the State, which was established for the purpose of cooperating in an effort to stem this vicious current. Such a situation appealed to every club and every club-woman both in the small town clubs and those in the rural districts whence the girls were decoyed, and also the clubs of the large cities where the poor victims were enslaved. By appointing committee members in all of the Federation districts, each chairman of such committee would in turn appoint a sub-chairman in each county who would make the appeal to every club in her county. Thus a network for the Traveler's Aid work was spread over the state. Once well organized the machine would work, and I could give my attention to some other field.

This same plan I worked for a score of years in various lines, some of which I will allude to as I recount my varied interests throughout the years.

To return to those early Berkeley days, one constant source of regret was that I had not been able to take a university course preliminary to the study of medicine. Going to college was not the routine matter in those days that it is now. It was not the fashion. Quite the reverse. Only serious-minded girls who really desired an education for its own sake went to college. Athletics and social prestige or college gaities did not figure then. With me the financial obstacle had seemed insurmountable. To finance four years in the university and three in medical college would have been too great an undertaking.

Therefore when I found myself unexpectedly located in the town-seat of our State University, I availed myself of some of the crumbs that fell from the master's table and took single courses whenever possible, throughout several years. The least work one could take as a special student which would count toward a degree was eight hours a week. Such an amount of time was for me utterly impossible, so I nibbled along on the crumbs for nearly twenty years. But such crumbs! Dr. "Joe," Professor Gayley, and other of the great lights shone just as brightly on me as on the registered students. Laboratory courses in chemistry and zoology also yielded as good food to me as to the enrolled class, and I trust was as well-digested and assimilated. Adding to this an "extension course" under my professorial husband, who for forty-two years has been my teacher of "natural philosophy" during our meals and in conversation, morning, noon and night, it may be that I can claim my share of university courses even if not the "degree." As to the disciplinary side of educational work, the training of a medical college may have supplied that.

Another somewhat unique piece of local social service requires a background. Dr. Shuey had returned after her unfortunate venture in Southern California and was established in Dr. Buckel's residence in Oakland. Dr. Fletcher, after a tryout for a year in Fresno, had settled in Alameda with her family clustered around her. Thus we four women physicians were near enough to work together when necessary, and relieve each other when one took a vacation. Among Dr. Buckel's clientele was the Frank Marshall Smith, or "Borax" Smith family living in their palatial home on one of the heights of East Oakland. One member of the household, Mrs. Smith's sister, was a confirmed invalid.

One year when Mrs. Smith was in poor health, they took Dr. Buckel to Europe with them and I was delegated to take care of the invalid sister. So Prince and I had the pleasure of visiting those park-like gardens twice a week for many months. The drive was refreshing and the gardens beautiful, and the opportunity to relieve Dr. Buckel gratifying.

Dr. Shuey was my mainstay whenever I desired to leave my practice either for pleasure or graduate work. Travel became increasingly a factor in my life due largely to Mr. Ritter's scientific needs. This arrangement with Dr. Shuey was particularly satisfactory as she was so thoroughly acquainted with Berkeley, many of my patients having formerly been her "families."

The local social relief to which I referred was this: Mrs. Smith conceived the idea of forming a Home Club for the purpose of studying problems concerning the home and bettering conditions pertaining thereto. Both husbands and wives belonged to this unique club. One of the first committees formed was the Milk Committee, whose purpose was to investigate the milk supply in the East Bay region and to try to secure pure milk. Dr. Buckel was chairman and Dr. Shuey, Dr. Fletcher and I the committee. Dr. Shuey and I were delegated to investigate all the dairies in Alameda and Contra Costa counties supplying milk to the cities and towns around the Bay. Such conditions of mud and filth as we found are indescribable. No wonder babies were ill.

Of course Prince was an important factor in this undertaking, as his contribution to this humanitarian work carried us many a mile.

Greatly was this work needed. Pure milk for babies was unobtainable and a bottle-fed infant was a source of sorrow to the baby, the mother and the family doctor.

It was winter. Mud was deep and the conditions we found in the dairies were unbelievably filthy and inimical not only to babies but to the entire community, both from the filth in the milk and the unhealthy conditions of the animals from which it was drawn. The dairy I remember most clearly was one in the hills back of Berkeley. The barnyards were in a hollow. The mud was deep and naturally covered with semi-fluid cow-dung in which the udders dragged and the tails swished. We waited to watch a milking. The milkers in filthy overalls and high boots drove the cows to a higher level in the barnyard and milked them without washing either the cows' teats or their own hands!

One dairy was found which was trying to carry out sanitary conditions. After fair investigation and interviews with dairy owners, the Club decided to sponsor this one dairy provided the owners would equip it according to the Club's requirements. This they could not afford to do at the price for which milk and cream were then selling. The Club then canvassed its members and friends and secured sufficient subscribers at an advanced price to enable the dairyman to make the requisite changes. Every effort was then made to induce the city authorities to require all other dairies to come up to this standard. Thus Oakland and Berkeley received their first certified milk, a matter they now pride themselves upon, that all milk is pasteurized and therefore safe. This was the first investigation of the milk supply in this locality, or in the State. Of course Dr. Shuey and I had simply added this duty to our routine work, and had to set aside certain hours for this purpose.

The early summer of 1893 found Mr. Ritter and me in the East. We went via Washington, affording me a second visit to that fascinating Capital. While Mr. Ritter was occupied in Cambridge and New York, I took the opportunity of taking one of the short summer courses offered to physicians at Johns Hopkins Medical School in Baltimore. Listening to the lectures and walking the wards for bedside instruction by such famous men as Drs. Osler, Howard Kelley, Welch, Llewellen Barker, and others was an inspiration as well as an opportunity to refresh one's self in the various branches represented by these men at the top of their profession. Whenever possible I took advantage of such opportunities to better fit myself for my work.

The following year, 1894, Mr. Ritter decided he must go to Europe for further study, especially in Liverpool with Professor Herdman, and at the famous Zoological Station in Naples, and also in Berlin. Naturally this plan delighted me, and making arrangements with Dr. Shuey to take over my practice, we were off for the accustomed fifteen months' vacation—accustomed, because University men having a year's leave of absence, usually combine with it two summer vacations from May of one year to August of the next.

The thrill of a first trip to Europe is indescribable and I shall not attempt it. Once launched into description of countries, one would be lost. Should I live another decade I might attempt to portray some of the grandeurs of nature: a sunrise over Monte Rosa as viewed from the top of Mount Pilatus in the Alps, the Muir Glacier in Alaska, Fujiyama in Japan, the Yellow River in China, the Blue Grotto of Capri, the Jenolan Blue Caves in Australia, the spouting Geysers in New Zealand, the fascinating South Sea Islands, to say nothing of all the grandeurs in my own country. Any one of these corners of the earth I can visit at a moment's notice by just pulling one of memory's strings, and like Jack-in-the-box, up will pop country, peoples, scenery and all sorts of recollections. I often quote the saying of some wiseacre: "Three-tenths of the joy of travel is in anticipation, three-tenths in realization, and four-tenths in retrospection." This I have found to be literally true. In retrospection the weariness of travel, the poor food, the discomforts of, for instance, a boat on the Pagsanjan River in the Philippines along with natives eating their succulent incubated eggs, all such revulsion of sentiments and aches of body are submerged and only the unforgettable joys and visions of wonderful scenery, architectural splendor, art galleries, and all the rest arise before one.

If we have been guilty of any extravagance in our otherwise simple lives it has been in travel, yet never have we taken a world-jaunt except those based upon some scientific call or need of Mr. Ritter's. Only three years ago he was asked to go to Java as a National delegate. I was eager to go but he would not. Finally to squelch my arguments he turned on me and exclaimed witheringly, "You need never expect me to take another long journey unless I am compelled to for scientific work!" Instead of being squelched I shouted with laughter. "You never went anywhere in your life except for scientific work, but thank the Lord your scientific work has carried you to almost every corner of the globe." The only exceptions to this statement which I recall at the moment were the three weeks in the Grand Canyon of the Colorado, and a summer's cruise in Mr. Scripps' yacht around the Caribbean Sea. But even these unusual islands and the glories of the Grand Canyon, the Yellowstone and repeated visits to Yosemite have always yielded scientific interests in flora and fauna as well as geological formations.

Please do not think that I have wandered from my subject. I have only been sailing to Europe, crossing an ocean for the first of many times. Here we are in England where we spent the summer, partly in London, partly in Liverpool, where there is an interesting University, with a more interesting Biological Laboratory on the Isle of Man.

In London I visited hospitals and found a surprising number of women physicians and surgeons carrying on excellent work. But most of my time was spent sightseeing. From England to Antwerp, such a night, up the Rhine to Switzerland and on to Italy. There were stops in Genoa, Pisa, Florence and Rome ere we reached Naples and work for Mr. Ritter. I was enabled to see the great hospitals of Naples, but no work. Having learned the art galleries, watched Vesuvius night after night as it illumined the sky with great sheets of red hot lava, and scanned the mountain of black lava with which it had buried Herculaneum, walked the ash-covered streets of Pompeii, visited Capri, Sorrento and bewitching Amalfi, I went back to Rome for a month while Mr. Ritter plodded. It was during this visit in Rome that I received the letter announcing my father's death.

Rome, Rome! I will say no more. Rome is still there, but it was not the same in 1926 that it was in 1894. After gorging on its wonders for a month, back to Naples. Just one incident, the ascent of Vesuvius. The crater of Vesuvius! It had seemed fearful from a distance, but a fiery molten mass of beauty when one stood on the rim and looked down into its depths, and dodged the lava flung into the sky. What a different world is this inferno from the snow crowned top of Jungfrau!

Back to Germany, via Venice, where we so nearly froze that Mr. Ritter's hands were covered with chillblains. Over the Tyrol, down to Munich, and later on to Dresden. In Dresden I remained several weeks and took hospital courses. Later on to Berlin, where I joined Mr. Ritter. He had gone there after a few days of sightseeing in Dresden. With the usual watchfulness of the German police, I was at once visited by two officers to ascertain why, if I was Mr. Ritter's wife, I had not accompanied him there. After an amusing, though exasperating cross-questioning, involving the marital history of two generations of antecedents, I was permitted to occupy the apartment which Mr. Ritter had secured.

A winter of hard study in Berlin followed for both of us, interspersed with operas, visits to art galleries and Sunday trips to the environs. The medical lectures and ward clinics were at seasonable hours, but for the surgical clinics, the doors of the operating room closed at seven in the morning, with no admittance if one were a few minutes late. With snow often several inches deep after a stormy night, few street cars running, and frequently not a droschke to be found, this was no joke, and unfortunately I was in wretched health.

In a laboratory class for blood analysis, the students had to supply the blood to be studied. One day mine was taken and soon there was a hullaballoo about some sort of serious anemia. The anemia was there all right, a severe one, but not a tropical form, just the result of the life-long sepsis, from which I had never given myself time to recover.

That year La Grippe became a world epidemic. The term Influenza had not yet become the style. To Americans it was grippe. To the one or many germs which produce this malady I have always been extremely susceptible.

I had tried every national variety in each country we had visited. Now came the German type and a mean type it was. The physician under whom I was studying internal medicine was called in and he watched me for some time after the acute stage of the illness was over. In addition to the anemic condition he found a seriously weakened heart, with "murmurs" calling for rest. After a severe lecturing he sent me off into the country to recuperate, pronouncing the dictum that I must lead a very quiet life and never attempt to practice medicine again.

I did take a month's rest because I could not do otherwise. The wheels would not go 'round. This vacation was spent in the Schwartz Mountains above Eisenach. We stayed at a little inn outside the gate of the Wartburg Castle where Martin Luther was so long in hiding, and where he threw the inkpot at the devil. The great inkstain is still there after four hundred years, so of course Luther must have thrown the inkstand.

Although I obeyed this mandate of the doctor, I disobeyed every other command, visited Paris and a few other places in France, returned to London for the summer, and when we reached home in August, went to work. My motto has always been, "I would rather die in the harness than surrender to invalidism."

CHAPTER 8

University Interests

ONCE MORE IN BERKELEY MR. RITTER BEGAN MORE VIGOROUSLY TO build up the new department of Zoology. He also inaugurated a series of summer sea-side laboratory courses which gradually developed into the permanent Biological Research Station at La Jolla. Before deciding on a permanent location he tried out various localities from Alaska to San Diego. Summers at Pacific Grove, on Catalina Island and San Pedro stand out prominently in memory. These few weeks were my resting time. The remainder of the year I labored hard.

Before attempting to illustrate what exigencies may arise in a physician's every-day work, it seems wiser to introduce another layer in the "plywood" of my life—that of my connection with the University. Again it seemed to be my lot to be a "starter," for I was the "crank" that turned over the machinery for several innovations in the lives of the women students. Although the number of women students had increased rapidly from three or four in each class in the '80s to as many hundreds in the classes of the mid '90s, they were still inconsiderable numerically, and not at all to be considered in the various activities enjoyed by the men students.

For example, the men had had a gymnasium and instruction in gymnastics for years. It was assumed to be beneficial to their health and therefore a necessity. But this argument did not apply to the girls. The idea seemed rather to be that regular gymnastic exercise would be detrimental to their well-being. I sometimes felt as if the masculine powers-that-be thought that women were made of glass and might break to pieces if they fell down. But the girls did not think that way.

In the passing years old Harmon Gymnasium had been enlarged to nearly treble the original size, with offices appended in the rear. This made the girls ambitious, until finally a group visited the instructor of gymnastics beseeching the privilege of using the "gym" part of the time. Reluctantly the instructor said, "Of course you have a right to part time in the gymnasium and I would be willing to give you instruction, but the boys use the gym for dressing for track practice—and—and—the only time possible for your use would be after they go home at five o'clock. I would be willing to give you one hour a week at that time." After the girls had expressed their gratitude for that crumb, he added, "But I could not possibly admit anyone to the class without a medical examination and there is no money for that."

Alas for his foxy loop-hole! He had not counted on feminine determination. When a woman wants a thing, she wants it. The girls talked matters over and a day or two later the same group called on me and told me their story, asking if I would be willing to make the medical examinations without pay. I readily consented. This was in 1891. The instructor gallantly allowed me to use the gymnasium examining room with its apparatus for the medical tests.

Thus the entering wedge was made for the vast amount of fine training of many sorts which the women students have enjoyed these later years in the beautiful Hearst Gymnasium. Until this present year I have never passed the palatial women's building and then old Harmon Gymnasium without a broad and somewhat sardonic grin. This year, 1933, the boys have come into their own splendid structure and poor old Harmon has been razed. But more than three decades have rolled by before that accomplishment.

The unsatisfactory arrangement outlined above continued for two or three years before Mrs. Phoebe Hearst came to the rescue. She was the one woman regent on that august board. She established her residence in Berkeley for a year that she might come into closer contact with faculty and students, and thus increase her knowledge of the institution, and also her efficiency as a regent. From this test developed many things, one of which was the Hearst world competition for an ideal university plan on the Berkeley campus.

But my story pertains to the girls' physical culture work only. Mrs. Hearst built Hearst Hall for the entertaining of students and other large groups. It was a characteristic Maybeckian building, planned by Bernard Maybeck, the architect of the Palace of Fine Arts in the San Francisco Fair of 1915. It was built so that it could be divided into sections and later moved onto the campus for a women's gymnasium.

Mrs. Hearst's interest in the women students was deep and abiding. She came to be known as their "fairy godmother." Only those benefactions with which I was connected will be noted. The first of these was my regular appointment through her influence, as medical examiner for women students, for which she assumed the payment of my salary for part time. This meant office hours every morning in the gymnasium, where girls could consult me about their ills of body, mind or "hearts."

The handful of girls who formed the original group had grown to two or three hundred. I had given my services for two years by which time the girls had demonstrated their determination to have gymnasium work. They had also proved that their health was benefited thereby and no disastrous results had occurred. Therefore after two years, the regents decided to pay a fee of two and a half dollars for each examination, for one year. But it was to Mrs. Hearst's generosity as regent and philanthropist that the women students owe the establishment of the permanent position of a woman medical examiner in the University. The boys had had a man physician for many years.

The girls were given work at Harmon Gymnasium, two hours a week after the first two years. They were allowed reasonable hours, during which time the boys were excluded from the building. This arrangement continued until Mrs. Hearst removed from Berkeley in 1900, at which time she gave Hearst Hall for a women's gymnasium. By this time physical culture was made obligatory for the girls. Unless they were excused by an age limit, all the women students had to pass through my hands.

Many of the young women were seriously interested in their physical well-being and wished to know more about themselves and about homemaking. Nothing of this sort was given in the regular university courses. Again a group of girls came to me and asked if I would give them lectures on hygiene once a week. Again I agreed and a time and place were arranged. Home sanitation as well as personal hygiene, which was largely physiology, were included in the lectures. This work was at first voluntary on both sides, but was finally made compulsory for first-year women, and credit given for the course. Since the establishment of so much health work and domestic economy in the curriculum this course has been abandoned, but it was the wedge which opened the way for the grafting of several strong branches onto the old university tree in later years.

My work grew and grew. Since I was the only woman on the campus to whom the girls could turn for any personal advice, such advice, perforce, spread and spread like spilled treacle. It was confluent but covered a large area. Every sort of personal problem was brought to me. On a few occasions hasty marriages were arranged after too ardent lovemaking, but the standard of morality was very high. There is no unselected group of a thousand people anywhere, any age, in which every individual is staunch and strong.

The few cases which came under my care were those of young people, weak, perhaps, but not evil. One was a freshman boy boarding in a family in which there was a young high-school girl. One day this girl came to my office for an examination. After making the examination my first question was, "Have you a lover?" "Yes," she faltered. "Bring your mother to me tomorrow." The mother admitted she had been culpable in leaving the young people alone after she had retired. Both were under legal age. Consent of the parents to their marriage was obtained. A quiet wedding occurred in Mill Valley, and the boy forfeited his college education.

Years afterward, during the war, in one of my lectures on Social Hygiene given under the War Department, one pair of eyes never left my face. I talked to those eyes as I discussed the necessity for social and moral training and protection while thousands of boys were huddled in camps and the sympathy and patriotism of girls was being appealed to. Tears streamed from the eyes of that fine-looking woman. When the lecture was over she came to me and asked chokingly in a whisper, "Dr. Ritter, don't you know me? I am G— W—." It was the unfortunate little high-school girl who had come a long distance to hear my lecture. Later when I lectured in her home-town, I paid her a visit and found a fine family in

MORE THAN GOLD IN CALIFORNIA

a lovely vineyard home. Her oldest son was a strapping youth, fortunately just too young to have been drafted.

I relate this incident because it typifies the other cases of college girls, and because of this chance aftermath. It has been such chance meetings with my college girls, such aftermaths, that have brought me compensation for the donation of part of my life to them in their college days.

Several times during my years of war-work lectures, women have told me that my course in Hygiene and Home Sanitation had meant more to them in their domestic problems as wives, mothers and home-makers than any other course in the University.

Pardon this bit of soul-balm, but such little crumbs washed back from bread cast on the waters of life bring a deep sense of gratification in the knowledge that one's work has been of real value in the lives of others. This is particularly true since I have always felt that I was considered a sort of pariah in the University. The innovation of an unwelcome course pushed into the fringe of the orthodox curriculum by scarcely acceptable women students caused some resentment in the faculty, when the work was considered worthy of any notice at all. Hence, finding it had been of practical value in helping the girls to work out their lives was a genuine heart-balm to me. So much better than flowers on one's grave.

One of the problems about which the girls most frequently consulted me during my University office hours was the problem of inexpensive living. I found malnutrition common among them and knew that many were skimping too severely. Extra nourishment, a full and better-balanced diet, was my most frequent prescription, but all too often the conditions under which the girls were living made this impossible. Finally, one day in the later '90s, a group of girls came and asked me if I could help them find a way to organize cooperative house-keeping. They thought that if ten or fifteen girls could club together and keep house they could live better without increasing their expenses, which they could not afford to do. Simple as the proposition seemed, obstacles to its practical carrying-out bobbed up on every side.

For weeks and months we turned the problem over, making inquiries as to its feasibility, but price of rental, lack of suitable houses with a sufficient number of bedrooms and furnishings for fifteen girls, made it

92

impossible. Our figures demonstrated that with less than that number the expense would be too great, even though a suitably furnished house could be found. Many a wakeful night I spent in pondering this problem, and finally decided that it could not be solved without monetary aid, and where was this to be found? Evidently, definite data as to existing conditions must be obtained, but how? Whenever I face a difficult situation I usually find that the one person whose aid I can depend upon is myself. Consequently I decided to visit every girl attending the University, who lived in Berkeley away from her own home. There were several hundred of them.

The University had not up to this time assumed any responsibility for the place or conditions in which the students lived. Having no dormitory system, this factor of education, the physical well-being of the students had seemed to be the concern of neither the regents nor the executive officers. I realized that in order to reach them with any plea one must have carefully collected, first-hand data. Hence my decision to seek it. As few of the girls were in their rooms until after recitation hours, most of my calls had to be made after my office hours, frequently after five o'clock. Thus it took months to complete my self-appointed survey.

One of my first reactions was to the unsanitary conditions existing in many of the boarding houses. Although the small town of Berkeley had by this time installed a sewage system and water supply in the more thickly populated districts, not all of the residences by any means had been connected with these sanitary systems. Outhouses still existed and sometimes nearby wells supplied the drinking water. In such houses bathing facilities were either definitely inefficient or entirely lacking. I also found that where conditions were the worst, the boarding-house keepers were the most reluctant to let me inspect them. I found I must have official backing as I could not get the requisite data alone.

Conferences with President Benjamin Ide Wheeler resulted in my being armed with an official document requiring the householder of any house in which students were living to permit me to inspect all sanitary conditions. If permission was refused the students would be required to find other living quarters. This was the thin entering wedge for the University's present list of accredited boarding-houses in which students are permitted to live. To be on this list is now an eagerly-sought privilege. Only a few months ago, while very ill, I was besought by an acquaintance to use my influence with the Dean of Women to permit a house owned by this woman to be placed on the University list of recommended houses for women students.

In passing, let me add that another result of this canvass was the establishment of the requirement that the two sexes live in separate houses. The mere fact of inadequate bathing facilities made this desirable. Again, my canvass caused the University to report to the City Fathers those houses which had not complied with the sanitary regulations of the town by connecting with the water and sewage systems. This in turn resulted in closer inspection of such houses by the town authorities and a general improvement. Wells and outhouses were prohibited within the area supplied by city water and sewage systems.

By this time Mrs. Hearst had come to Berkeley to live and our association had become very intimate. She was keenly interested in all problems pertaining to the girls, so when I reported to her that I had found girls living—cooking, eating, sleeping and studying—in small attic rooms or sunless basements, with one small window in either case, and all sorts of desolate conditions, she agreed with me that something must be done to remedy the situation. I told her of the girls' desire for cooperative house-keeping and of my dream of some sort of clubbing-together scheme for them. She instantly approved. "But," I added, "I do not know how to work it out. I want to study the living conditions of women in other universities and colleges." "Good," she replied. "If you will go East this summer and make the survey I will pay your expenses."

Accordingly, in the summer vacation of 1900, I visited as many women's colleges as possible from Wellesley near Boston to Bryn Mawr in Philadelphia, and also co-educational institutions from the Universities of Chicago and Wisconsin to Cornell in New York, about a dozen, all told. In Smith College at Northampton, Massachusetts, I found the cottage system, which most nearly suited our needs but was far more elaborate than was possible here. Discussions with the deans of women in all the institutions visited were helpful to me and aided in bringing about some of the regulations I have referred to.

On my return, equipped with more data and ideas, Mrs. Hearst offered to furnish two club houses to test the efficacy of my plan. In the autumn of that year, 1900, the "Pie del Monte" and "Enewah" Club Houses were started with fifteen girls and a house-mother in each, paying their own expenses pro rata, except as to room rent which varied according to size and location of the rooms. To cover the cost of rental, the house was divided on the basis of so much per room. Naturally the large front rooms were assessed for more than the smaller back rooms, and the third-floor rooms for less than the second-floor. Two girls occupied each room which was furnished with twin beds, separate bureaus, chairs and study-tables.

These two club-houses were a decided success and led to a new era in the life of many women students, and later men students also. But the added work had been arduous and told heavily on my strength, bringing nearer the inevitable crash.

The greater part of the following year, 1901, I spent in a sanitarium for heart cases in Santa Barbara. In 1903 the club-house project was again taken up. I quote here the first page of the minute-book of the "Club-House-Loan Fund Committee of the University of California."

Berkeley, Dec. 4, 1903.

President Benj. Ide Wheeler issued a call for the meeting together of ten persons to consider the matter of helping to form clubs of college students in order to help those who at present are living in an unsanitary way: some in garrets, some in sheds in back yards, and many doing their own cooking and not supplying themselves with wholesome food.

The temporary committee was composed of the following persons:

Dr. Mary B. Ritter
Mrs. Benj. Ide Wheeler
Professor Jessica B. Piexotto
Mrs. Maude W. Richardson
Mrs. May L. Cheney
Professor Wm. Carey Jones
Professor C. H. Rieber

Professor James T. Allen

Mr. Warren Olney, Jr., 1891

Professor Geo. C. Edwards.

These appointees met Dec. 4, 1903, at the home of Dr. Mary B. Ritter, with the exceptions of Prof. Jones and Mr. Olney.

Mrs. Ritter was elected chairman and Mr. Edwards, secretary.

It was moved and carried that the trustees aim to secure $5000 with which to furnish 5 clubs, said sum to be obtained by subscriptions by the individual members of the committee.

Mrs. Richardson was appointed a purchasing committee of one, for the small task of buying everything from an egg-beater, spoons and forks, to parlor furniture, curtains and rugs for a family of fifteen! Professor Edwards served as secretary for four years, when Dr. James T. Allen succeeded him. Dr. Allen is still secretary, with twenty-six years of service behind him, and more ahead. My chairmanship ended only because of our removal to La Jolla in 1909, but I am still a member of the Board. I was succeeded by Mrs. Cheney who is chairman to this day.

Of that original committee appointed thirty years ago, half of the number are still active members. Two have been removed by death, Colonel Edwards and Professor Jones. Dr. Rieber was transferred to the University of California in Los Angeles. Mr. Olney, an attorney of San Francisco, after contributing his legal services in drawing up a contract form and otherwise advising us as to legal requirements, resigned from the Board since he was unable to attend meetings. After Mrs. Richardson had served eighteen years, in which time she furnished about thirty club-houses, exigencies in her family caused her to resign. The loss to the committee was a serious one, but if ever any volunteer worker deserved the praise, "Well done, good and faithful servant," she merited it. But not more so than Mrs. Cheney and Dr. Allen who have been chairman and secretary for twenty-four and twenty-six years, respectively. Dr. Allen once laconically remarked, "No one ever gets off this committee except by death."

In 1906 Miss Lucy Sprague came to the University as the first Dean of Women. She was appointed on the Club House Loan Fund

Committee, December the seventh, 1906. Later the deans of men were made *ex-officio* members of the Board. A representative of the California State Federation of Women's Clubs was also added. Miss Lucy Stebbins, the second Dean of Women, became a member of the Board, May twentieth, 1911.

That entry in the minutes of the Board of Directors that the money for furnishing the Club Houses should be secured by subscriptions, the individual members of the committee to be the solicitors for the same, sounds innocent enough, but alas! the weary toil and the trials and tribulations it involved. The plan was that the Board should loan to each club the equivalent, in furniture, of one thousand dollars without interest, the same to be returned in annual installments of one hundred dollars. The first thousand was raised relatively easily, by begging. The first club to receive this loan was the "La Solana."

Raising the money for the second and third clubs was extremely difficult and brought various woes in its trail, some of which seem highly amusing in retrospect but were most vexatious at the time. In consequence, it became evident that some more stable source of supply must be found. Two such came to our aid.

The first was the California State Federation of Women's Clubs. The incoming president, Mrs. Bulkley, resided in Berkeley. A proposition that the State Federation should espouse this cause and raise money among its members for housing students was laid before her and she consented to present it to the next convention of the Federation, meeting in Sacramento that year, 1904. The Federation agreed to raise one thousand dollars for a club house, and did so during the regime of Mrs. Bulkley, who later represented the Federation on the Club House Board and also served for several years as house-mother in one of the clubs.

The plan of the Federation was to pass the responsibility for collecting the money through the District and County officers to the individual clubs, asking each member to give ten cents a year. This was carried on until the Federation had donated five thousand dollars. I was for many years State Chairman of the Club House Loan Fund in the Federation, and made this plea many times each year to clubs and conventions.

Another friend came to our rescue. Mrs. Margaret Fowler of Pasadena first gave one thousand dollars for a single Club House, and later gave five thousand to the University for the housing of women students. This sum was handed over to our Board by Miss Sprague, Dean of Women.

Although the collection of this amount covered a period of many years, it has enabled the Board to continue to establish club houses for both men and women students until up to the present time, forty-two such groups of students have been aided by the establishment of club homes. Of these, twenty-three club houses are for women and nineteen for men. Four or five of them became sororities or fraternities after their indebtedness for furniture had been met. At the present writing the club houses furnished for student homes are scattered all over Berkeley. After the furniture in a house was paid for, the Board had no further jurisdiction over it unless, as has occurred on several occasions, the members requested another loan for an enlarged group.

These forty-two club-houses seem to have met the pressing needs of students, for such club-house applications have been relatively few in recent years. Any estimate of the number of individual students assisted through the Club House Loan Fund Committee during the thirty years of its existence is extremely difficult, as the personnel of each group varies constantly. Seniors graduate each year and freshmen enter. A modest estimate makes the number thus assisted run well toward ten thousand. To indicate the universality of such housing needs in earlier days, one item of interest may be the fact that the present President of the University, Robert Gordon Sproul, was a member of one of the first men's club-house groups, and its secretary for several years.

An unanticipated outcome of an instance of bartered labor is vouched for by Mrs. Cheney. During one summer four club-houses were furnished, two for men and two for women students. At the opening of the college year all of these groups were invited to President Wheeler's residence to meet the members of the Board and to learn their responsibilities as house-holders in the University circle. Informal discussion followed and the students were invited to ask any questions or make any criticisms about the furnishings. After some hesitation one boy rose and said, "We boys find that the Committee has provided us with two dozen unhemmed napkins. We fellows don't know much about hemming napkins, but we hear that the girls want the floors in their houses painted. Now I propose that if the girls will hem the four dozen napkins for the two men's clubs, we will paint their floors." The exchange was accomplished, and after college days were over, five weddings among those exchangers resulted. While the Board had no intention of serving as a marriage bureau, statistics show that marriages between college students rate very high as to success, so perhaps the Board served society better than it knew.

My husband is not given to words of laudation, but once when I was ill and feeling very much of a failure, he said, "If you had never done anything but initiate that Club House Loan Fund plan, your life would have been worth living."

As I re-read the minutes of the Committee for the past twenty-four years during which I have lived elsewhere, and note their valiant and self-sacrificing work, I wish hereby to give them the credit for the successful carrying on of this arduous but soul-gratifying labor of love for the students. I can however, honestly lay claim to having been the "starter" in this student activity inasmuch as I conceived the plan, made the initial survey, and with the financial aid of Mrs. Hearst and the official consent of President Wheeler furnished two successful club-houses before the formal committee was called together. It was the success of these two club homes which resulted in the formation of a permanent Board under the University authorities.

After twenty-two years of residence and work in Berkeley, my husband's labors necessitated our migration to Southern California. Although I remained on the Club House Loan Fund Board and attended the meetings whenever possible, the burden for the past quarter of a century has been carried by the valiant Board, half of whose members have served during the entire thirty years of its existence.

I must refer to one organization of the women students, the Prytanean, because it came into existence in my home with me as consultant. Credit for its formation is due to Adele Lewis. As a junior, in 1900, she conceived the idea of an organization of women students which would be of service to its Alma Mater and an honor to its members.

Early in the Fall semester she and Agnes Frisius, president of the Associated Women Students, came to consult me about the plan. I approved enthusiastically, realizing the need and value of such an organization. We three worked out a scheme and a tentative constitution. It was decided to invite all the heads of women's societies to meet at my home and become charter members of an unnamed infant organization. The naming of the infant was so difficult that it became humorous, and I imagine was somewhat of a nuisance to the Greek authorities who were consulted.

I was naturally the first honorary member. The next two, as I recall, were Mrs. John Fryer and Madame Paget, women especially devoted to the welfare of girls. The Prytaneans met in my living room until it was outgrown.

Discussion centered about the first project to be undertaken. My survey of the living quarters of the girls and the need of some place where sick students could be cared for were foremost in my mind. Instances of similar needs among the men students many times presented to the president by their physicians verified my report. A committee consulted President Wheeler, who cordially approved their idea of working toward a hospital for women students.

The Prytaneans attempted to raise funds for the project but found it too great an undertaking at that time. But slowly the plan developed and five years later it became the honor and privilege of Dr. George Reinhardt to establish the University Infirmary. That same year, 1905, I was forced by ill health to retire from the University.

In its thirty-three years, Prytanean has enrolled nearly four thousand student members, beside about one hundred and twenty-five honorary members. Once a Prytanean, always a Prytanean. A strong daughter society has been recently organized in the University of California in Los Angeles.

In 1931 the splendid Cowell Memorial Hospital superseded the Infirmary. To the first struggling effort to care for sick students, Prytanean had contributed over six thousand dollars; and has since raised a Prytanean Loan Fund of over fifty-five hundred dollars.

In the first Prytanean Booklet President Sproul writes: "The past record of the Society justifies confidence in its future ... fine work." And

Dean Lucy Stebbins says: "I would assure all Prytaneans that their found-ers' conception of the union of honor and service has weathered the years. It has outlived classes and survived the clash of tradition and innovation. It has animated all past endeavor and present promise. Together honor and service are the spirit of Prytanean."

Of the several hundred "infants" I have assisted into this world there is none of whose career I am more proud than of Prytanean.

Doubtless my readers are wondering where the practicing physician was during all these years of social service of one sort or another. My reply is, hard at work. These activities were my recreation, dare I say? It must be remembered that they were spread over a period of twenty years in Berkeley, and probably the number of hours per week spent in social ser-vice work did not greatly exceed those spent by many modern physicians at golf. When I accepted part-time work in the University on salary from Mrs. Hearst, I deliberately cut off my more distant practice, particularly maternity cases. But I had done ten years of hard practice before that occurred.

CHAPTER 9

Medical Practice

HOW CAN ONE WRITE OF MEDICAL PRACTICE? VISITS TO PATIENTS' bed-sides and the routine of office hours, while always interesting to the physician, would for the most part make dull reading. Only illustrative cases can be told in a brief account of years of work. I will relate a few experiences, mostly to show by contrast the advantages given the physicians of today, both in diagnosis and treatment, by the advance of other sciences. Bacteriology has made tremendous strides since that time; physics has contributed the X-ray, fluoroscope and dozens of other aids to the knowledge of existing conditions which in the 19th century could be only reasoned about.

Anti-toxins were then unknown. The only immunization commonly in use was vaccination against smallpox. Diphtheria and typhoid were deadly foes, and very prevalent. Now the cases are so scarce that some physicians have never seen a typical case.

Of enzymes, only those of digestion were discussed in our lectures in physiology. They were too recent to have been mentioned in our text books. Now seven or eight are recognized. Those dormant endocrines which make or mar our lives were then unknown. Now they are so familiar that whether or not one needs thyroid extract is a common subject over the tea-table. So on and on. "Medicine" now-a-days is virtually a different science.

At that time there were no hospitals in Berkeley and very inadequate hospital service in Oakland. It was not then the fashion for expectant mothers to be taken to hospitals, whereas now almost every obstetrical case goes to a hospital, and the physician is not called until labor is well advanced. All of my several hundred maternity cases were attended in their homes and often I had to attend to all the sanitary preparations such as sterilizing, and sometimes even to fixing the bed. Trained nurses were few and far between. A neighbor or at best a practical nurse was all the help I had. Many times I had to wash and dress the baby, not only the first time, but for successive mornings. And for the pre-natal care, the accouchment, and visits for ten days after, the regulation fee was twenty-five dollars—when one got anything.

Rather recently I read a book called *One Day in a Doctor's Life*. It began at one in the morning with a birth, and ended at midnight with death of an aged patient. Between times were cases of every sort, both physical and mental—tales of woe that are poured into a doctor's ears. The family doctor sees more skeletons in closets than the priest. Simply to list the burdens laid on that doctor's mind, heart and body in that one day, would fill this page. Yet it was not an impossible story, though such congested days seldom occur. A doctor could not long survive with twenty-four hours of work every day. By the end of forty-eight hours of such congestion the human machine is thoroughly fagged, yet such strains are not so uncommon as one could wish.

Two cases—one surgical and one medical—may well illustrate my remarks on the lack of X-ray aids in diagnosis. As I watch modern practice with the X-ray relied upon for verification of almost every condition in surgery, from broken bones to a suspected tooth, and from any and all chronic conditions of the internal organs to the progress of an acute tuberculosis, I wonder how we dared set bones or venture a diagnosis of any sort forty or fifty years ago. Seeing that we did, how was it that any of our patients lived?

The cases which I remember had always some unusual feature which stamped them on memory's tablet. In the following case it was the touch of humor as well as the difficulty caused by the initial neglect of the parents, which stamped the picture on my mind.

An eleven-year-old son of a Welsh gardener who worked by the day for the townspeople went out one late afternoon to bring in the cow. Bossy was playful, or hungry, and started to run as the boy loosened the rope by which she was tethered. His foot was caught in a loop of the rope and he was dragged for some distance over a rough field. How he got to the house I do not know. I was not called until the next morning about nine o'clock, at least sixteen hours after the accident. I found the boy feverish and suffering greatly. His entire left leg was swollen to twice the size of the other. Being of a stocky build and muscular greatly impeded diagnosis, but by the senses of sight, touch and hearing (crepitus or grating sound of broken bone) I recognized a fracture of the shaft of the thigh-bone. I sent at once for Dr. Eastman, a Berkeley physician, asking him to bring the anaesthetic, and splints for a fractured femur.

The boy was under the anaesthetic for more than two hours. To reduce the fracture (or set the leg) accurately in that condition of extreme swelling and inflammation was extremely difficult. Of artificial visual aid we had none, and the conditions rendered the sense of touch almost nil. We could get the leg into proper shape only by using the other as a guide. Oh, how we had to pull against those inflamed, contracted muscles to get that knee-joint down to correspond with the other leg! Dr. Eastman held it in position while I bandaged and applied the splints. A cast could not be used until the swelling was reduced.

It was a little after ten when Dr. Eastman arrived with the needed accessories and it was nearly two before we left the patient. I cautioned the mother not to give the boy any dinner but said that he could have a few sips of water when the post-anaesthetic vomiting ceased, or if he were very hungry she might give him a few teaspoonfuls of milk. I would return after office hours.

When I arrived about five, the patient looked surprisingly cheerful. I asked if he were hungry. "No." "Did you take any milk?" "No." A flush and dropping of the eyes aroused my suspicions. "What did you have?" "A piece of cherry-pie." I called the mother in. After a severe reprimand, she whined, "You didn't tell me not to give him cherry-pie!!!"

This story served me often as an adroit reproof to recalcitrant patients. Suffice to say, the boy's leg was neither shortened nor deformed despite the lack of X-ray, but what a help that would have been!

Another condition which would now be diagnosed by X-ray and probably relieved by surgical operation was a case of ulcers of the stomach and intestines. A lovely young woman patient, who has been a life-long friend, suffered from a chronic indigestion of years' standing. I diagnosed it as gastric ulcers and treated the case mainly by diet. There were never any hemorrhages and in course of time the ulcers apparently healed. At any rate, this same patient, no longer young, and a chronic invalid, had many and careful X-ray pictures taken of stomach and intestines three or four years ago. Scars of former ulcers showed clearly. When Miss B. saw the pictures, and the physicians showed her the cicatrices, she exclaimed, "Why, that is exactly what Dr. Ritter said was the trouble forty years ago!" "Forty years!" retorted the doctor somewhat scathingly. "How could she? There were no X-rays then!" Miss B. insisted such was the case, and brought the radio-graphs for me to see. There were the scars beautifully delineated. She told me of the above conversation which riled me a bit and I retorted, "Please tell that young man for me that it is true we had no X-rays forty years ago. We had to use our brains." I will admit that was a cutting remark but the incident well illustrates the handicaps under which all physicians, previous to the twentieth century, had to labor. Many diagnoses could not be verified then as they are now. Doubtless more mistakes were made than now, but we did have to use our brains, all of them, all of our five senses and perhaps a sixth sense of what the Scotch call "canniness," more than is necessary in modern practice.

In this connection may I be forgiven for relating one of the most gratifying compliments I ever received? The professor of English in the University was called to Yale. His wife, an invalid, had been my patient ever since I succeeded Dr. Shuey. Accompanying a lovely farewell gift from my patient came a note from the professor which surprised me greatly, but which I treasure to this day. The closing sentence read, "We never expect to find again such a combination of devotion to duty, skill, and good horse-sense." I was nearly bowled over that the precise Professor C. should use such a homely phrase as "good horse-sense." When it came to devotion to duty I think I honestly earned the compliment, and perhaps the horse-sense or some sort of an uncanny "sixth sense" I may lay claim to. As to the skill, when I look back, I am filled with a sort of horror at my temerity. How dared I, with so little skill, attempt such battles with life and death?

To illustrate pre-immunization treatment of diphtheria and typhoid fever I will relate a case of each, the most severe cases I had to deal with.

The minister's little eight-year-old daughter had diphtheria. She had been ill several days and the attending physician, a homeopath, had "given her up,"—said he could do nothing more. I was sent for. Such a picture I never witnessed before and hope never to again. The nostrils seemed solidly plugged with diphtheritic membrane which extended down over the entire fauces and tonsils. The child was almost *in extremis*. I sent at once to the Children's Hospital in San Francisco for two of their finest graduate nurses, those rare trained nurses. And how we three worked! The Lord was on our side and the child did not die of paralysis of the heart as so often happens.

Of anti-toxin nothing was known. We could only stimulate the patient and try to kill the membrane. The poor little child lay there almost moribund. Every fifteen minutes of the twenty-four hours, that membrane was sprayed with solutions to destroy it. One solution I recall was tincture of iron, recall because of a pun made by the convalescent child. When the membrane had been cleared and the patient was apparently going to live, the day nurse, on coming on duty said "Oh, I see you've been washed, Florence." "Yes," Florence replied. "I've been washed and sprinkled and ironed." A pretty good pun on the iron spraying, I thought.

To those nurses I want to pay a tribute. At first neither of them slept, then six hours off and six to eight hours on duty; only rest enough to keep going. They were heroic. I saw the patient from four to six times a day— and night, and it being a poorly-paid minister's family, we knew there was no monetary compensation for any of us. But I had compensation thirty years later when a fellow-passenger on a trans-Atlantic steamer came to me and said, "I am Florence H. Do you remember when I had diphtheria?" Could I ever forget it? She was then a teacher of singing in a Southern California school. With her on the steamer was her husband, a professional organist, at the head of the Music Department. With them was a fine son in his early 'teens. They were enroute to Europe for a year of study in music and language. Could one ask for better compensation than to have saved such a life?

And now a sketch of the worst case of typhoid fever I ever had to battle with. In the summer of 1898 typhoid fever was prevalent. Typhoid immunization was a thing of the future. At that time one simply waged a battle to maintain the patient's strength through a weary struggle for the weeks it took for the disease to run its course. I was the physician of Miss Head's School, where a pupil, a frail girl, apparently little ready to fight such a battle, came down with the dreaded disease. Yet one thing which can never be measured is individual endurance. Often the seemingly-frail will stand a long siege where an active, robust person quickly succumbs. So it was in this instance.

The patient was quarantined in the attic, which meant three flights of stairs (beside the high outside steps) for me to climb on every visit and for weeks that was three, four or more times each day and night. Again two splendid nurses were installed, and how we fought! How many gallons of orange juice and strained white of egg were poured by the teaspoonful between the teeth of that raving, delirious girl, I cannot even guess. At that time, reducing the temperature by cold immersions was a common practice. There being no conveniences in the attic, this was impossible, so often, very often, cold sponges were substituted.

There was another virulent case near by, a strong, athletic daughter of a San Francisco physician. As the father was in Europe, half a dozen of his confreres came from San Francisco to try to save the life of his daughter. Valiantly they fought and from day to day I would hear of the most modern methods they were trying. This often discouraged me, gave me a feeling of decided inferiority, but I struggled on, endeavoring by constant watching and devotion to forestall every crisis.

I was recently reminded by Dr. H. B. Torrey, then a student assistant of Mr. Ritter's, of an incident which I had forgotten. He said that one day while I was working on this case, I came home late for dinner. I sat down at the table but could not eat. I buried my head in my hands and muttered, "This girl must not die." I think this was just after the death of the doctor's daughter. Apparently her hold on life had been less than that of my patient, though she had been seemingly stronger. But I had an advantage in watching my patient morning, noon and night instead of seeing her once a day. Anyway, after a struggle of weeks and weeks, the girl recovered.

I really think that the same dogged determination which prompted the five-year-old child, regardless of spankings and being shut in a dark smoke-house, to insist, "I don't want to wear that hat," had something to do with the surprisingly small death list that fell to my lot. I will illustrate this later in the case of a newborn babe.

To indicate "the day in a doctor's life," I well recall being summoned from this case where life was hanging by a thread, at about five o'clock one morning to go to the residence of Mrs. Little, my former home. At this time we were living in our own home which we had built on Durant Avenue near Telegraph. I went to the very room I had occupied before I was married and by noontime there was ushered into this world Mrs. Little's first grandchild, the first-born son of John and Ada Little Merriam. Home to lunch, back to the typhoid patient, off for visits to other patients, office hours, again up all those flights of stairs to the attic sick-room, dinner, a bedtime visit in the attic—that was my day before my weary muscles and brain could seek rest. "All in a day's work" in a doctor's life.

Shall I mention the monetary side of medical practice? To me money was never the paramount question. The poorest patient received the same devoted care as the richest. Little Florence received just as much attention as this well-to-do-girl. It was the life I was battling for. But when I was asked by this patient's family for my bill, I sent one for five hundred dollars to a brother who was executor of his father's large estate. I received a partial payment check with a reference to the size of the bill. This wounded me greatly. I wrote him that if his sister's life was not worth that amount he might reduce the bill to what he considered was equitable, but that as for me, had another cipher been added to the amount it would not have been adequate recompense for what my devotion to his sister had taken out of my life. I received an abject apology and the full amount of the bill.

I cannot conceive of a conscientious physician refusing to serve any worthy person because of his lack of ability to pay for the service. Every physician expects to carry a large percentage of non-paying patients on his books, yet his practice is his means of earning a living. His education has been expensive and his overhead is heavy, therefore he expects his clientele to be as faithful in paying for his work as they would be to an attorney who had saved a piece of property for them, and he resents it when he finds his leniency abused. I would never sue for a bill; the money was not worth the ordeal, yet I still have on my books, long unopened, accounts of hundreds of dollars against some of the elite of Berkeley, who could attend every opera but never had money for the family doctor. And these very people are the ones most prone to call the doctor out into a storm in the middle of the night for some trifling ailment.

* * * * * * *

The most arduous and ofttimes the most heroic part of the family doctor's life is that of ushering new lives into the world. At any rate it was the most fatiguing part of my duties, since it usually meant a night of labor for me as well as the patient. In those old-time horse-and-buggy days, when the father or other messenger had to come for the doctor, and the horse had to be harnessed, the doctor was usually sent for at the earliest evidence of approaching accouchment. Often it was a false alarm, and equally often a weary, dreary waiting through the first stage of dilatation where very little could be done for the sufferer except to give hot sitz-baths and occasional whiffs of chloroform. Frequently I was in attendance eighteen hours, and sometimes more. The lack of trained nurses and of telephones made it necessary to be close at hand. Occasionally I would run away to make a call or two but soon returned.

As noted before, I usually had to do all the sterilizing and sometimes oversee the arrangement of the bed. And bed it was, never a delivery-table. I always used chloroform to ease the pains, but never had an anaesthetist unless the case was a very severe one. Thus this delicate responsibility was added to my cares.

Perhaps it was to this unsparing devotion to duty, as Professor C. wrote of me, that I can lay claim to the heart-balm of never having lost a woman in child-birth, nor had a case of "puerperal fever." To be sure my practice was not large as compared with those of doctors of the present age of autos and hospitals, nor did it extend over a long period of years.

Of my several hundred cases about three-fourths were normal and uninteresting to a layman, but birth, the advent of a new life, is never uninteresting to those vitally concerned. Aside from the sentiment there are always enough dangers lurking around the corner for both mother and babe, to keep the attending physician on the alert. Of the remaining fourth of the cases, probably twenty per cent were sufficiently difficult to require instrumental aid to nature. Possibly four per cent were really dangerous from one cause or another, and one per cent a real battle for the life of mother or babe, or both.

Three cases in this last category I will try to relate; I say try, because it is impossible to completely translate the situation into words. But these three cases illustrate different sorts of dangers which may occur to test the physician to the utmost. At any rate in these illustrative cases my skill and strength were tested almost to the limit.

Three times in my practice I was faced with that dread spectre, post partum hemorrhage—a menace to life which occurs so quickly and is so violent that a few minutes may turn the balance between life and death. One account will explain all such instances.

The one I relate occurred in a lovely home on Piedmont Avenue. The people were almost complete strangers to me. Having had a severe ordeal in a former delivery with the attendance of a male physician, they turned this time to me. All went well until after the baby was born. The uterus had seemingly contracted normally. With my back turned toward the mother while I cared for the baby, I turned, at an exclamation from the nurse, to see that deathly pallor of approaching death on the mother's face. Her eyes were uprolled in unconsciousness. I rushed to her side and felt her abdomen. The womb had relaxed almost to the size of the parturient uterus. The fundus reached almost to the diaphragm.

Quickly I dropped on my knees, grasped the fundus with my left hand and inserted my right hand and arm inside the uterus. Never shall I forget the feeling of that hot blood striking my arm with the seeming force of a garden hose. Closing my right hand firmly, with my left hand outside the abdominal wall, I grasped the clenched fist inside and thus forced the dilated uterus to contract on my fist. As the uterine muscle contracted I gradually withdrew my right arm which had been inserted nearly to my elbow, reaching almost up to the patient's diaphragm. Inch by inch my clenched hand was lowered until withdrawn. Meanwhile I was directing the nurse and husband as to methods of restoring the mother to consciousness.

How long I was there on my knees, exerting all the strength of my left hand to force the uterus to contract, I do not know, but to the best of my memory it was nearly two hours before I dared slacken my hold on that slowly-contracting womb. With the least relaxation of my left hand I could feel the uterine muscle relax also, so I had actually to hold her life in my hand until Nature and medicine had time to stimulate the natural, strong uterine contractions.

During the first part of this battle my own heart almost stood still. The fell destroyer had gotten such an advantage that it seemed doubtful if the patient could be snatched from his grasp. When at last the advantage seemed on my side, there was still a long and weary tussle.

Oh, what I suffered mentally, and how my body ached as I knelt on the floor in a cramped position, using all my muscular power to hold that flaccid uterus in the grip of my left hand. At last the danger passed, the mother slept quietly and I went home utterly exhausted.

Years afterward, when my own health was seriously broken and I had been for nearly a year in a sanitarium, I met this lady on the little Berkeley train. She said to me, "Dr. Ritter, I simply cannot conceive of you being ill or nervous or anything but a tower of strength—cool and calm." I thanked her, and was glad that she had not been aware of the tortures of hell which I had suffered in both body and mind during that two-hour struggle for her life.

The next case illustrates a totally different situation, one in which the danger to the child was greater than that to the mother, although the peril to both was greatly increased. This was an instance of faulty position of the foetus *in utero*. When I was summoned I found what I had suspected, an almost transverse position of the foetus, that is the child lay nearly crosswise of the mother's body instead of head downward as is normal. As the pains or uterine contractions began, the breech of the child was forced downward and the head upward, the reverse of the natural position. In such cases Nature has no chance to do her part in moulding the head of the unborn babe to enable it to pass through the pelvis, the diameter of which is usually slightly less than that of the head of the child. Neither can Nature bend the chin onto the chest and thus present the crown of the head as the entering wedge and rotate it to fit the longest (diagonal) axis of the pelvis. Nor can Nature use the head as the dilating wedge in the mouth of the womb itself.

This case was a primipera—the first baby of a fine young couple, both of whom had been my personal friends before their marriage. They are still among the most prominent people in this community. My personal interest in the parents may have added zest to my determination to save their child, but I am not sure. A life is a life and must be saved if possible.

Realizing that version and manual extraction, breech first, would be necessary, with an instrumental delivery of the after-coming head, both requiring complete anaesthesia of the mother, I sent for Dr. Buckel to assist me. The child was unusually large and was doubled up like a partly closed jack-knife, the feet reaching nearly to the head. The breech was too large to enter the pelvis. All I could do was to reach up into the uterus with my right hand, and using my forefinger as a hook in the right loin of the child, try to bring the breech down into the pelvis. This was a long and wearying process. Dr. Buckel and I worked for two or three hours, taking turns at the attempted delivery and the anaesthetizing. Version and delivery are not matters of brute strength, but of skill, as co-workers with nature, directing and aiding her efforts.

Finding that it was to be a long and difficult struggle we sent for my good friend Dr. Eastman, so that Dr. Buckel could give her entire attention to the anaesthesia.

For two or three hours more, Dr. Eastman and I worked by turns to bring the babe's breech down into the channel of the pelvis by using our forefingers for traction. Gradually this was accomplished sufficiently to deliver the body of the child, releasing first one leg and then the other, then one arm at a time. But that large, unmoulded head was yet to be delivered.

The delivery of that after-coming head was a more difficult operation than any I had ever witnessed in an obstetrical clinic, and here was I responsible for the lives of two human beings. Were such a thing possible as sweating blood, I should have done so. Dr. Eastman and I took turns in applying the forceps to force the head as slowly and gently as possible into a position where it could be made to enter the bony canal. This too was a long and tedious task. The child was larger than average and the unusually large head was of the round, brachy-cephalous type—a so-called "square head."

The peril to the child's life became momentarily greater. The cord was wrapped three times around the neck, causing danger of strangulation. After what seemed eons of time, the after-coming head was forced through the pelvis, Dr. Eastman and I taking turns in pulling on it until our arms were weary. At last it came but the child was apparently dead. Ordinary means of resuscitation were of no avail. Dr. Eastman said, "You cannot revive that child. It is dead." "This splendid baby has got to live!" I replied. "If you and Dr. Buckel will attend to the mother I will work on the baby."

Alas, there were no pulmotors to be sent for. It was a case of performing artificial respiration and using every possible means to resuscitate the moribund child. An occasional faint gasp would encourage me, only to be followed by seemingly absolute lifelessness. The other two doctors insisted it was a hopeless endeavor, but the obstinate determination of that stubborn child who would not wear her hat resulted at last in victory.

The faint gasps came more and more frequently and finally there was a faint wail with several successive respirations. The minutes seemed hours though in reality it was less than half an hour—but such a half hour, fighting face to face with death! The child's color improved—a stronger cry—blessed sound—and more regular breathing, until finally a smart slap on that poor abused breech caused that fine baby to let out a yell which was the sweetest music I ever heard. Soon the child was warmly wrapped and laid in his crib, able to breathe for himself—which he has continued to do these forty years.

That seemingly lifeless baby is now a prominent business man in the Bay region. I met him with his wife and mother since our return to Berkeley, and as I looked at his square forehead and unusually large head I shivered inwardly, while outwardly smiling, as he told me he had been brought up with the understanding that he owed his life to my persistence.

The third case which I will cite illustrates two things—first, one of the most deadly foes to motherhood; and second, the reason why physicians cannot "heal themselves."

One of my patients, the wife of one of the University professors, and again a personal friend, had a history of scarlet fever in her early 'teens which was complicated by acute nephritis, leaving her kidneys permanently damaged. They were able to function normally under ordinary circumstances but could not stand the added work and pressure forced upon them by gestation.

Uraemia is one of the conditions carefully watched for in every case of pregnancy because of the double load placed upon the kidneys by having two organisms from which they must eliminate certain virulent poisons, the natural results of body metabolism. If the kidneys are in any degree abnormal, there is danger of failure in this eliminating process which goes on every minute of the day and night, just as do breathing and heart-beating. The result of such failure causes more or less uraemic poisoning which is liable to end in toxic convulsions.

This woman, though seemingly in normal health, had crippled kidneys as an aftermath of nephritis. She was extremely desirous for children and was willing to hazard her life for that purpose. Before coming to California she had twice attempted to have a child, both attempts culminating in eclampsia, or puerperal convulsions, before the child was advanced enough to be viable. She came to me with her story, adding that she was going to try again to bear a child and wanted to place herself in the hands of a physician in order to be put in the best possible condition before the undertaking. This plan was carried out. When her entire system was apparently functioning normally, she entered upon her perilous venture. All went well for nearly five months.

One very stormy day in winter I came home at the end of my day's work with a severe cold on my lungs. I ached from head to foot and by the time I got to bed had a temperature of one hundred and two degrees. I had my housekeeper make hot flaxseed poultices for my chest and put a hot water bottle at my feet. The rain was still coming down in torrents and from my warm bed I said to Mr. Ritter, "I wouldn't go out tonight for Queen Victoria!" I did not go out for Queen Victoria, but I did go for Mrs. L—.

Sleep had come to my weary brain and body and I was far away in the Land of Nod when the doorbell clanged that ominous call to duty. My first waking thought was, "I simply cannot go out for anyone tonight!" It was one o'clock in the morning; the rain was pouring down and a cold wind blowing. I opened the window and spoke to the messenger. It was Professor H—, who said, "Mrs. L— is very ill and Professor L— asked me to come for you. He wants you to come as quickly as possible." I was terror-stricken both for the patient and myself. There was no chance of getting help from San Francisco, as I had counted on doing in case of serious trouble, since the ferry boats had stopped running. It seemed to me it was a choice of the patient's life or mine. I fully realized the danger of the exposure to myself, but how could I desert Mrs. L— when I knew how great was her peril? I replied, "Get my horse and buggy and I will be ready."

All that cold, dreary night and until noon the next day I worked over my patient. The dreaded convulsions were avoided by the previous care and dieting and the expeditious emptying of the uterus. Dr. Eastman helped me, and in twelve hours the imminent danger was over for the patient—but not for me. I was able to visit her once more in the late afternoon, but by the next day I was down with pneumonia.

Do you wonder that I resent having people remark with a smirk, "Physician, heal thyself?"

A month of serious illness followed, but the end had not yet been reached. From this terrific exposure and the consequent strain of pneumonia on my already weakened heart, I never fully recovered, and my heart collapse was brought much nearer. Yet I never regretted my decision. How could I have done otherwise? Well, I could not, though wiser heads than mine might have been able to do so. That devotion to duty which was so dominant a factor in my make-up, drove me to do it. John Whittlesey's prophecy—"Duty will be the death of you some day," nearly came true on that occasion.

Before closing this chapter I must pay a tribute to motherhood. Mrs. L— was an educated woman who fully understood the gravity of her danger in attempting to have a child. She realized that the chances were ninety-nine to one against her bearing a living child, and the peril to herself was extreme. However her desire for a child was so great that a few years after this failure she made all her plans to attempt it again. This time she was kept in bed most of the time; her diet was carefully censored, and every known means used to keep the kidneys functioning normally. Before the fatal period of about five months of gestation, as demonstrated in her previous experiences, she was put in Dr. Charlotte Brown's private hospital in San Francisco and an incubator made ready to care for the probably premature foetus, if it could be carried to an age when it was possible to keep it alive. Thus guarded she retained her babe until nearly seven months of pregnancy passed. Both mother and child survived—the latter spending several weeks in an incubator. That tiny, tiny baby is now an attorney of fine physique and intellect, and in every way a splendid specimen of womanhood. But to the heroism of her mother, what adequate tribute can we pay?

To descend from the sublime to the ridiculous, dare I for the sake of contrast with present-day practice and prices, remark that the joint fee of Dr. Eastman and myself in the case narrated was fifty dollars? Dr. Eastman had taken the after-care of the patient while I was battling with pneumonia. Apropos of fees, in only a few cases did I ever charge one hundred dollars, the usual fee now-a-days for a normal obstetrical case. One instance was a case of difficult instrumental delivery in which the mother was a primipera over forty years of age, a tense, muscular woman. Her family, also my dear friends, were wealthy. Instead of objecting to my large bill, the husband wrote a note to accompany the promptly-paid check, saying, "There should have been another cipher added to that check,"—but he did not add it.

The date of that night's struggle (a night when I had to forego the lovely engagement-announcement party of Berkeley's foremost poet) is graven not only on my memory but also on the handle of a lovely silver sugar-bowl, the gift of the mother. The date was October 2nd, 1891.

Apropos to the subject of mothers and babies, another phase of the problem was infant feeding. After the survey of dairies made by Dr. Shuey and myself, it was evident that all milk was contaminated with filth, so it is no wonder that bottle-fed babies were a sore problem to both mothers and doctors. Since then such progress has been made in the science of feeding babies, the discovery of all the vitamines necessary to health, the general and immediate pasteurization of milk now required by the Bay cities, that I wonder any babies lived in the 1880s and 1890s.

Home sterilization of milk was virtually impossible after it had traveled for hours about the streets in huge milk cans, been poured into the milkman's quart measure used for all customers, and again poured into open pans where it sat in warm pantries as ice chests were almost unknown. Naturally the patent infant foods were in great demand. These were good when properly modified by the addition of other ingredients necessary for a balanced food regimen. But the regulation of the baby's food was a thorn in the flesh of the 19th century family physician. Specialists and pediatricians had not yet made their appearance hereabouts.

Hence it was as common to find cases of malnutrition in the homes of the well-to-do as in those of the poor. In fact, being able to purchase artificial foods containing an undue proportion of carbohydrates made rachitis (rickets) and other forms of malnutrition all too frequent in those homes. I will cite three of such cases, all in professors' families, where I was called in to care for babies not belonging to my own list of several hundred.

One was a roly-poly baby, too fat, yet evidently ill and undernourished. She was fretful, and when lifted, cried out with pain. A diet of too much sugar and starch and not enough proteids and vitamine-containing foods was producing scurvy. Another was apparently up to the standard weight but examination showed a typical picture of rachitis—"the pigeon breast," "rosary ribs," and swollen bleeding gums. The third was breast-fed, but the mother's milk was utterly inadequate and I never saw a child more nearly starved. It looked like a little mummy, simply skin and bones, with the skin drawn tightly over the facial bones.

In all of these cases I gave a formula for modified milk rich in cream, for regular feedings, plus a teaspoonful of orange-juice after certain meals, and a half spoonful of scraped meat juice at others. Also the juice of certain strained vegetables at times.

A week or ten days after my first visit to the starving baby, the father, a chemist, came one evening to ask if there was any danger of the baby gaining too fast. I quieted his fears by telling him there need be no concern until the child had fully attained the normal weight for his age. This baby, then several months old, weighed seven pounds. At the end of three months it had reached the normal weight for its age—fifteen pounds.

These cases are not thrilling, but they round out the story of the daily routine of a family physician's life. Now-a-days each group which I have illustrated would require the services of two or more specialists.

CHAPTER 10

Keeping Pace with a Biologist

ANOTHER LAYER IN THE PLYWOOD OF MY LIFE CAME THROUGH MY marriage to a biologist. The "ply" furnished by my husband was of solid oak, firm and enduring. I use the term biologist purposely and use it in its original and broad sense. The word is derived from the Greek *bios*, life, and *logos*, laws of, or science. Thus biology is the science of living things. William Emerson Ritter is not a zoologist only, but a biologist, since his interest is in all animate or living nature.

While his scientific research has been on the animal side of living things, his interest and his joy in inanimate nature is also broad and deep. In the great outdoors nothing fails to give him both pleasure and material for study. I remember one summer when he kept me busy finding the many varieties of the lowly mosses on trees which he was studying at the time. His professorial title should be the old fashioned "Natural Historian."

Inevitably, comradeship with him has greatly broadened my own appreciation of nature and given a different bent and color to my life. My husband's scientific enterprises have determined the course of our lives. A brief survey of the way these interests have grown seems the easiest method of outlining this layer in our activities. In this chapter I deal especially with a decade mostly in the nineteenth century although it laps over two or three years into the twentieth.

Our first scientific outing began the day after we were married. It was that trip to Coronado and San Diego in 1891, when we went in search of the queer blind fish living under the rocks below Point Loma. I have already referred to the fact that in this search we hung our boat on the anchor-rope of a huge dredge, and but for the cool head of Mr. F. C. Turner we should probably not have been rescued and this tale would not have been told.

The following year, 1892, the biologist took his first group of students for a seaside summer-schooling. Pacific Grove was the field chosen for the first station in his proposed survey of the coast before selecting a permanent site for a marine biological laboratory. That site finally proved to be La Jolla, California, but the decision was not reached for more than a decade.

A movable tent laboratory was erected with the intention of using it wherever the summer work was located during the progress of the survey, but it was used only once more in the summer of 1893 at Avalon, Catalina Island.

Beside the students, a Berkeley teacher, Juliet Lombard, a personal friend, went with us. Memory fails me as to the students and their work but a vivid memory both of sight and sound lingers concerning one exploit of this novice. One day we all went collecting on the rocks at low tide. Juliet was particularly amused by the tiny side-walking crabs. With her usual enthusiasm she thrust her arm down into a hole between the boulders. Unfortunately for her a large-clawed crab lived there and instead of her catching the crab the crab caught her finger with his huge claws. Such yells as rent the air and such an expression of pain and terror as was on her face! She seemed bound to the rocks by her lusty foe, but before we could reach her she had dragged her captor from his hole, still clinging to her finger. Her release was soon accomplished, leaving this novice at shore-collecting a sadder and wiser woman.

At the close of the college year in May, 1893, Mr. Ritter returned to Harvard to take the examinations for his degree of Doctor of Philosophy. I spent the time at Johns Hopkins Medical College in Baltimore.

July of the same summer found us at Avalon, Catalina Island, a place so charming that we left our dismantled tent laboratory stored in the basement of a church, hoping to return another summer, but such did not prove to be the case.

Our student group consisted of senior and graduate students in zoology. The latter were largely the same throughout these wandering years, as they were pursuing their studies for higher degrees and acting as instructors for undergraduates. There is no record of the students on the summer trips and the groups varied so that it is impossible to recall the personnel except when some incident fixed an individual in my memory. Those whom I most vividly remember in the earlier years are Samuel J. Holmes, Mr. Ritter's first assistant, Frank Bancroft, Harry Beal Torrey, Alice Robertson and Harry Horn; and later, Calvin Esterly and John Bovard. Three of these became professors in the University of California after obtaining the coveted "Ph.D." elsewhere. Dr. Holmes is still in the department of zoology and is an authority on eugenics. After fifteen years service Dr. Torrey, an associate professor in zoology, and also librarian and investigator in the growing marine laboratory, resigned to accept a call to Oregon. In 1927 he took a medical degree at Cornell, New York, and is now a professor in Stanford University.

Frank Bancroft after attaining his Ph.D. returned to his Alma Mater as assistant professor where he remained until called to the Rockefeller Institute, New York, in 1910. He died in middle life. Harry Horn became a physician, but his life also was cut short. Alice Robertson later became professor of zoology at Wellesley College and remained there until her death.

The summer at Avalon, 1893, was especially pleasant owing to the beauty of scenery and the agreeable company. I recall more of the late afternoon pleasures than of the work, with the exception of one incident when a student emptied out a pail of water containing some minute specimens, tornaria, for which Mr. Ritter had been searching for years. He was keeping them alive in a pail of sea-water while watching their development. I will draw a curtain over the scene. Mr. Ritter's disappointment was the greater as no more could be found.

The beauty of the sea-bottom, the warm water for swimming are characteristic of Avalon. Most of our boys were fine swimmers and stunts became the order of the day after five o'clock. Diving off the end of the pier and staying under as long as possible became a competitive stunt, as well as swimming races. The diving contest excited particular attention.

Even we who knew of the competition were sometimes alarmed as the length of time extended, and rescuing boaters at times started toward the spot where the divers had gone down, only to see them come up sputtering and panting for breath.

In this group I recall two boys, now prominent citizens of Berkeley. One slim youth, now rounded out in form and fortune was Dr. Thomas McCleave, whose black head would sometimes disappear in the distance, but he always came back. Fred Koch, a San Francisco high-school principal, was a special stunt swimmer, as were also Frank Bancroft and Harry Horn.

This particular summer one young woman student added greatly to our pleasure. Julia Morgan, now a notable architect, was at that time undecided whether to choose architecture or biology for her life work. The former profession won and she spent eight years in Paris studying at the Sorbonne and elsewhere.

Our party at Avalon was honored by the presence of one of America's leading zoologists, Dr. Edmund B. Wilson, professor of zoology in Columbia University, who had been invited by the University of California to lend the weight of his knowledge and experience to the solution of the problem of a location for a future marine laboratory. As all the students had been drilled in Professor Wilson's text book, *The Cell*, they were ready to bow to him as an authority on these elements of life. But aside from his established reputation as an investigator and writer, Dr. Wilson proved to be a charming personality, and his humor and his stories added gaiety to our lively as well as studious group.

Being anxious to explore the shore of the island, Mr. Ritter arranged for a small group to make an excursion to the Isthmus, as it was called, a place where the island is narrowed on both sides by the inroads of the sea. A Finnish skipper with a large sailboat was hired for a trip of several days. Camping was the only method of living since there were no habitations. Professor Wilson and two or three students, with Mr. Ritter and the skipper, made up the party.

They set sail early one fine calm morning—so calm that it was difficult to make progress. All were wishing for a good wind to fill the sails. In early afternoon they got more than they desired. A stiff breeze came up, making the sea very choppy and pitching the boat around in such a way that the skipper became frightened and while steering the boat with one hand, pointed the forefinger of the other into the wind to keep off the "evil eye" which menaced them. Some of the passengers were too seasick to care what happened. Professor Wilson was invulnerable to that malady but not to the resultant loss of the beans, a large pailful of which had been supplied as the chef d'oeuvre of the camping rations. The boat had been shipping seas until a goodly pool had splashed into the bottom of the boat. With one heavy lurch the pail of beans was upset near Dr. Wilson's feet. His first impulse was to save their staple food. Instinctively, as he sat with coat off and sleeves rolled up to catch anything floating by, he stooped over and with both hands scooped the spilled beans back into the pail, salt water and all, thus spoiling the flavor of the beans which had not yet been emptied from the pail. Mr. Ritter cannot to this day recall, without a hearty guffaw, that picture of the eminent scientist scooping up the beans and brine.

A rather startling incident occurred when a whale came up to blow, right alongside the boat. He showed no interest whatever in the scientific party, but they were greatly interested in him, not as a zoological specimen but as an undesirable visitor. Had he risen a few feet to the leeward there would have been a spill of something beside beans into the brine. Dr. Holmes avers that he and Harry Horn were the students on this trip and that when danger of being submerged was the greatest, Harry Horn valiantly drew his mighty "22" and popped at the monster of the deep, who did not deign to flip a fin at that flea-bite. The superstitious skipper thought that the devil himself was after them but his fears only lent zest to the adventurous scientists whose trip was pronounced a decided success as far as their explorations and collections were concerned.

While in the summer of 1894, Mr. Ritter and I were en route to Europe for fifteen months of study, Sam Holmes, Frank Bancroft and Harry Horn, with a camping outfit, explored the coast to the north as far as Eureka.

In 1895 a group of six, headed by Assistant Professor H. P. Johnson, established themselves at San Pedro, a place which had attracted the attention of the biologists on their trip to Catalina.

No summer work was planned for 1896, but hearing that two young geologists were to explore San Clemente Island, Mr. Ritter suggested to Harry Torrey that he go with them, and gave him for his expenses the entire budget for sea-side work, sixty-five dollars. His only experience had been the previous summer's work at San Pedro, but he packed three cases with collecting materials from glassware to axes, paid his steamer fare to Catalina and return, and his share of a private boat to take them to Clemente Island and return for them in three weeks. He also paid his share of the camp mess and all trivial expenses out of the sixty-five dollars. He returned with a fine collection and all of the laboratory equipment intact, breaking neither a bottle nor an axe, and handed Mr. Ritter twenty cents surplus for next year's expenditures. There was no expedition in 1897.

The problem of expense was an ever-present one. Such expeditions were expensive, and although President Martin Kellogg and Professor Joseph Le Conte were in heartiest sympathy with the project, the University's funds were limited. For the first summer in Pacific Grove two hundred dollars had been provided for the erection of the tent-house laboratory and incidental expenses. Microscopes and other necessary laboratory equipment had been loaned by the University.

But when the distances to objective points became longer and the expense of travel necessarily greater, the students and poorly paid instructors required financial assistance. Certain friends including Mrs. Hearst aided in raising funds to add to the University's allowance for the summer scientific work, but with the growing interest and increasing number of students and instructors the task of raising money became greater and greater. One of the surprises of my life has been the way in which business men have responded to the scientific interests presented to them by the leader of this cause, a man with a vision, but one who could never directly ask anyone for a dollar.

For the four years from 1896 to 1900, expenses and seashore work were kept at a minimum, but the department of zoology and the spirit of work grew. One great acquisition came through securing Dr. Charles A. Kofoid of the University of Illinois as assistant professor of zoology. Professor Kofoid had had wide experience in aquatic research, and with Mr. Ritter made a strong team to carry forward the seemingly impossible ambition. But he did not come to California until the beginning of the new century and account must first be taken of the waning 19th century.

In 1897 we built us a house, and besides the vexations of building, there came unthought-of additions to the complexity of life. The student housing problem in Berkeley was a serious one. The University had grown much faster than the town. Anyone who had unoccupied rooms was appealed to as in war-time to sacrifice comfort to loyalty to the University.

Scarcely were we in our new home on Durant Avenue near Telegraph, then a residence street, when there came an appeal to Mr. Ritter from an alumnus, Henry O'Melveny, a prominent attorney in Los Angeles, who had helped to raise the money for the San Pedro summer work, urging him to take a freshman, Sayre Macniel, into our home for one year, as a personal favor. At first I was horror-stricken and full of "no's," but the pressure was heavy, so for Mr. Ritter's sake I yielded, and we had a delightful addition to our family. The next year another request came from another patron of the San Pedro station, and again we had to repay the kindness shown us there.

When these boys could settle themselves elsewhere I breathed freely. But it did not last. Two young unmarried faculty men who had been dispossessed of a home by Mrs. Charles Palmer's illness came begging for a home with us. I absolutely refused, but who could resist the pleading of Charles Noble when he said, "We will not make you any trouble. Please try us for a month. We have nowhere to go." "If Josie is willing, I will agree," I said, "but it lies between you and her. I can take no additional cares." A dry smile. "We can trust Josie's cooking." Thus Charles Noble and Lincoln Hutchinson added delight to our table-talk for another year. But for my faithful housekeeper all this would have been impossible.

In 1898 came our first trip to Yosemite, a trip to which I had looked forward with keen relish for the glorious scenery, the mountain air, congenial companionship and freedom from care and ceaseless work. The spring had been unusually hard, due to a small but virulent epidemic of typhoid fever. I have described my record case in the chapter on "Medical Practice." If anyone ever needed rest and recuperation, I did. For one blessed week my anticipations were realized, and then, through the thoughtlessness of a gossipy woman my dreams were rudely destroyed by that three a.m. human hoot-owl, and I was forced into an orgy of exhausting work, the story of which is told in my illustration of a doctor's vacation.

Mr. Ritter was fortunately enabled to do some exploring of Puget Sound in the summer of 1899 while on the Harriman expedition.

The last summer of the century brought an unusual experience. Mr. Ritter and I were planning a vacation in the mountains when he was invited to join the Harriman Alaskan Expedition. The railroad magnate, E. H. Harriman, was ordered by his physician to take a complete rest. To do this it was necessary that he should go beyond the reach of telegraph wires. Telephones were still confined to larger towns and the radio had not yet been invented. Mr. Harriman decided to go hunting for big game and chose Alaska as his field of operations. As he wished his family, his wife and four children, to accompany him, it was necessary to engage a large sea-worthy vessel. So he chartered a coast-wise steamer, the *George W. Elder*, and had it refitted for the needs of his family, his photographers, and his guests, among whom were his family physician and their pastor, or "Dominie," as he was called on shipboard.

Having chartered this steamer capable of carrying hundreds of people, it seemed wise to make it count for more than a pleasure trip. Dr. C. Hart Merriam, chief of the Federal Division of the Biological Survey, was called into conference with the result that forty scientists (biologists, geologists and geographers) as well as artists and writers were invited to accompany the expedition as Mr. Harriman's guests. The idea was to include a representative of every vocation that could be benefited by a visit to this little known region. Mr. Ritter was chosen by Dr. Merriam as an expert in marine zoology. Thus began years of friendship with the Harriman family. John Muir and John Burroughs were the writers selected to describe this region unknown to most of the party, but familiar to John Muir.

The expedition was gone almost three months and discovered many uncharted glaciers by following up unfrequented inlets of the sea. The Aleutian Islands were visited and a brief call made on the Siberian shore. This gave Mr. Ritter the opportunity to survey the Alaskan coast-line from Victoria, Canada, to the Shumagin Islands, and resulted in excluding the northern coast from his purview of a future marine laboratory site. It required years for the scientific results of this expedition to be published. This was done at Mr. Harriman's expense, under the direction of Dr. C. Hart Merriam of Washington, D.C.

The proceedings of the distinguished party were not confined to study and research alone. The young people of the Harriman family, with some friends of their own age, had to be amused. When the same group of fifty or more people are thrown upon their own resources for recreation for three months, it naturally follows that all their various talents will be brought out. Each and every one had to produce a stunt, sedate scientist, writer and artist as well as the laity.

One day Mr. Ritter chanced to see John Burroughs hanging onto the ship's railing and trying out a mild clog dance in preparation for the evening's entertainment. Instantly there occurred in him a most interesting example of what I call muscle-memory. In a flash he recalled something which he says he had not thought of for full twenty years. I certainly had never heard of it in the fifteen years of our intimate association. As a boy in his early 'teens he had learned to "jig" from a negro youth brought home by one of the neighbors, after the Civil War. All the boys at school had tried to learn this difficult stunt from their colored playmate, but Willie Ritter alone was pronounced proficient. He had danced jigs, pigeon-wings and double-shuffle during schoolday parties, but presumably had completely forgotten it after leaving home for the Normal School in Wisconsin.

Immediately upon seeing John Burroughs practicing by holding onto the railing, he started to dance. He says he could see no difference in his agility due to the lapse of years. His muscles had retained their memory of early boyhood's strenuous training. He not only brought down the house that evening but had to establish a class in "jigging."

He later used the same talent in electrifying many a gay household party among our intimate university friends. I especially recall one such party. We were spending the week-end at Mrs. Hearst's beautiful hacienda at Pleasanton. How many delightful memories I have of visits for days at a time in that charming place. Seemingly this was a dignified and sedate party, but somehow, Saturday evening, the lighter side of life was dominant. In the spacious music-room, fitted with a stage for concerts, and an enticing dancing floor, the somber music of Handel's Largo drifted later into modern jazz, although that term was not yet current. Whatever the name, a negro melody resulted in a "cake-walk" in which Agnes Lane, a niece of Mrs. Hearst, and Mr. Ritter led off.

Then someone who knew of Mr. Ritter's accomplishment called for a jig. "The Irish Washerwoman" was struck up, followed by the "Fisher's Hornpipe" and the "Arkansaw Traveler" to the rhythm of which he danced his various "steps." To me the funny part was seeing white-haired, philosophical Professor Howison, who with his wife, was among the guests, patting the "jig time" on his knee, apparently completely absorbed in the muscular rhythm.

A jolly evening that, the thorough relaxation of which was beneficial to all, even serious-minded Professor Howison. And how Mrs. Hearst laughed! Dear Mrs. Hearst! How much those years of intimacy meant to me. Christmas has never possessed the same joy since she left this earth. Her Christmas box was always the first to arrive, days ahead of the gift-giving day, and how enticing it was, requiring considerable self-control to leave it unopened until the festal morn. May I add that Mr. Ritter at seventy-five years of age can still jig?

Having been left behind when Mr. Ritter set out with the Harriman party, and feeling the need of a vacation, I decided it was my opportunity to see Alaska too. So Dr. Charlotte Brown, Juliet Lombard, Mrs. Charles Huggins and I made up a party and took a steamer soon after the expedition left. In fact we missed them at Sitka by only a few hours. Not to be outdone by the millionaire party with which Mr. Ritter was voyaging, we found ourselves fellow-passengers with John D. Rockefeller and family. The son, John D. Jr., and daughter, Edith, afterward Mrs. Harold McCormick, were young people around twenty years of age. The senior Rockefeller proved to be affable and friendly. I well recall sitting on a deck ventilator with him for a couple of hours, discussing the welfare of the world; and also playing a game of "duck on rocks" at the foot of the great Muir Glacier.

* * * * * * *

The opening year of the new century took me East again on the exploratory trip among women's colleges, as the guest of Mrs. Hearst who later returned to her palatial home in Washington, D.C., where I visited her a few days after the inspection of colleges had been completed.

While in New York I spent a week-end with the Harriman family, going with them to their lovely country place at Tuxedo. Saturday morning Mr. Harriman was fretting because he had to go all the way to the city and spend an hour in a doctor's office to have his throat swabbed. Hesitatingly, I offered to do it. "I'm afraid you wouldn't reach the spot," he responded. "The trouble is very far down." "I think I can reach it. I can but try." When Mr. Harriman, with weeping eyes caught his breath after the swabbing, he said, "When you go after a thing you get there."

Alas, the throat, sore so far down, proved to be a malignant growth which caused his death a few years later. Mr. Harriman was lovable and devoted in his family relations, astute and perhaps relentless though he was in business. We had some fine drives over his great estate while he described the hillside roads he intended to build with a four or five per cent grade. Before I left, Mr. Harriman said at table one day, "I wish you might have gone on the Alaskan trip with us," and the children echoed, "We do too!" The compliment from the reticent financier I greatly appreciated. He was not given to laudation.

With one of Mrs. Hearst's secretaries assisting me, the pair of club-houses for which Mrs. Hearst provided the money were furnished and ready for occupancy by the opening of the college year.

During my absence Mr. Ritter spent the summer classifying and describing the collections which he had made on the Harriman expedition in Alaska the preceding year. This was a long and arduous task and occupied his research time for several years.

* * * * * * *

The winter of 1900 and 1901 was a hard one in every way. Influenza was rife and I had always been an easy victim to that elusive germ. Having had an attack early in the winter, I was not in condition to cope with the increased amount of work caused by the epidemic. A young physician, Dr. Eleanor Stow, a cousin of Dr. Shuey, had located in Berkeley. I turned over as much of my work as possible to her and later in the winter during an especially severe attack of my dread enemy, I too became her patient.

Not having allowed myself time in which to fully recover from the first attack, the second one was especially virulent. An ear infection occurred and the abused heart dilated to an alarming extent. Dr. Stow called Dr. Philip King Brown, a heart specialist of San Francisco, in consultation. Both decided that if I were to live I must be removed from Berkeley. Dr. Brown had a sanitarium for heart cases in Santa Barbara and proposed my being carried there on a bed. But he said to me, "There is a chance for you to recover but I will not undertake the case unless you will promise to obey orders for three years." I promised, and while I may not have obeyed all his orders, I was under his care for eight years, until we went to La Jolla to live.

To describe a life-and-death struggle is impossible. The memory of those days and weeks, dragging on into months is very clear, but why recall them? Suffice it to say that Miradero, the name of the fine home of a rich Boston woman, then converted into a sanitarium for heart cases, was a place where both nature and man's handiwork gave every assistance to recovery. Beautifully located on the hill slopes of Santa Barbara, a short distance beyond Mission Canyon and the old Mission Church, the beauty of scene added greatly to my own native strength and determination to live.

At first I was unable even to turn in bed. So constant were the nurses in attendance, that one day I jokingly said to the superintendent (another of those fine early-day graduate nurses of the Children's Hospital, and a personal friend), "Do you think I am going to steal something that one nurse always comes in as another goes out?" She smiled and said, "We are only watching to see that you do not steal away from us."

To the splendid nurses and physicians, combined with the quiet of Miradero and the treatment received there, I feel that I owe my life. That I could have weathered the gale in Berkeley seems very doubtful, since it would have been impossible for me to have been entirely free from care. In Miradero, in addition to the constant medical attention, there were all the accessories of a German Spa. At first I was given very light massage to improve the circulation, and later Nauheim baths with increasingly heavy massage to stimulate the heart's action.

One thing which this as well as other illnesses has taught me, is that the fear of death is a phantom which disappears when the danger is great.

One's very weakness seems to dispel the dread one ordinarily has of death. Although I fully realized the seriousness of my condition, I had no intention of dying.

An incident which doubtless would not have occurred in any sickroom save that of a physician patient, who understood her own condition, pertained to the visit of one of America's foremost heart specialists, Dr. Richard Cabot of Harvard Medical College. Dr. and Mrs. Cabot were visiting Dr. Brown. The two physicians entered my room one day during my convalescence and Dr. Brown said he would like to have Dr. Cabot examine my heart. After doing so, the famous specialist turned to his host and said, "This heart is larger than an ox-heart." "Ox-heart," Dr. Brown replied, "It was the size of my head when she was brought here!" "Well," Dr. Cabot said, "if she lives, as apparently she is going to, the good Lord has some further use for her. There is no other excuse." I can only say that I hope these succeeding years have in a slight degree repaid the thirty-year extension of life which has been granted me.

I spent the spring and summer of 1901 at Miradero, and returned there the two succeeding summers for a few weeks of rest and treatment of Nauheim baths and massage to strengthen the heart muscle.

CHAPTER 11

The Quest of a Southern Site

THE EXPLORATIONS OF THE COAST FROM ALASKA TO CATALINA ISLANDS for a Laboratory site threw the balance of preferment in the southern scale. Both Catalina and San Clemente Islands were too inconvenient so it was decided to seek a mainland site. With the opening of the new century, San Pedro Bay was the first selection.

San Pedro was in many ways attractive for biological work and during the first summer seemed likely to be the choice for a permanent location. The littoral fauna was rich and diversified, and Los Angeles friends of science and of the University contributed generously to the support of the laboratory and to the marine investigations. A grand total of about two thousand dollars was raised for the first summer's work, including the University contribution, a minor portion.

In a report to the president, Mr. Ritter says, "Detailed comprehensive, continuous and long-continued observation and experiment are necessary. These are the two golden keys that will lead us farthest into the mighty arcana of the life of the sea." Alas, "continuous and long-continued" work of any kind is costly and this necessitated a permanent and endowed laboratory for which no funds were available.

The sum raised for the first summer enabled exploration at sea to be added to the usual shore work. For a laboratory, a small and ancient bathhouse on a sand-spit was rented and reconstructed. An open gasoline launch, the *Elsie*, forty feet long, with an engine of fifteen horsepower, was rented for the work at sea. A hand-winch which required four men to operate was provided for hauling the dredge and trawl. A sounding-machine and an apparatus for taking sub-surface samples of water were improvised, the funds not permitting the purchase of even the least expensive manufactured articles. A total of eighty-five stations were located for work on the sea bottom in depths not exceeding one hundred fathoms. The principal localities were off San Pedro, around Catalina Island and San Diego. Numerous visits were made to each of these marine stations. The *Elsie* was very active for the three months from May 15th to August 15th, 1901. Professor Kofoid had charge of the work at sea. Shore courses in marine zoology and botany were given in addition to the usual laboratory investigations.

Added to the regular staff of the department of zoology of the University was Professor W. J. Raymond of the department of physics, who had charge of the hydrographic work. Two graduate students, Miss Alice Robertson and Calvin O. Esterly, were then beginning their careers in biology and remained identified with the station for many years, contributing to its success.

Calvin Esterly obtained his doctorate at Harvard in 1907 and was made professor of zoology in Occidental College, Los Angeles. The same year he continued his work with the Biological Research Institution and was made non-resident member of the staff in 1910. In 1909 he married Ruth Orgren, one of my favorite university girls. Dr. Esterly continued his work in both institutions until death in 1928.

In the second year at San Pedro several disquieting conditions arose. In searching for a permanent laboratory site in San Pedro Bay, the increase of industrial activities menaced many of the best collecting areas of the shore. The attendant increase in population likewise brought an added menace of contamination of the shore waters. A very minute quantity of sewage is devastating to the lowly creatures living on rocks or in shallow waters.

A third disquieting feature was the virtually impossible task of raising funds to build, equip and endow a permanent laboratory by the method of personal subscriptions. Financing sea-work in 1902 had failed.

In the exploration of 1901 Dr. Kofoid had been greatly impressed with our friend, Dr. Fred Baker, who was positive that not only was the variety of collecting areas greater near San Diego, but that the community would support the work. Dr. Kofoid returned enthusiastic over the biological merits of the more southerly locality. Correspondence with Dr. Baker resulted in a decision to test that region during the following summer. Mr. Ritter's great "finds" of goby fish and amphioxus on our nearly fatal wedding trip made him eager to complete his ten years of coastal survey at this terminal of the state. Although this had been included in his original plan, Dr. Baker's enthusiasm added zest to the quest. The difficulties looming in connection with San Pedro Bay also made it imperative to investigate the remainder of the coast.

Although naturally enthusiastic about anything pertaining to San Diego, Dr. Baker had had occasion to know whereof he spoke. By vocation a physician, he was by avocation an amateur conchologist and had collected shells on practically every inch of local coast. Being also an expert sailor of small boats, he knew all the mud flats and rocky shore. In passing, let me add that his avocation has filled his years of retirement with unceasing interest. His collection represents the globe and is valuable as well as interesting. Part of it is on exhibition at the San Diego Natural History Museum, and he gave another set to the Scripps Institution at La Jolla. This interest and collecting experience added weight to his advice. His standing in the community made his promise of financial backing also worthy of serious consideration. So it was that in the summer of 1903 the marine investigations were carried on at Coronado, which later led to the choice of La Jolla as a permanent site.

Dr. Kofoid's cooperation was of inestimable value both to Mr. Ritter personally and to the cause in general. With him had come his talented wife and they have both been for thirty-two years acquisitions to the University faculty and "faculty wives," as well as to the community at large. At the same time our circle of intimate friends has been notably enriched by their inclusion. The Kofoids thus became members of the summer group in 1901, and continued as such until the itinerant colonies were no more. Our migratory summer expeditions ended in 1905, when the permanent station was located at La Jolla.

The two summers at San Pedro were enlivened by the presence of a bride each year. In 1901 Frank Bancroft brought his wife, Dr. Eleanor Stow, to the summer colony; and in July, 1902, Harry Beal Torrey enriched his life and our scientific group by marrying Grace Crabbe, another of my favorite university girls.

In the summer of 1902, after a few weeks at Miradero Sanitarium for a second course of Nauheim treatment, I spent most of the summer-session period at Mt. Lowe, as I was not equal to the primitive house-keeping of the summer colony. Various members of the party visited me there. I especially recall a week's visit from Dr. Alice Robertson, one of Mr. Ritter's assistants.

Mr. Ritter planned to come up on the mountain for week-ends, but once, due to a belligerent sting-ray he made an unintended visit of two weeks. The sand beaches were infested with these well-armed creatures which bury themselves deep enough in the sand to hide their forms, and severely punish any unwary person who steps on them by thrusting a long, sharp and poisonous tail-barb into the foot of the victim. There were several cases of wounds of this sort but Mr. Ritter's was the most serious. In his case the barb went entirely through his foot and poisoned him severely. He was on crutches for some weeks and too ill to work for a fortnight, during which time I had the unexpected pleasure of his company. "It's an ill wind—."

* * * * * * *

With Dr. Baker's enthusiastic and efficient assistance the laboratory equipment for biological research was removed from San Pedro to San Diego for the summer work in 1903. The boathouse of the Coronado Hotel was secured for a laboratory which afforded more commodious and well-appointed quarters than any previously extemporized. Likewise better living facilities for the colony were more easily obtained.

Dr. Baker had secured sufficient financial backing to assure two months' work in the summer, and also for the Christmas vacation in order to test the location in the winter season. A small schooner, the *Laura*, was rented and outfitted with the meagre apparatus for marine work. It was placed in charge of an intelligent Portuguese fisherman, Manuel Cabral.

The business affairs of the laboratory were handled by the San Diego Chamber of Commerce. This arrangement was for immediate exigencies only, and in the autumn the Marine Biological Association of San Diego was created and duly incorporated under the laws of the state. The articles of incorporation provided that the Station should later be transferred to the Regents of the University of California. The Board of Directors consisted of prominent business men, two of whom are still on the advisory board of the Institution, having thus served thirty years. One of these is Julius Wangenheim, an alumnus of the University and president of a local bank; the other, faithful Dr. Fred Baker. Professor William E. Ritter was made Scientific Director, and Miss Ellen B. Scripps and E. W. Scripps were members of the Board of Directors.

This branch of the University was known for twenty years as the Scripps Institution of Biological Research of the University of California.

Dr. Baker had enlisted the interest of Miss Ellen Browning Scripps of La Jolla and Edward Wyllis Scripps of Miramar, both of which places were suburbs of San Diego. Here begins a story of the deepest friendships of our lives. It was their interest which determined our residence in La Jolla for fifteen years.

Never shall I forget my first glimpse of Ellen Browning Scripps. It was on our first survey trip to La Jolla. We went out late one Saturday afternoon to spend the week-end in order that Mr. Ritter might explore the shore in that region. On the little rattling La Jolla train I noticed a small, inconspicuous, plainly-dressed woman who attracted my attention because she was so different from the other passengers. I studied her as she sat diagonally across the car and a little in front of our seat. I decided she had the plainest face I had ever seen, yet it was attractive. We stopped at a station. She looked out of the window and quickly rose, went to the door and waved to three small children seated in a buckboard drawn by an old white horse and driven by an aged negro. As she waved and smiled at the children whom I later learned were those of her brother Fred, her face lit up with such a sweet expression that I exclaimed, "Oh, how beautiful she is!" The plain features were illumined by a spirit of such grandeur that they were transformed. This was a fitting introduction to the character of the woman who became a most intimate friend and associate for a quarter of a century.

Mr. Ritter's first ride to Miramar Ranch is unforgettable. Mr. E. W. Scripps lived unto himself on a ranch of three thousand acres on a broad mesa in the foothills. When he wished to interview one or a dozen men it was his habit to summon them, whether they were in San Diego, Cleveland or New York. One day he asked Mr. Ritter and Dr. Kofoid to come out to Miramar for an interview. He sent his oldest son, Jim, with an auto to get them. Although automobiles were rare in those days each adult member of the Scripps family had one. Jim's was an open touring car. The two scientists, neither of whom had ever been in an auto before, were seated in the rear. Jim was an eighteen-year-old dare-devil who sized up his passengers as highbrows and decided to give them the ride of their lives. They started out through the sage-brush across the canyons and mesa for the seventeen-mile drive over a deep-rutted wagon-road. Jim's pace was the car's limit, often rounding corners on two wheels. He made no concessions to the "profs" on this occasion, and confessed later that he drove so fast he could not keep the machine on the rough road. To stay in the car each man on the back seat held desperately with one hand to the arm of the seat, while with the other he clung tightly to his hat. They bounced sometimes a few inches and often a foot, according to the depth of the ruts, and their occasional contacts with the seat were almost violent enough to cause concussion of the brain. Neither scientist expected to reach his destination intact. Dr. Kofoid insists that, failing to round a curve, Jim plunged out across the sage-brush and jumped a ditch, the momentum of the car being sufficient to carry it across. All three lived to tell the tale of their hair-raising experience, and Jim enjoyed recounting the joke at the expense of the two university professors.

The interview with Mr. Scripps was interesting as well as history-making. This millionaire newspaper man later made the biological station his protégé.

The chief pleasure of the summer was sailing with Dr. Fred Baker. How he could handle a sail-boat! Skimming over the waters of the bay with the boat often at an acute angle was a special delight to me. Had I been born in this day and age I should doubtless have chosen aviation as an avocation at least. Visiting with hospitable Dr. Charlotte Baker in her home on Point Loma was another pleasure.

* * * * * * *

During the years between 1901 and 1904, Mr. Ritter had diligently tried to persuade me to give up all outside work, but that to me seemed impossible. It would have been like cutting off my own limbs. After returning from Miradero Sanitarium in the late summer of 1901, owing to my depleted strength it was necessary to relegate most of my outside medical practice to Dr. Stow Bancroft. But I carried on office practice, and my work as medical examiner of women students and my lectures on hygiene, which Dr. Shuey had taken over during my absence.

In 1903 President Wheeler formed the Club House Loan Fund Committee of which I was made chairman. I continued in that position as long as we lived in Berkeley. My work in this capacity was largely executive, aside from the difficult task of raising money. Of this I did my full share, but the organizing of groups of students, the selecting and furnishing of houses, was carried on by committees.

In the summer of 1904 fate abetted Mr. Ritter's cause and made it impossible for a considerable time for me to continue my usual activities. On the return trip from the second summer of the biological group in Coronado, Mr. Ritter and I decided to take a few days' outing in the Santa Cruz Mountains, since he had had no respite from work during the summer. We therefore stopped in San Jose where my brother's family lived, and he and his wife outfitted us with a horse and open buggy and the accoutrements for a brief camping trip. It was very brief—one night. We drove up a canyon in the mountains where the headwaters of the Guadalupe Creek form a lovely stream. We selected a charming site on its bank and had our picnic supper and slept out under the stars. Such joy! After a bacon and coffee breakfast, we started to drive down a steep grade along an embankment some thirty feet high—or deep.

Apparently there was something wrong with the harness: the breeching was too loose to take the weight of the buggy on the horse's haunches. The horse, a beautiful chestnut mare highly prized by my brother, began to "act up" and sidled toward the precipitous bank. I tried hard to pull her back into the road. In obedience to the bit she turned her head, which prevented her seeing the precipice, and she continued sidling toward it. Mr. Ritter jumped from the buggy to try to reach her head, but before he could do so I screamed, "We're going over! We're gone!" And so we were. The horse fell and slid down the thirty-foot bank to the rocky creek below. No such slow and easy method for me! I was hurled out of the buggy-seat and felt myself gliding over the horse's back. The next instant my left shoulder collided with the rocky creek-bed. With my usual ambition I had got there even ahead of the horse. But in a moment I felt her hot body against my back. The buggy had caught in the trees on the bank and the horse had somehow slid out of most of the harness. She began to struggle and I realized that I must get out of her way or I should be crushed. Exerting all my strength I succeeded in rolling over, thus increasing the distance between us. The horse too had rolled on her back, and I never saw an animal with so many feet pawing the air. It seemed to me she was a centipede as she made such desperate efforts to right herself.

By this time Mr. Ritter had dragged me out from under those flying feet. But his effort to help me revealed the fact that I was badly injured. To my immense relief my brother's prized mare had no broken bones. Fortunately a farm house, serving also as an inn, was located on the stream a quarter of a mile farther up. Help was summoned and I was carried there. The only telephone in that region was at the New Almaden Quicksilver Mine in another canyon several miles away, and the only saddle animal available was a mule. On that Mr. Ritter crossed the range and phoned to my brother to bring a doctor and nurse, and help to get me down to civilization. Meantime I spent a day and night of agony in that wayside inn.

By the greatest good fortune the home of my beloved friend and nurse, Sarah Adams Badger, in the Willows six miles south-west of San Jose, was about the nearest possible place to which I could be taken. My brother brought his wife and this competent nurse with him. They arranged a bed in an open wagon and I was laid on that and carried about sixteen miles down that mountain road to the home of my friend where I was destined to remain many weary weeks. The less said about the agony of that ride the better.

"Badge," as I called my friend, had been a senior nurse in the Children's Hospital Training School for Nurses when I was an interne there eighteen years previously. We had become devoted friends at that time, and when I was operated on by Dr. Charlotte Brown she and Kitty Estep were my nurses. During the years she had often nursed crucial cases for me, and I had made frequent visits to her delightful home in the midst of a prune orchard. A more advantageous place in which to recover from a severe accident could not have been found.

Due to the uncompromising stones which checked my thirty-foot flight, and the pressure exerted by the horse's body, my collar-bone and four or five ribs were fractured, the latter in three places. That terrible ride resulted in a severe pleuritic inflamation, and my sufferings were extreme. The shock too was excessive. After pleurisy set in I could not change my position, and every breath was extremely painful. But one of the clearest memories I retain is of the exquisite pain in my heels after lying flat on my back for days. This was finally relieved by circular pads of absorbent cotton and gauze which the nurse and my sister made for my heels to rest in. I had always supposed that the old jingle about old Dan Tucker who "died of a toothache in his heel" was a myth, but I decided from my experience that it could easily have been an actual fact.

As it was physically impossible for me to return to the University in time for the opening of the college year in August, Mr. Ritter took advantage of the situation and without consulting me submitted my resignation. Of course it was inevitable, but I have always used the very bad pun that "My husband resigned for me but that I have never been resigned." It was a severe blow to me but I have to acknowledge that it was the part of wisdom. However I continued the Club House Loan Fund work until we moved to La Jolla in 1909, and also resumed medical practice as soon as I was physically able. Dr. Eleanor Stow Bancroft succeeded me in the University position.

In the autumn after my accident, Mr. Ritter was to attend a conference of the American Association for the Advancement of Science at the St. Louis World Exposition at which he was to deliver an address. I was so depressed over having to give up the university work and being as yet unable to resume my practice that I determined to go with him. This meant having a drawingroom on the train in order that I could lie down most of the time, and a wheeled chair at the exposition in St. Louis that I might be able to see some of its sights. This served as a mental diversion which expedited recovery.

CHAPTER 12

A Transitional Half Decade

DURING THE SECOND SUMMER AT CORONADO IN 1904, IT HAD BEEN decided to spend the following summer at La Jolla. It was the intention to locate there permanently if a suitable laboratory could be provided, with adequate financial support. Although it was desired to make it a community affair, the Scripps family was relied upon as the chief source of revenue.

Dr. Baker collected a thousand dollars with which to build a small laboratory in the village. The building was ready for occupancy on the arrival of the University party in June, 1905. It was situated in a flat area now known as the Ellen Scripps Park, owing to its later development by that community benefactress. The building was sixty by twenty-four feet, and contained three laboratory rooms, a small library and reagent room, and a public aquarium-museum. This cheaply constructed laboratory was built in full confidence that it would have to serve only a few years before it would be replaced by a permanent and commodious one.

This was an epoch-making period. It was Mr. Ritter's ambition to establish an institution in which there should be a permanent staff of salaried experts selected to carry on certain lines of research year in and year out. The common idea of a biological research laboratory was a place where trained persons could go to obtain facilities for individual research, entirely unrelated to any other work in the same laboratory. Mr. Ritter's idea was to lay out fields of work covering as many problems of the sea as possible and to employ specially trained workers to solve these problems, according to the usual custom in astronomical observatories.

In order to inaugurate this work in a small way, Mr. Ritter installed one all-the-year resident biologist and began immediately to pay the summer workers.

Since it was necessary for him to be on the ground during the work of organization, he secured a leave of absence from the University for this purpose and also that he might increase his knowledge of marine laboratories in the Occident and Orient. He had also been asked to give a paper at an oceanographic conference in France the following autumn.

From a report to the president of the University, written in 1901 at San Pedro, I quote: "The future marine station must be for physical, chemical and hydrographic, as well as for strictly biological research. The work must go on every hour of the day and every day of the year." At that time there were no funds for putting these large conceptions into execution, but in the report the following year, the man of vision writes: "For the rest, like Elijah of old, we stand before the Lord, hungry but full of trust, and therefore expecting the ravens, laden with bread and meat, to appear at any moment."

With the removal to San Diego the ravens had appeared with at least some crumbs of bread and enough "meat" to enable Mr. Ritter to install the resident naturalist to carry on continuous work. The first incumbent was Mr. B. M. Davis, the head of the biological department of the Los Angeles Normal School. He was willing to accept the position for one year on the small available salary with the consideration that half of his time might be devoted to his own biological researches. At the end of the year a position of greater responsibility and compensation lured him away, though with regret on both sides.

Our recreation periods during the seasons at La Jolla were the visits at Miramar Ranch, in that great Spanish-type house, built around a patio about one hundred by one hundred and fifty feet, with an old Italian marble fountain in the center and bronze dogs guarding the various entrances to the vine-covered corridor surrounding the patio. A house of thirty-six large rooms, with ten suites of two or three rooms and bath each, made a delightful place in which to refresh one's soul. Mrs. Scripps and I became great friends. She was an enthusiastic horse-woman and kept a stable of fine Kentucky horses. Memories of numerous excursions to San Diego to matinees; of trips into the mountains for several days, come trooping into my mind. As the years rolled by Miramar became a second home to us.

One summer when Mr. Ritter was ill, Mr. Scripps sent a large auto fitted up with a mattress on which the patient could lie and we were taken to Miramar for a month of recuperation. By this time the roads were very different from the one on which Mr. Ritter took his first ride to Miramar. Since automobiles necessitated good roads, Mr. Scripps accumulated a road outfit and either built new ones or transformed the old country roads. The result was that good roads radiated from his home in every direction. These were for public use as they traversed the county between all important local points. This he did at his own expense for his own convenience, but it was a community benefaction as well.

Years later he loved to tell this joke on himself. When paved highways came into vogue he was on a committee to induce local county districts to vote to have the county cooperate with the State in building them. At one meeting a farmer rose and said, "I have misgivings about supporting any scheme of Mr. Scripps for road-building. Just look at what he's done. Every road he ever built runs to his own Miramar Ranch!"

The importance of extending the sea-work over a greater portion of the year became more and more clearly recognized. This need was met in 1904 when an arrangement was made with Mr. Cabral, the fisherman-collector, to run his own fishing boat, the *St. Joseph*, three days a week during the summer period and at intervals throughout the remainder of the year.

Before the summer was over, Mr. Scripps gave his pleasure yacht, the *Loma*, to the association, with another gift of fifteen hundred dollars for refitting her with a propelling engine and scientific gear. This boat was admirably adapted to the station's sea-work. Having been built for a pilot-boat it was sturdy and suitable for dredging and trawling and was seaworthy for the long trips. The area covered was from Pt. Conception above Santa Barbara on the north, Catalina and San Clemente Islands on the west, and the Coronado Islands and the coast of Lower California on the south.

The scientific part of the sea-work was supervised by Mr. Clarence W. Crandall, head of the biological department of the San Diego Normal

School. Mr. Crandall was also secretary of the Biological Association at this time. Now that the Station possessed a boat of its own, Mr. Crandall fitted himself to pass the necessary examinations for a captain's papers. He conducted the sea explorations for several years before becoming an official of the Institution.

Unfortunately the *Loma* was wrecked virtually in her own door-yard when she ran onto a sunken rock near the lighthouse on Point Loma when Captain Cabral attempted to save time and distance by running between the kelp-beds and the Point. The scientific equipment was salvaged but the boat was a complete loss. This occurred in July, 1906, while we were in the Orient.

A gift of fifty thousand dollars from Miss Scripps being available, plans for a new boat were soon under way. The *Alexander Agassiz* was launched August 16th, 1907, with Captain Crandall as her master.

We had remained in La Jolla until January, 1906, when we sailed for the Orient. Mr. Ritter arranged to have Dr. Kofoid, the assistant director, take charge of the sea-side work during our absence. This same summer Dr. Torrey made a trip through Japanese waters in the United States Fisheries Steamer *Albatross* on a collecting expedition under Dr. David Starr Jordan.

Our first stop was in Honolulu, where we spent a month with our dear friend, Agnes Crary Weaver, and for the first time enjoyed the semi-tropics.

During the month Mr. Ritter made a trip to the Island of Maui to climb the crater of Haleakala. He and a friend rode up the mountain on horseback, intending to spend the night on the edge of the crater to watch the effects of the full moon on this monstrous cavern. The wind was blowing a gale and it was freezing cold at that altitude. They were clad only in linen suits and had brought no overcoats nor blankets. They had only sandwiches for a picnic supper. The moonlight scene was grand, but by the wee sma' hours the piercing cold had chilled them to the bone. To keep from freezing they had to cuddle up close to their horses' backs, using them as wind-breaks and their saddle-blankets as partial covering.

We reached Japan the latter part of March and after a few days of sight-seeing set off on a three-day jinriksha trip with an extra ricksha for luggage, and two coolies to each vehicle. As we were entirely off the tourist routes we were forced to stop in characteristic Japanese inns. We conformed to the national customs as far as possible but when it came to sleeping on the padded matting floor with two futons (heavy quilts) under us and one over us, with the wooden neck-rest for pillow, I resorted to strategy, and by pantomime succeeded in getting five futons for mattresses, and used our traveling rugs for pillows.

Our distal point was Masaki Rinkai Jikkin-jo, or the Biological Laboratory of the University of Tokyo. It was located on a beautiful but isolated point sixty miles south of Yokohama. Here we were met by Professor Ijama, who spoke English fluently and was dressed in European clothes. But when we entered his house for dinner, we found our host in Japanese garb, sitting on a floor-mat ready to have the meal served on individual tables six inches high. Off came our shoes at the door and we accommodated our limbs to the unaccustomed squatting position on the cushions assigned us. We remained at the station several days when we were summoned back to Tokyo for the cherry blossoms.

The return trip was made by boat, three lusty oarsmen sculling us the length of Odawara Bay. The day was clear and the mountains stood outlined against the sky with Fujiyama rising to twice the height of the others. Peerless Fuji! Rising solitary to its majestic height it dominates everything in Japan. This day we saw the mountain from three sides, and were taken to the point near Ayama, where this perfect snow-capped cone can be seen unobstructed for over twelve thousand feet from the waters of the bay, and its image reflected in clear outline in the same waters. This double view of flawless Fuji is a sight not to be duplicated.

We settled at Seiyoken Hotel, Uyeno Park, in a grove of cherry trees with many score of tall stone lantern monuments for the dead and a great Dai Butsu in the hotel grounds. We were within walking distance of the Tokyo University where Mr. Ritter was working. As this was a strictly Japanese hotel where tourists came only for meals, a student who spoke some English was assigned us as interpreter. Professor Mitsukuri, a Johns Hopkins man who had visited us in Berkeley, was head of the biological department of the university. He kindly arranged that American beds should be secured for us.

We were scarcely settled before that fatal day of April 18th, 1906—a day of cataclysms. Mr. Ritter came home at noon, reporting that an earthquake was recorded on the university seismograph, which was supposedly located some four thousand miles across the Pacific Ocean. While eating luncheon, Mr. Ritter was called to the phone by the United States Embassy and was told that San Francisco was destroyed and everything within a hundred miles was in ruins. Eager to learn details I took the train to Yokohama where I knew Americans would assemble, in hope of catching steamers for home. Upon arrival I found that the Pacific cable was broken and only the most exaggerated and unverified reports were circulating.

By a strange coincidence, during that same luncheon, a message had come from the Steamship Company stating that the liner on which we were booked for Europe in June had been sunk in the Indian Ocean; and also a letter from France with the information that the Oceanographic Conference to which Mr. Ritter had been summoned was indefinitely postponed. Thus our plans were changed and we decided to continue our journey only to China and the Philippines and return to California in the autumn. Meantime we had an anxious month before receiving definite news as to the extent of the damage in San Francisco and environs. The last report had been that Berkeley and Oakland were sunk beneath the waters of San Francisco Bay.

One disappointing factor in the change of plans was the relinquishment of an invitation to visit Mrs. Hearst who was living in Paris that year. A compensating feature was an additional four months in the Orient. After the close of the university, we traveled the length and breadth of Japan having many wonderful experiences.

In June we went to the Philippines, encountering so severe a typhoon in the China Sea that we had to run away from it. This change of course carried us to the west of Formosa, an island as large as California. It was a fortunate change since our ship had all it could do to weather the storm even in this more sheltered channel. Only one man and I appeared on deck that day. It was the most terrible storm I ever experienced. Oh, how that old ship did creak as it was twisted and wrenched by the terrific seas. The rain came down in sheets and the spray from the lashed seas so filled the air that one could not see the waters, which resembled a boiling cauldron. The gigantic waves struck the boat both forward and broadside, causing it to career dangerously. It was impossible to stay on deck as the water rushed over it.

To pass by the Philippines and China with scarcely a word seems sacrilegious, especially when they deserve many chapters. We had three months of such unusual sights and experiences as only the Orient can afford, especially when kind friends proffer the open sesame. General David P. Barrows was then minister of education in the Philippines, and Dr. Dean Worcester was in charge of the natives on the smaller islands.

Through Dr. Barrows' influence we were permitted some trips into the interior which otherwise would have been impossible. A never-to-be-forgotten three-day trip was that up the Pagsanjan River with Dr. Brink, first assistant director of education, who was making the rounds of native schools in remote provinces. My diary reads: "Left the house at 6:30 in a carromato (Philippine carriage) for the Passig River Station. Met the Brinks and took a covered banca (canoe) out to the middle of the river to get on the boat to Pagsanjan. The river was alive with carabao wallowing in the mud and water, and natives floating in the stream—all of them trying to cool themselves. The scenery was beautiful, mountains all around, and the banks of the Pagsanjan River lined with cocoanut and banana trees and giant bamboo. We reached our destination at 3 p.m. Toward evening we walked up a hill which overlooked rice-fields on the river side and fifteen million cocoanut trees on the land side. It was moonlight and we Americans rowed out on the river between the cliffs covered with fern-trees, and sang old plantation songs.

"Next morning a great treat awaited us, a canoe trip up through the rapids. Oh no, we must not wear our regular clothes, just semi-bathing suits furnished by our hosts. We soon learned why. Our canoes or bancas were dugouts made of small logs about a foot wide. Each held one passenger seated flat in the bottom. We were warned not to move or there would be a spill. Two bancheros, each with a short paddle, steered the frail craft, one sitting on the bow, the other on the stern, their feet in the water. Six bancas with twelve bancheros made up our fleet. We soon entered a gorge with precipitous cliffs from three hundred to five hundred feet high, covered with tropical foliage, large trees, palms, tree-ferns and wild calla lilies. Monkeys frequent the trees, their native haunts. The bancheros jumped out and hauled the canoes through the rapids. Over the steeper rapids and small falls we too had to climb out and scramble on all fours from rock to rock, or use the canoe as a foot-bridge.

"As we neared the three-hundred-foot waterfall, the cliffs overhanging and nearly meeting above our heads, a thin sheet of water trickled down upon us. We reached our destination, and after feasting our eyes on the scene, started down stream. Mr. Ritter's canoe brought up the rear of the single-file fleet. We suddenly found he was not with us. Two men started back in search of him. Only his head was above the water, all else was submerged. His six-foot stature saved his life. Explanation? The two bancheros began fighting with their paddles, tipped over the canoe, and continued the interesting fight regardless of their helpless passenger. The canoe was sunk. No pity need be wasted on Mr. Ritter's drenched condition as one is drenched with perspiration if not with water. The white teachers go swimming at five in the morning and at ten in the evening, and at least once during the daytime for brief periods of coolness."

From here, Mr. Ritter went farther into the mountains on a horseback trip with the educational inspectors, while I returned with the ladies to Manila. On the homeward boat trip we had pigs, goats and natives on the deck of the small craft. At noontime the natives jumped overboard and dug frantically in the warm sand for a much-prized delicacy—eggs buried for weeks, incubated and rotted. That horrible odor added to the smell of the livestock, together with the most audible sucking of the decayed embryo chicks was more than my stomach could stand.

Mr. Ritter returned to make a trip with Dean Worcester through the southern islands and coral reefs. On the Island of Mindoro they found the wild Mangan race living in cabins built on posts, which they reached by bamboo ladders, drawing the ladders up after them for protection from enemies.

During Mr. Ritter's absence I visited some American teachers in a northern province whom I had met on our steamer-trip from Japan. The native children in these American schools were neatly clad and averaged well in appearance and intelligence with children in similar schools at home. I also visited the son of the native chieftain of the Province, who was a very rich man. His son had formerly cut a wide swath at the University of California, with an allowance of five hundred dollars a month and a beautiful saddle-horse. He and his bride lived in a fine house over their stable. The parlor was furnished with Louis XVIth upholstered chairs and heavy but magnificently-carved Philippine ebony tables and settees. The old chief, in his airy shirt with ruffled tail, worn outside his trousers, was out under the trees enjoying an exciting cock-fight. Every rich man has a prize cock, and many poor men also.

We saw only the fringe of China, principally the coastal cities. In Macao, the Monte Carlo of the Chinese, with its famous gambling place, we spent hours hanging over a balustrade watching the concentrated gamblers at their play. Hongkong the double city, squalid on the lower level and beautiful on its heights, had to be ascended in sedan chairs carried on the shoulders of three coolies. The view was wonderful in the sunset hours. At Amoy, the treacherous port with a tide that rises and falls thirty feet at times, a former student of Mr. Ritter's greeted him. The pirate-infested river leading to Canton proved unexciting to us. We preferred it so, as our steamer wound its way among the thousands of covered sampans on which families live for generations, seldom going ashore. The narrow streets of the city through which our sedan chairs were carried with difficulty—one way traffic at that—gave glimpses of stupified people lying like logs against the walls on either side, transformed by the curse of opium.

Northward through the Yellow Sea to Shanghai with its foreign and native cities; the former did not attract me and the latter rather frightened me. Being alone in this strange city, I decided to return to the steamer after one day's experience, and continue on to Japan and friends.

Arriving there, we had six weeks more to spend in visiting unusual places in the land of the Rising Sun. Of Nikko the beautiful, Kyoto the ancient capital, Nara with its wondrous temples, and all the other oft-described places, I shall say nothing except that they deserve their reputations.

Our journeyings are always tinctured with biological interests and one such led us into remote districts of great beauty, with Shinto temples at Ise where the emperor worships his ancestors. The simple majesty of those Shinto temples is a refreshing contrast to the highly ornate, colored Buddhist temples of the cities. The contrast in location is equally great, being in remote forests of camphor trees, and cryptomerias, which are closely related to our giant redwoods.

Mr. Ritter had been invited by the president of the Mikimoto Pearl Company to visit their fisheries. This required another two days' jinriksha-trip along the most wonderful coast of southeastern Nippon. The pearls are grown by a remarkable combination of masculine inventiveness, feminine endurance, and oyster reaction. Beds of oysters are reared at a depth of about eighty feet. Women divers perform the remarkable feat of swimming down to this great depth, too deep to reach by diving. They dive as far as possible and then swim downward, select young oysters and bring them up in baskets. The masculine technicians then implant a grain of fine sand inside the mantle of each baby oyster, after which the women return to the strangling depths and plant the doctored bivalves which respond to the irritation of the sand by covering it with layer after layer of pearl substance. The pearls grow along with the oysters for about three years when again the women descend to the beds and bring up the matured crop. There are beds enough to keep up the business of sowing the seeds and reaping the harvest of pearls the year round.

But what about the lives of these women? It is pitiful to see them pant when they come up from their deep immersion which, it is said, shortens their lives. In the meantime they live the daily round of housekeeping and bearing and rearing children. They lay off only a brief period for child-birth and then resume their diving. The husbands and fathers are considerate enough to care for the babies and small children while the wives and mothers are earning the livelihood by this strenuous and unusual labor.

Another semi-biological and beauty-seeking expedition off the beaten tourist route was from Kyoto to Lake Biwa over the steep, rugged Mt. Hieizan. This almost precipitous mountain is famous for the great Buddhist temples hidden in the huge forests. The trail is so steep, with hundreds of stone stairs in such narrow defiles, that one wonders how the materials for the temples were ever conveyed there. Three of us women hired kagos with three carriers each to take us over the mountain. The kago is a flat basket swung from two poles carried on the shoulders of the men. They are made for small Japanese women who are accustomed to sitting on their feet. The comfort (?) of an American woman, twirled up in such a position for an all-day trip, can be more easily imagined than described. The ascent was so steep that often the bottom of the basket scraped on the stony stairs, adding more discomfort, but the grandeur of the scenery paid for it. Memory fortunately retains only the beauties; the aches and pains are soon forgotten. It was nine long miles up and down that precipitous trail to Lake Biwa and for this the sturdy carriers charged the huge sum of fifty-five cents each. Leaving us there they retraced their weary steps. Lake Biwa is all that is claimed for it in beauty of scenery, and the display of fireflies in the evening defies description.

Another unique mode of travel completed the round trip back to Kyoto. We took a boat across the lake and at its mouth entered upon the most unusual ferry-trip of our lives, six miles in a tunnel-canal through the heart of the mountains. This wonderful engineering feat shortens the distance to Kyoto many miles, and provides an easy route for freight as well as passengers. A walled-in tunnel pierces the mountains, connecting again with the circuitous outflowing river. Along the sides of the canal run two cables for pulling the boats by hand. The flickering torches carried by the boatmen furnish the only light. Weird enough! It was a fitting climax to a series of memorable experiences.

Just as we were about to sail homeward, I was invited to participate in the first Young Women's Christian Association Conference ever held in the Orient. It was to convene in a mission school in the suburbs of Tokyo, that city of one hundred square miles. Being a member of the Pacific Coast Branch of our National Young Women's Christian Association, it was incumbent on me to be present. Hence we deferred sailing another month.

One hundred and fifty-five girls from twenty-six schools from the most northern to the most southern parts of Japan were there. The conference lasted three days and it was an inspiration to find such talented young women, some of them remarkable musicians. One fine pianist had recently returned from seven years of study in Paris. Another, a sweet-voiced singer, had been trained in the United States. Many of the Japanese teachers were graduates of Bryn Mawr, Wellesley and other American colleges.

While I was occupied with the conference, Mr. Ritter made use of the opportunity to go with Professor Mitzukuri of the Tokyo University to visit the government turtle, eel and carp farms. Fish-rearing is a science in Japan as it is in our country.

The teachers of a Quaker mission school in Sendai urged me to visit their school, and offered many inducements, among them a visit to the biological station and some of the finest coast scenery in Japan. One inducement appealed to Mr. Ritter and the other to me. As we had not visited this extreme northern end of Hondo and had unexpected time on our hands we decided to go, and were well repaid.

The scenery was all that was claimed for it, equaling any of the pic- turesque shores of Japan. My diary reads: "Hundreds of pine-clad islands dotted the surface of the Bay of Matsushima, all precipitous, rocky hills with scraggly artistic pines clinging wherever they could gain a foot-hold. Most of them were mere rocky points protruding twenty, thirty or fifty feet out of the water, with one lone storm-beaten tree, or at most two or three, clinging tenaciously to their rocky base. It was a glorious sight. We sailed through the archipelago to Shiogawa, a great fishing region. Large Japanese junks filled with whale meat in chunks as large as could well be handled, was a novel sight—and smell. The junks were filthy and the whale meat was odoriferous to say the least. It was thrown out on the dirty wharf and carried away in dirty carts! Where?"

Mr. Ritter was interested in the eel and fish traps, the latter made of bamboo-fencing which served as seines.

An interesting feature of Sendai was the Military Hospital where eighteen hundred wounded soldiers and fifteen hundred Russian prison- ers had been cared for after the Russo-Japanese War. Several hundred of those permanently injured were still in the hospital. The hospital for countless orphaned children appealed more keenly to me. I naturally visit hospitals wherever possible.

Back to Yokohama for a few days of shopping and packing and fare- wells to friends. Then one last ricksha-ride over a famous route, final shopping, and aboard the steamer to watch the shores of beautiful Japan fade from sight as evening approached.

Those lovely green shores of Japan and the Philippines! I have not noted the number of days in my dairy reiterates, "rainy day," "showery," "pouring rain." Such verdure necessitates frequent and heavy rainfall. But one can be comfortable in a ricksha with a rain-coat and umbrella, regardless of the elements.

Four thousand miles of most pacific ocean, much of it calm as a mill-pond; a stop at Guam; a few days in Honolulu; and headed homeward on seas less pacific—to see—what?

Home again in September, 1906! Everything seemed changed as a result of the April earthquake and fire. As we entered San Francisco Bay we faced only blackened ruins instead of the familiar city. It was a heart-sickening sight. It was difficult to get from the dock to the Berkeley ferry. Not a friend or acquaintance to be seen; a striking contrast to the jolly party that had bidden us farewell eight months before. Never did I so keenly feel the brown hills and dust-covered streets of the unpaved road-ways, so great was the contrast to the brilliant greens of the moist tropics.

Berkeley was filled with strange faces. We had sold our home before going away for a supposed two-year absence. The apartment we had engaged at Cloyne Court had been given to homeless San Franciscans. Homeless ourselves and stranded, our friends the Kofoids took us in for a few weeks until we could make other arrangements. After a few months of unsettled life we secured an apartment at Cloyne Court and made that our home until we moved to La Jolla in 1909.

PART II:
BIOLOGICAL PIONEERING

CHAPTER 13

Pioneering in a Biological Laboratory

DURING OUR ABSENCE IN THE ORIENT IN 1906, DR. KOFOID HAD CAR-
ried on the laboratory work at La Jolla. I quote from Mr. Ritter's official
report:

"During the spring and summer of 1906 while the Scientific Director
was absent from the United States, the conduct of affairs devolved upon
Professor Kofoid as Assistant Director, and the period proved to be one
of special importance for the station in that, largely through his initia-
tive, three biologists, Professors E. L. Mark of Harvard University, E. B.
Wilson of Columbia University, and H. S. Jennings of Johns Hopkins
University, were invited to La Jolla at the expense of Mr. E. W. Scripps,
primarily as advisers on certain matters of policy, particularly on the question then being considered, of locating on the land afterward acquired for
the station's permanent site."

We spent the summers of 1907 and 1908 in La Jolla. The steady
growth of the youthful station is noted by the following excerpts from
the same report: "The scientific staff during the summer sessions averaged
fifteen persons on the payroll, and from four to six visiting investigators.
A few of these visitors remained several months. Each summer series of
free lectures on scientific subjects were given. For these not only our own
staff but the visiting scientists were pressed into service." Regarding the
payroll, I may add, this referred to the assistants only. The director never
received any compensation other than his regular university salary.

By 1907 a permanent laboratory was a matter of serious discussion.
The same old problem of sewage contamination made it necessary to seek

an unpopulated area and to own sufficient land to control the purity of adjacent shore waters.

To Mr. Scripps belongs the credit of what at first seemed an extravagant solution of the problem. San Diego was a large land-owner, due to the huge grant of land given for a city by Mexico when she was sovereign. For a nominal price a pueblo of one hundred and seventy acres was secured two miles north of La Jolla, with an ocean frontage of one-half mile for a Marine Biological Station. The agreement was that Miss Scripps should expend ten thousand dollars in building a public roadway through this and contiguous lands belonging to the city. This road became the highway between San Diego and Los Angeles via the Torrey Pines and Del Mar.

The long anticipated transfer of the institution to the University of California resulted. This transaction and the expenditure of a large sum of money to build a permanent reinforced concrete laboratory brought to a focus the problem of the scientific director becoming a resident. Mr. Scripps was quite insistent that Mr. Ritter give all his time to the Research Biological Institution of the University of California, as it was then named. As all my interests were in Berkeley, this was a particularly severe blow to me. For Mr. Ritter to give up his teaching and sever himself from his university associates was also a hard wrench. It was finally decided that he should remain on the faculty of the University and return each year to give a brief course.

The fact that plans for our new home on Piedmont Avenue, next door to Professor Gayley's residence, had been completed by Julia Morgan, gave an added pang to this change. I had to extinguish the fire of my enthusiasm as a home-builder by paying for the never-to-be-used plans and selling the beautiful site. Years after when Piedmont Avenue, the pride of early-day Berkeleyans, became an avenue of fraternity and sorority houses, my grief was assuaged.

Beside being torn from various boards of organizations in which I was working in and around Berkeley, I could foresee years of pioneering in order to turn that large tract of arid land into—what? A permanent and growing marine biological station and a home-site for its scientific staff and employees was the answer.

At this point I insert another quotation from Mr. Ritter's report regarding the relation of the station to Miss Scripps and Mr. Scripps, its main supporters.

"What these two have done in a monetary way is shown under the other captions. The fact of fundamental importance to be brought out here is that whatever has been accomplished has been by earnest, thoughtful, sympathetic cooperation between those, on the one side, possessed of technical scientific knowledge and experience but no material resources; and on the other side, those possessed of large material resources but little of the technical knowledge and experience requisite for such an enterprise, the common meeting ground of the two parties being great faith in the efficacy of natural knowledge toward the highest good of mankind. By cooperation I do not mean that one party furnished merely the money and the other party merely the technical experience. Such a conception is altogether too small for the sort of cooperation that is being practiced here. The truth is that one party furnishes the money primarily, and secondarily solicitude, sympathy and keen intelligence in the general development of the institution, while the other party furnishes technical knowledge and experience primarily, and secondarily thoughtfulness, care and judgment in the business management."

Another quotation is apropos: "Into the general working plans of the station are woven the suggestions, the ideas, and the activities of Professors C. A. Kofoid and H. B. Torrey in so intimate a way that surely without them the institution could not have been exactly what it is; indeed could not have been at all without services quite like theirs. To Professor Kofoid's extensive knowledge of laboratory plans, construction and equipment, to his skill in working out details for such purposes, and to his ability in devising mechanical appliances, are largely due the laboratory building and some of the most important apparatus used on the *Agassiz*. Professor Torrey also took an important part in planning the laboratory building and the *Agassiz*; while his special efforts have largely produced the library, not only as it now is but as it will be in its fuller development."

In June, 1909 we removed, bag and baggage, to La Jolla which was destined to be our home for fifteen years. A freight-car conveyed our household goods and gods to our new home. For the first year this was a large and pleasant house situated directly over the caves on a sheer cliff three hundred feet high. The view was magnificent, and our time was fully occupied.

Beside his biological work, Mr. Ritter was intensely occupied in writing an extensive philosophico-biological treatise which I had the pleasure of reviewing and typing several times. Other occupations outside my domestic duties came my way, testing my ingenuity. In reading Mr. Ritter's report written in 1911, I was surprised to find this brief summing up of my two years' work:

"Nor would the list of those whose labors have contributed most to the institutional upbuilding and operations of the station be in any wise complete without reference to the vicarious activities, official and scientific, of Mrs. William E. Ritter, wife of the scientific director."

These "vicarious activities" in developing the new site for the enlarging institution were three-fold. First, the building. While a San Diego architect with the aid of the scientists had planned the laboratory, and a contractor-builder did the actual construction, an overseer of the work was necessary as the architect's visits, owing to the great distance, were infrequent, and automobiles for common usage were still in the future. It fell to my lot to be this overseer or go-between architect, contractor and owners. I had had no experience in building aside from watching the erection of our home in Berkeley, but I had a keen and accurate eye and could read the specifications intelligently and listen to directions from both architect and scientific director.

Hours each day were spent on the job, two and a half miles from our home. For this as well as another activity some means of transportation was necessary, a means that could carry me over the entire one hundred and seventy acres of rough mesa and canyons, as this barren tract must be planted with trees.

One of Mr. Scripps' pastimes during the years had been the transforming of his arid three thousand acreage into a forest of eucalyptus trees, orange and lemon orchards, and cactus, as well as domestic gardens. For this he had large green-houses for propagation. He generously offered to supply twenty thousand eucalyptus seedlings of different varieties for the Station's bare land. Supervising the planting of these trees and five hundred Monterey pines fell to my lot, beside the laying out of ornamental gardens.

I purchased a stout Stanhope trap and harness and Mr. Scripps provided a horse for my equipment. Employing a student of horticulture and two or three workmen, I spent much of the winter of 1909 and 1910 driving over that unbroken land. This, with overseeing the building of the laboratory, left me no time the first year for loneliness. Unfortunately it was a dry year and eleven months passed with scarcely any rainfall, causing a heavy loss in our would-be forest. But the sturdy eucalyptus groves on the mesa are the living monument to that first year's work. The Monterey pines could not withstand the long drought, and alas, my ornamental garden over which I had worked so hard, was the site chosen for the next laboratory building. The spring of 1910 brought us back to Berkeley for Mr. Ritter's short course of lectures.

On our return to La Jolla we knew we were to be faced with another domestic problem. It was necessary that Mr. Ritter should be on the ground at the new Station. Where and how should we live? More ingenuity as well as activity was needed. The laboratory, tank-house, aquarium and garage were the only buildings at the Station. Being built for the future, the laboratory was large enough to house all the scientific work on the lower floor. I was faced with the problem of converting a future lecture-hall, six laboratories, a library and apparatus-room into a residence with all of its requirements. There was nothing but bare walls and scores of windows; not a closet nor any housekeeping conveniences.

While in Berkeley I lay awake nights and figured out a plan even to the placing of the furniture in the living-room (the lecture hall), so huge a room that our later commodious director's residence could have been placed in it and have left sixty-five square feet of unoccupied floor space.

This was the plan. Four laboratories were converted into bedrooms, one into a kitchen and the sixth end-room into a dining room. The future library became Mr. Ritter's library and study, and the apparatus room was transmuted into bathroom and laundry. The building was piped with gas and water, but the heating apparatus even for bath and laundry had to be invented. So spacious a residence was never mine, before nor after. Everyone who entered that huge living-room exclaimed over it. It was arranged

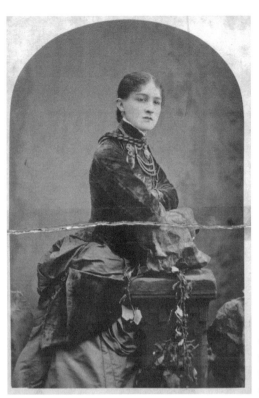

Mary Bennett Ritter: The school ma'am who thrashed five big boys, circa 1882.

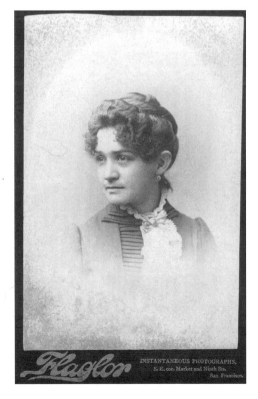

Mary Bennett Ritter graduation head shot, 1886

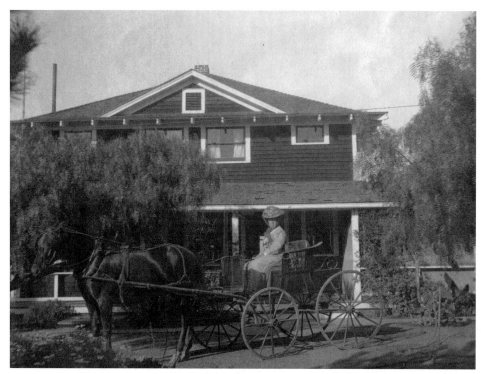

An undated photo of Mary Bennett Ritter with her horse and buggy. WILLIAM E. RITTER PAPERS. SMC 4, BOX 5, FOLDER 7. SPECIAL COLLECTIONS & ARCHIVES, COURTESY OF UC SAN DIEGO LIBRARY.

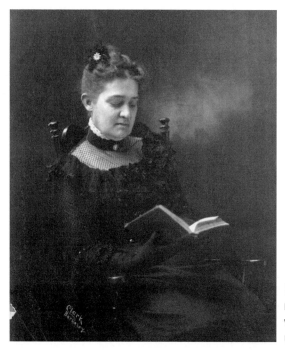

Mary Bennett Ritter reading, 1908. PORTRAIT COLLECTION POR, RITTER, MRS. W. COURTESY OF THE BANCROFT LIBRARY, UC BERKELEY.

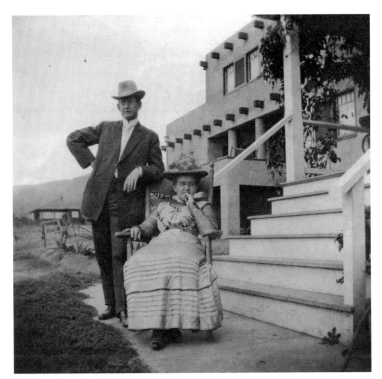

William E Ritter, founder and first director of the Scripps Institution of Oceanography, shown here with his wife Mary Elizabeth Bennett Ritter. Circa 1908. DIGITAL COLLECTIONS. COURTESY OF UC SAN DIEGO LIBRARY. HTTP://LIBRARY.UCSD.EDU/DC/OBJECT/BB1673363V

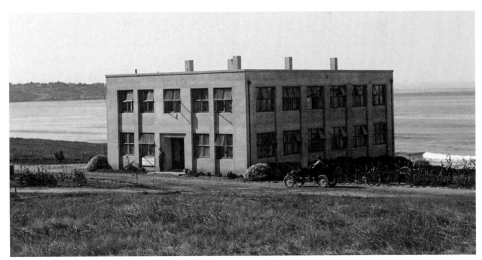

Close-up of Marine Biological Association of San Diego with William Ritter standing on the steps of the George H. Scripps Laboratory waiting for his wife, Mary Bennett Ritter who is driving an automobile towards the building. 1910. DIGITAL COLLECTIONS. COURTESY OF UC SAN DIEGO LIBRARY. HTTP://LIBRARY.UCSD.EDU/DC/OBJECT/BB2936351D

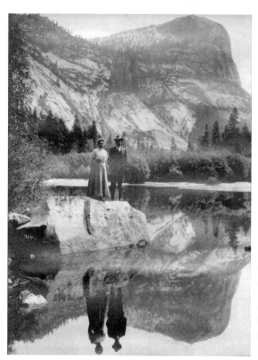

The William E Ritters, Mirror Lake, Yosemite 8 a.m. after a two mile tramp, June 23, 1912—their 21st wedding anniversary. DIGITAL COLLECTIONS. COURTESY OF UC SAN DIEGO LIBRARY. HTTP://LIBRARY.UCSD. EDU/DC/OBJECT/BB80215922

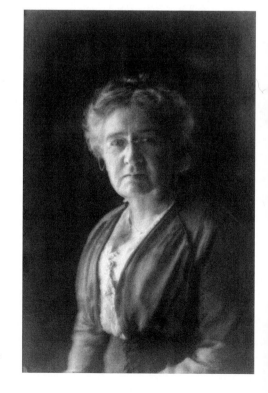

Mary Bennett Ritter: War Lecturer 1917–1918. WILLIAM E. RITTER PAPERS. SMC 4, BOX 5, FOLDER 7. SPECIAL COLLECTIONS & ARCHIVES, COURTESY OF UC SAN DIEGO LIBRARY.

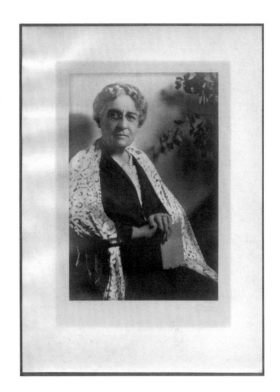

Mary Bennett Ritter: My first leisure years, Washington DC, 1925–1927.
WILLIAM E. RITTER PAPERS. SMC 4, BOX 6, FOLDER 1. SPECIAL COLLECTIONS & ARCHIVES, COURTESY OF UC SAN DIEGO LIBRARY.

MARY B. RITTER, M. D.

BERKELEY, CAL.

Office and Residence
2434 DURANT AVENUE
Bet. Dana St. and Telegraph Ave.

Office Hours:
10 TO 12 A. M.
Tel. Dana 51

For _Mrs. Turner_

℞ Chrysarobini   ℥ī
  Ac. Salicyli   ℥ī
  Etheris   f ℥ī
  Ol Ricini   ♏
  Collodionie q. s.   ℥ī

N. S. Apply to patches with a stiff camel's hair brush.

M. B. Ritter

Prescription by Dr. Mary Bennett Ritter on office letter head. MSS 71/3 BOX 24. COURTESY OF THE BANCROFT LIBRARY, UC BERKELEY.

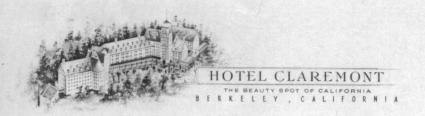

HOTEL CLAREMONT
THE BEAUTY SPOT OF CALIFORNIA
BERKELEY , CALIFORNIA

Whereas my husband, William Emerson Ritter, having proved by his use and care of a certain blue and gray lounging-robe during the period covering several months when said robe was loaned to him that he has the necessary qualifications to put said robe to its proper use, I hereby give the above mentioned robe to him for his use and pleasure.

Mary B. Ritter

Mary B. Ritter

An undated note from Mary Bennett Ritter dedicating a bathrobe to her husband. MSS 71/3C BOX 18. COURTESY OF THE BANCROFT LIBRARY, UC BERKELEY.

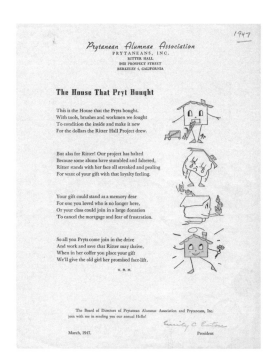

Ritter Hall Fund-Raiser, 1947. MARY
BENNETT RITTER HALL COLLECTION. CU-201.1
BOX 2. COURTESY OF THE BANCROFT LIBRARY,
UC BERKELEY.

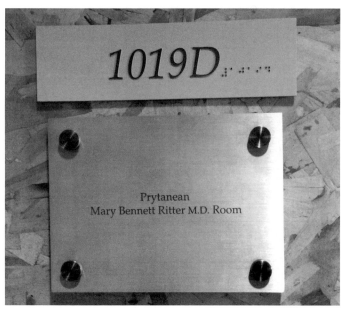

"Prytanean Dr. Mary Bennett Ritter Conference Room." 2015.
University Health Services, Tang Center, University of California,
Berkeley." PHOTO BY CAROLINE M. COLE

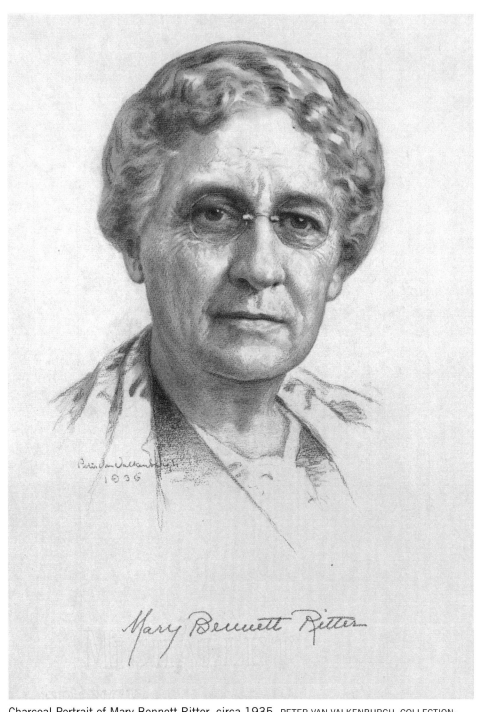

Charcoal Portrait of Mary Bennett Ritter, circa 1935. PETER VAN VALKENBURGH. COLLECTION: PORTRAITS OF EMINENT CALIFORNIANS. FEDERAL ART PROJECT. COURTESY OF THE BANCROFT LIBRARY, UC BERKELEY.

as three units—living-room, sitting-room and library. The partitions were not evident, but the effect was.

A large skylight in the roof which caused a disastrous glare, I covered with brown canvas, giving a soft mellow glow in the room. The general reaction to the uniqueness of the room was typified by that of my niece, Ruth Bennett, a lovely girl of seventeen who spent the summer vacation of 1912 with us. It was her first trip from home. She told me afterward that when she arrived in the late afternoon and entered the solitary stone building set up on the cliff overlooking the whole Pacific Ocean, and went up the broad concrete stairs with the thud of the surf in her ears, a flood of homesickness swept over her. But as she came into the large living-room, softened by the glow of the setting sun, the beauty and hominess of it filled her with a delight which overcame all sense of loneliness. Before her month's visit was ended she served as bridesmaid in that room for the second wedding that disrupted our household arrangements.

This isolated residence soon proved that more rapid transportation was necessary for the frequent trips to San Diego, eighteen miles distant. I therefore acquired an open Buick and essayed the province of Institution chauffeur. Nothing was delivered to us at the Station. For everything we ate or used, even milk or a paper of pins, a trip to La Jolla had to be made over three miles of rough road and a long grade. The Buick fulfilled all needs, but like all cars at that time it had to be cranked, as starters had not then been invented. The lights were small, wobbly, uncertain oil lamps. When we later acquired acetylene lamps and tank we felt greatly elated, but for the deadly crank a substitute could not so readily be found. What havoc that crank later wrought!

Not all of my time was devoted to the Institution. There were club affiliations, local and State Federations. La Jolla had a small but vigorous woman's club, and I was still an official on the State Federation Board. In the summer of 1910 I was elected president of the Southern District comprising the six counties south and east of Los Angeles. This gave me plenty of occupation.

It goes without saying that I could not do so much outside work and the inside work as well. Neither my tastes nor training had been kitchen-wise, so I always turned that necessary department over to some more efficient person. In Berkeley I had been blessed with an almost perfect servant who lived with us from the time we began housekeeping until we sold our home and went to the Orient twelve years later. The grief at parting and the feeling of general disruption had been mutual, as she tearfully said to me, "Doctor, you are breaking up my home."

In La Jolla it was impossible to keep a person of the regular servant class; it was too lonely a life. So someone who could be interested in our sort of life and work had to be found. The first year in the village we were fortunate in securing a young girl who wished to live in La Jolla but could not find employment in her own line of book-keeping. She filled the position most satisfactorily for a year, but young Cupid was flying about and settled on our roof-tree, and she married a rising young grocer in the village. So it came to pass that I began what seemed to be an amateur but successful matrimonial bureau, as I married off three young culinary assistants in succession.

When we moved out to the lone laboratory, the problem was serious. It simply meant finding someone who could be incorporated into the family life and yet competent to run the house while I ran all out-doors. Appealing to friends far and near for help, my college mate Dr. Fletcher came to my rescue. She wrote me that her niece, Nettie Cadman, who was then in training as a nurse, was breaking under the strain and would be glad to come to me for a year, for the change of climate and occupation. This young woman I had first met twenty-two years before when I ushered her into the world. She was the dilatory baby whose mother I took for a drive with Prince to "hurry things up," when Prince took the bit in his teeth and hurried them up to such an extent that I had to pick up a strange youth to prevent a runaway. Gladly I accepted her services.

Nettie was not to lack companionship of her own generation as two young teachers, Edna Watson and Myrtle Johnson, former students of Mr. Ritter, were with us.

As the distance to La Jolla was too great for them to walk back and forth I took them into our spacious laboratory home. Myrtle was working toward her doctor's degrees; Edna had received hers in May of that year. At Mr. Ritter's request she had come to help him with a difficult piece of work on which he was engaged. This work later evolved into the *Unity of the Organism*, but at that point of its evolution it required an amount of delving into the ancient philosophies and the translation of modern ones that called for more time than he could afford to give.

Edna Watson, now Dr. Bailey, had the same philosophico-biological trend of mind as Mr. Ritter and had been working with him intermittently since her college days, making her better fitted to help him than anyone else. She wrote years later that Mr. Ritter was at that time wrestling with "the disease of dissatisfaction in about equal degree with all varieties of subjectivistic metaphysics on the one hand, and all varieties of materialistic metaphysics on the other.

"Restoration to spiritual health came at last in the organismal conception of life combined with the natural history method of philosophizing."

Alas, a more virulent physical disease was soon to engage all of his attention, and this happy comradeship for Nettie proved of short duration.

During the latter part of November, the annual meeting of the District Federation was held in San Bernardino. Mr. Ritter and a driver took me there. Mr. Ritter had a severe cold and on the way home became seriously ill. I was not informed for two or three days and when I reached home I found a desperately sick man with what proved to be pneumonia and pleurisy. He had injured the pleura (as was found later) in trying to crank the auto when the gas tank was empty, the night before the San Bernardino trip.

Then began a battle for his life that exceeded in mental and physical strain anything ever endured by either of us. For six weeks the patient grew steadily worse. The case was a complicated one baffling physicians and nurses. Two nurses, day and night, aided me in caring for him. A La Jolla physician and one from San Diego were in constant attendance. In addition to the lung involvement, meningitis or inflamation of the membranes covering the brain developed, causing delirium. For a month he scarcely recognized anyone. He raved about the creatures he saw in the room, golden bats and weird fancies of all kinds, some beautiful and some terrifying. We could catch only occasional words, and at times there were cries of terror as he visioned something in the room. And that room! His bed had been brought into the sitting-room section of the huge living-room that we might have the benefit of the small stove to relieve the wintry chill as there was no way of warming the laboratory-bedrooms, and this was one of California's worst winters. Following the eleven months' drought of the previous year, Jupiter Pluvius was making up for lost time. It poured a deluge. The casement windows, thirteen of them in that huge room, leaked horribly. We had to take up all the rugs, and one day we had to wear rubbers while the janitor scooped up the water in bucketfuls and then steadily mopped up the incoming flood.

I rarely wholly undressed, and though I was supposed to sleep at night, I was up every two or three hours and slept only when nature was exhausted. For about six weeks I felt as if I were standing on the edge of an open grave, but I would not despair though I could see my husband was steadily losing ground and that the complications and confusing symptoms were baffling the physicians.

One night when I came out in the wee small hours to see how he was, I found that the nurse had recorded, "Cheyne-Stokes respiration." That to me meant the death-knell, the occasional faltering breathing of the last day or two. I had never heard of a patient recovering after "Cheyne-Stokes" set in. I turned furiously on the nurse and whispered, "That is not true! I will not have it!" "Oh yes, Dr. Ritter, it is true. There have been several attacks of it." "It is not true! I cannot have it so; he has got to live!" I replied through clenched teeth. How I longed for Berkeley and for the medical aid to be had there; the keen diagnostic acumen of Dr. Herbert Moffitt and the skill of Dr. Philip King Brown.

In the early morning visit of the doctors they too tried to cover up their anxiety, but I could see they expected the end. When Miss Scripps and Mr. Scripps came I wailed, "Oh, if only we were in Berkeley!" "Is there anyone there who could help?" asked Miss Scripps. "Yes, Dr. Moffitt could find out what the trouble is," I said. "Send for him," they both exclaimed. So Dr. Corey, the local physician, telegraphed for him. Back came the reply, "Out of town. Returns tonight." A telegram was sent to Dr. Corey's son in the university: "Meet Dr. Moffitt at train and have him take train from same depot for San Diego." The youth met the train but Dr. Moffitt answered the message by saying, "I cannot go to San Diego. I am just getting home from a long trip to a patient's bedside. I must be at my office tomorrow." "But you must go," the boy pleaded. "Professor Ritter is dying!" "What! Professor Ritter?" "Yes." "I'll go! Phone my house. I'll go anywhere for Will Ritter!" They had been college mates.

Boarding a train bound for Los Angeles, he started to save the life of his friend, which he did. The fast train to San Diego did not stop at Miramar, the nearest station, but Mr. Scripps wired the president of the railroad of the dire emergency, and the train was stopped to let Dr. Moffitt off. Mr. Scripps' car met him and brought him to our bleak laboratory home.

It was late in the evening and how it was raining! Dr. Moffitt's first words were, "What! Are you in such a desolate place as this?" It did look desolate, that lone concrete building on a bleak coast, in pitch darkness and a pouring rain. But the next day when the sun came out he changed his mind.

What relief he brought to my troubled soul! After examination he said, "Of course that is Cheyne-Stokes respiration. You know it is, and you are only trying to hypnotise yourself to keep up your courage. But you need not despair. I saw one case in a German hospital that recovered after Cheyne-Stokes had set in, and I believe Will Ritter will be a second case. He is strong, has never been ill nor abused his health in any way, does not drink nor smoke, and with all this fresh air I believe he will live after we remove the focus of infection and relieve the pressure on the lungs."

With his wonderful diagnostic skill, Dr. Moffitt had differentiated a double pneumonia plus a purulent pleurisy, and it was this focus of infection that had caused the meningitis. In the morning the three physicians agreed that removal of the pleuritic effusion was necessary. A quart of thick fluid was drawn off, when the patient collapsed and they had to stop. Later another quart was removed and another collapse occurred. It was estimated that about one more quart remained, but it was deemed safer to leave that for nature to absorb rather than risk another such drain on the patient's strength.

Dr. Moffitt remained with his patient eighteen hours and without doubt saved his life. In the morning the physician-friend tried to rouse his old-time college-mate from his delirium. He spoke loudly, and shook his shoulder, saying, "Ritter, don't you know me?" Repeating the question, the patient opened his wild eyes, stared blankly, then fastened them on the doctor's face. One could see a glimmer of intelligence, and finally he whispered excitedly, "Herb, Herb Moffitt! You here?" Then unconsciousness recurred.

A third pneumonic infection had just set in, hence the third terrific rise in temperature. For another eight days the struggle went on—rising temperature, continuous delirium and oft-repeated attacks of Cheyne-Stokes respiration. But fresh courage had been infused in all the attendants and the lungs had been relieved of the terrible pressure as well as the constant source of infection.

Finally the crisis was passed, and rationality and strength gradually returned, although the patient was left with a solidified lung. After eight weeks of the life and death battle, Mr. Ritter was sufficiently strong to have a barber relieve him of his heavy beard. What a ghost of himself he was when that hirsute growth was removed.

Then came the long convalescence. It was necessary to get the patient with infected lungs away from the moist air and continuous rains into a warm and dry climate as soon as possible. With the aid of friends and the use of the Scripps' auto, I took Mr. Ritter to the Imperial Valley. We remained in El Centro two months when the heat drove us to Redlands the first of April. Two more months in the lovely Wissahickon Inn, located in an orange orchard where one was allowed to eat his fill of oranges straight from the trees, brought healing strength and renewed energy.

During the spring months, in these two counties within the Southern District of the State Federation of which I was president, I stole away sometimes in the afternoons to give talks at the clubs. Since Mr. Ritter was by that time able to walk about a little, being left to his own devices was beneficial to him. It was also refreshing to me beside enabling me to carry on, to a certain extent, my neglected official duties.

By June the call of the University library was too strong to be resisted. The patient had become impatient and would go back to some intellectual pursuit, and I was anxious to have Dr. Moffitt's further advice. So we returned to Berkeley for the summer vacation.

Dr. Moffitt's dictum was that at least another year of watchful care would be required on account of a serious and menacing solidification of the upper half of the left lung. Egg-nogs, cream and other fattening foods every three hours was his prescription. This was begun in Berkeley and faithfully continued at La Jolla where we returned late in August, nearly nine months after the illness began.

We returned to Berkeley again the following summer, and again Dr. Moffitt examined the patient. The lung had not cleared up as he had hoped and he prescribed another two years of the same treatment. However he remitted the night-feedings though extra nourishment between meals and at bed-time must be continued. This order was conscientiously followed, but it was not the patient's conscience that worked so vigorously, in fact he often rebelled. But the glass was always on hand, and the reminder, "You know what Dr. Moffitt said," usually caused it to be emptied. Even at the end of the three-year period he was not entirely free from the tyranny, but the frequency was gradually lessened and at the end of five years Mr. Ritter was pronounced thoroughly well and sound. It had been a long slow convalescence, but how well worth while; and instead of being left a semi-invalid he was fully restored. And now at seventy-five, he is so hale and hearty that he is always mistaken for a younger man.

The young nurse-in-training, Nettie Cadman, who had come to us for a change of climate and occupation, never returned to her hospital career nor to her maiden home. That same winged Cupid again sought us out in the treeless biological station, and the huge laboratory living-room and the corridor adjoining made a lovely setting for the wedding procession and ceremony when she married the young contractor who later built the director's residence from the plans drawn and supervised by the director's wife. The rooms were beautifully decorated with flowers sent by Mrs. Scripps, flowers which filled her own large car and a small truck.

I was thankful to have had this young woman to run the house during Mr. Ritter's terrible illness, since after her marriage I was forced to try the kind of material sent by an employment agency. The first one was a negro woman who from sheer loneliness ran away in the night. The next was a Chinese cook who stood it a month before seeking the amusements of San Diego. With such riff-raff we managed to survive while our new home was building, which was in 1913 when the laboratory work and staff had grown to such an extent that it became necessary to relinquish the laboratory home.

Previous to Mr. Ritter's illness I had had plans drawn for a home on a point near the laboratory, but the bids on the plans had been beyond our means. Having a long lease on the land we had thought to build the house on the Station's property, but after the lesson learned by Mr. Ritter's desperate illness we decided not to tie up our small means in so isolated a location.

It was finally decided that a moderate sum should be set aside for the director's residence, but the sum was not sufficient for the architect's plans, and having twice paid for unused plans, I decided to draw my own. Here fate brought us another thoroughly satisfactory household member, only to have the satisfaction terminated by another onslaught of Cupid, this time a war romance. But that belongs to a different story.

Thus ends our "pioneering in a biological laboratory."

CHAPTER 14

The Half Decade—1913–1918

WHAT A TOPIC! THE HALF DECADE 1913–1918, FILLED AS IT WAS WITH devastating war, fall of empires, change of dynasties and world upheaval. With such a background how futile it seems to follow the chronicle of two individual lives and one relatively small institution. But such is life in the gross and in the concrete. The daily round of life goes on whatever happens. I can but continue with our individual efforts and the small part we played in aiding world conditions.

These were years of growth for the Biological Institution. The inconveniences of having to live in the village of La Jolla and be transported back and forth to the laboratory every day made it imperative that cottages for the workers and their families be provided. Mr. Scripps was willing to furnish money for these if they were built very simply. Beside, the business had grown to such an extent that it was encroaching heavily on Mr. Ritter's time—and mine. The only assistant residing on the place was a janitor who was man-of-all-work.

Mr. Ritter's scientific work was being crippled by the administrative duties, a fact which irked him exceedingly. One of Mr. Scripps' hobbies was that it was poor policy to try to fit a "round peg into a square hole," so he objected to having the time of a scientist usurped by the details of business administration.

Finally it was decided to find a square peg to fit the square hole of the business side of the growing enterprise. A man must be found who could attend to business matters; supervise the daily routine of transportation and other details; superintend the future building operations;

and carry on the scientific work at sea as Captain of the *Agassiz*. Such a square peg was secured in the person of Wesley Clarence Crandall, who resigned from the San Diego Normal School to assume the position of Business Manager of the Biological Institution in February, 1913.

The first addition to the plant was twelve board cottages. These were built during Mr. Ritter's summer work in Berkeley. They cost Mr. Scripps about one thousand dollars each, and were truly masculine in their planning and lack of conveniences. So I determined to draw the plans and to supervise the building of our new residence, with Mr. Crandall handling the business side of the arrangement. We employed a thoroughly reliable contractor and builder, John Morgan, and the house was built by daylabor, which proved to be a most satisfactory arrangement. A week before Christmas 1913, we moved into our new, commodious, two-story house of eight rooms, pushed out of the laboratory by the growth of the Institution's staff and volume of work.

From my personal point of view the domestic upheaval caused the most pressing activity. Having no adequate help at the time, I sent to the San Diego employment agencies for a competent and able housekeeper. A woman, large enough to move mountains, came to the house. Her size seemed a guarantee of her physical strength and she was recommended as a marvelous cook. With Christmas only a week away this was a necessary qualification. It was my custom to gather in all the lone or lonely members of the colony for Christmas dinner, and for this post-moving and post-settling festivity, fourteen were enrolled.

My gigantic helper soon began to show signs of fallibility; her back was weak, her feet hurt. In fact she was obviously not fond of hard work and soon developed "spells." She would frequently disappear for periods of rest. But I was crossing a river, a deep one, and could not "change horses in mid-stream."

I had felt disturbed because Mr. Ritter had reserved some eight hundred volumes as a gift to the laboratory library; but before I had unpacked all the remaining heavy books from the many boxes and arranged them in our living-room on the twenty-eight feet of book shelves five feet high, and a large bookcase in Mr. Ritter's study, beside a case in the hall for the overflow, I wished he had doubled or trebled his gift. Such is the book-acquisitive instinct of an omniverous student.

With the aid of Mr. Crandall and the laboratory janitor, pictures were hung, beds set up and furniture arranged in time for the Yuletide festival. Thank goodness we had outlived the days when carpets had to be taken up and tacked down. All our floor-coverings were rugs, one of my collecting hobbies.

During the preparations for the Christmas dinner the cook periodically disappeared, and once I found her asleep on the floor of her room. She could not get up because of her back, she said. I urged her and helped her up, and finally dinner was prepared, the guests came and went, but there was evidently something wrong with the culinary artist.

After dinner she disappeared, leaving the unwashed dishes piled in great disorder. I went to her door; it was locked—no answer. Thinking she was tired I let her sleep. But when evening passed and morning came with no cook in sight, I became alarmed and had her door forced, fearing she might be ill or dead. We entered to find her—dead drunk! And what an array of bottles I found! This was before Volstead days.

This trivial incident led to important consequences as it brought about the most skilled domestic arrangement we ever experienced. For me, there were five years of trained supervision of household affairs; and for the new member of the family, a complete change of occupation as well as of life-history.

After finding the cook drunk, I telephoned to San Diego to have her removed, and then I called the Y. W. C. A. for help. No more employment agencies for me!

Years before, as a member of the Pacific Branch of the National Y. W. C. A., I had added my efforts to the founding of the San Diego Association, and had kept in close touch with the flourishing organization. In consequence, the secretary paid special heed to my S. O. S. call for help—help—help! She had no one. "Then you must find someone," I said. "Someone who can cook. Send me someone without fail!" I was desperate with that sick (?) woman upstairs, that muddle in the kitchen, that still expanded Christmas dinner-table standing there.

The secretary had responded to my desperation, so when an hour or two later a fine-looking young woman came to get a room in the "Y," she was met with the question, "Can you cook?" She smiled and said, "Yes, I think I can." "Well, Mrs. Ritter wants you." "But I do not want Mrs. Ritter! I do not want work. I am visiting California and only came in on today's train to see San Diego." "But Mrs. Ritter needs you greatly. Won't you go to her if only for two or three days?" After considerable parleying the young woman agreed to succor the distress of the unknown Mrs. Ritter, and a few hours later there walked into my upheaved house, a teacher of domestic science in an eastern school who was taking a leave of absence for rest.

Suffice it to say, Bertha Wilson walked into our lives and was a member of our family for five years, the years of the war when we kept open house for the soldiers at Camp Kearny, the sailors from Point Loma, and the aviators from the Coronado Aerial Station.

For these five years my house ran itself as far as I was concerned. The teacher of domestic science reigned supreme until she walked out of our living-room, the war-bride of an officer who was at the same time assistant professor of French of the University of California, Mr. Alfred Solomon.

This third onslaught of Cupid on our domestic arrangement was a severe blow, but I could only be thankful for the able, professional headship of our household during those tragic and soul-racking years of the World War. But that onslaught was three years ahead, and meantime there was another epoch of building for me.

One day early in 1914, Miss Scripps sent for me and placed a challenge before me. The building used by the La Jolla Women's Club had been sold some time before and the small club had been meeting in a room in Miss Scripps' basement. She told me that she was willing to furnish the money for a home for the club if I would take the entire charge of the construction, relieving her of everything but signing checks. I was even to sign the vouchers. She also stipulated that I should reconsider my refusal to be club president, and assume that duty and build up the club membership until it could support its new building. As much as I disliked to refuse Miss Scripps, I did so firmly, saying I could not possibly assume another responsibility. "You mean your work for Mr. Ritter and the Institution?" "Yes," I said. "My husband needs every spare hour of my time for typing and reading manuscripts and other duties. He would otherwise have to take much time from the Institution's affairs." "We will discuss that later," she said after I had made a side remark about the Institution having the services of two people for one salary.

The following Monday afternoon Mr. Scripps dropped into Mr. Ritter's study at the laboratory for his almost daily talk. These discussions of the two men embraced almost every topic "in the heavens above, in the earth beneath or in the waters under the earth," from the scientific standpoint; as well as almost every topic pertaining to the human race, from the ethical standpoint. So constant were these discussions, and so close and deep did their friendship become during this decade, that Mr. Scripps' secretary and I each dubbed them "David and Jonathan" without either of us being aware of the other's nickname.

Regarding the relations of these two men, Dr. Kofoid wrote years later: "There grew up from the very first a close and ever enlarging intellectual attachment and personal friendship between Dr. Ritter and Mr. Scripps. The attachment between the men rested upon a mutual understanding of certain rather deep-seated motives which guided these two men, who otherwise differed greatly in almost all particulars. The one was a masterful, dominating man of affairs, with a largely assumed indifference to culture and refinement, but withal with the keenest of intellectual grasp of the world's thought and life, and, under the mask of realism, a great idealist. The other came from the academic shades with the aspirations of the idealist and a program devoid of all immediate practical implications. The two had this in common, both were inquirers, both were earnestly seeking the truth, and both were believers that the truth, science, would set men free, if men could only come to know the truth."

In the course of their conversation on this particular Monday, Mr. Scripps said, "Look here, Ritter, you need a secretary. It is not good business policy for you to devote your time to outside details, and it isn't fair for Mrs. Ritter to have to do all your typing and editing and to look after outside affairs too. She ought to be free to do club work and attend to other women's doings. Now you find a secretary who can understand your scientific writings and do your typing, and I'll pay his salary." Then he added half sheepishly, "Sister Ellen has some project she wants Mrs. Ritter to help her about."

I laughed when Mr. Ritter related this conversation to me for I knew what had happened. Mr. Scripps religiously spent Sunday afternoon with "Sister Ellen," and this was Monday. Never before had Mr. Scripps been so solicitous for my welfare. Supervising the construction of the laboratory and our residence, and also the planting of his gift of twenty thousand seedling eucalyptus on the mesa had never disturbed his tranquility as being unfair to me. It wasn't. I was doing only my share of what fell to the lot of pioneers, as my own mother and thousands of other pioneer women had done.

However, out of that Sunday afternoon visit of the devoted brother and sister came two changes in the uneven tenor of our lives. One was my undertaking to fulfill the mission imposed upon me by Miss Scripps, and the other the search for and selection of a scientific secretary for Mr. Ritter.

Temporary arrangements were effected while the search for the ideal secretary was made. After several months the choice fell upon Frank E. Thone. Mr. Thone was an alumnus of Grinnell College, who was doing graduate work or his degree of Doctor of Philosophy. Being in need of money to continue his university work, he was glad to accept a position where he could be in a scientific atmosphere and yet have time and library facilities to continue his own studies. So Frank Thone came into our circle and has never left it. This remote plan of Miss Scripps to build a club house resulted in changing the drift of Dr. Thone's life work, as he became one of the writers on the staff of Science Service, a later development of the David and Jonathan friendship.

My task with the La Jolla club lasted four years, but I did not entirely desert Mr. Ritter's work. When Mr. Thone began his duties as secretary I was in the midst of editing and typing the first volume of *The Unity of the Organism* and Mr. Thone wished me to work with him in making corrections of the manuscript. So for two hours daily we two secretaries sat on opposite sides of the table-desk in Mr. Ritter's study in our home and read and discussed the text, sentence by sentence, and phrase by phrase.

Many a time, after puzzling our brains over some difficult expression, Mr. Thone would say, "Here, you make that cut; I would not dare." Of course all of our work had to be resubmitted to Mr. Ritter. Sometimes our changes were accepted, sometimes not; but the hundreds of pages of manuscript had to be gone over again and again. From the typing part of it I was graduated. I am wondering how many hundreds of pages I had typed during those first five years in La Jolla. One huge volume that was never published in that form I did over three or four times as the author changed the text. Frank Thone stayed with us until April, 1918, when he enlisted and answered to the call of duty.

It was fortunate that the "domestic economy" of our lives was in able hands when I undertook the task Miss Scripps assigned me, or I should have been unable to give the necessary time to the project. My part was to help plan and supervise the construction of a reinforced concrete building, and also to develop a small club whose revenues were less than one hundred dollars a year into a large club undertaking the support of a club-home which cost one hundred and twenty-five dollars a month for janitor alone.

Miss Scripps' idea had been to erect a simple cottage-like building to cost about seven or eight thousand dollars; but before the architect had finished his plans we were launched upon the construction of a forty thousand dollar concrete building. The architect was the one who had built our laboratory, the La Jolla library, a gift of Miss Scripps to the town, and the Bishop's School, to which she had been a liberal contributor. Knowing of further day-dreams of the town's benefactress, he insisted that the club-house be of concrete, in keeping with the other buildings then in existence as well as those yet to come.

Perhaps this is a good place to tell a sombre joke on Mr. Scripps. When our first laboratory building was under consideration he had said to Mr. Ritter, "Ritter, I want you to get my sister Ellen so deeply interested in this project that she will forget her age. She is seventy-one, and our family drop off at seventy-one or seventy-two years, and I know Ellen is thinking about it. I want her to become so absorbed in something that the next two or three years will pass before she realizes it. So I am going to urge her to build this laboratory in memory of our brother George."

Then he added, "She was so poor in her younger days that she has never been able to feel rich. Now I want her to give away all her surplus money instead of leaving it for me to attend to. I know she has made me executor of her estate, and I want her to make her benefactions during her own life."

He persuaded her to build the Memorial Laboratory for George H. Scripps who had had scientific tastes, and thus hurdled her into an orgy of building and giving that caused her brother to utter words of warning later, all to no effect. She had truly learned the joy of giving, and the pleasure of building seemed to fascinate her. She was still building Scripps College, one of the group of Claremont Colleges, when she passed away last year (1932) at ninety-six years of age, while her brother followed the family tradition and was snapped out of life at seventy-two years.

Miss Scripps was eighteen years old when the youngest of the clan, Edward Wyllis was born. Her baby brother was laid in her arms and she adopted and reared him as her very own. His mother, her stepmother, was an invalid, so she largely took the mother's place in the child's life, and the bond was never broken. The life-long association of this brother and sister was unique. Beside mothering her little brother during his early years, Ellen was his only teacher and inspirer in his early youth.

Being among the earliest graduates from Knox College, Ohio, one of the first to admit women students, it was she who instilled the idea of college training into Edward's mind. To earn money for it he took a position as "printer's devil" in the office of the *Detroit News*. This was after the Civil War, and imbued with the war-time spirit, both became newspaper writers and later established a small paper of their own, the forerunner of the Scripps-McRae chain of newspapers over the United States, and the source of their fortune. This was no get-rich-quick fortune, but one built up by unusual brain power, business acumen and vision.

Ellen Scripps was the originator of "feature writing" and was always a partner and business associate of her brother whose genius she recognized when others considered him only a queer boy, and later a freak.

Edward Wyllis Scripps was a born experimentalist—as much as any explorer or laboratory scientist. He was also a believer in the common man, and it was for this class that he established his penny papers. But whenever his luxurious imagination prodded him into dubious projects he carried them, as he did everything, to his sister Ellen for her opinion; and he listened to her advice. Thus for thirty years this close intimacy of sister and brother, business partners and intellectual companions, continued unbroken.

Mr. Scripps spent the last two years of his life on his yacht, dying suddenly during one of his cruises off the coast of Africa.

The club-house was many months in process of construction. Miss Scripps gave an extra five thousand dollars for the furnishings, which included not only seats, tea-tables, dishes and an entire culinary outfit, but also beautiful hangings for windows and stage, and several Oriental rugs.

To support this expensive club-house and its gardens was no easy task for the small village club. Annual dues had to be raised from one to five dollars, and at the same time it was necessary to treble the membership to have even a working basis. In addition, pay entertainments of all sorts, lectures, and concerts were given. Outside as well as home talent was requisitioned. A pageant representing twenty-six Shakespearean plays was given by the club; the Greek play *Agamemnon* was also staged. This meant hard work for all of us; and all took part; even Miss Scripps, who was leader in the Greek chorus as well as in the pageant.

Having the only good hall in the village, we counted on rentals as one source of revenue. But alas, another day-dream of the woman who had learned to give materialized, conferring a great blessing on the community but largely reducing the club's source of revenue. This occurred when Miss Scripps bought up two blocks of properties opposite the club-house, had sixteen houses moved off onto vacant lots, and gave the City of San Diego *carte blanche* to build playgrounds for La Jolla, with a community-house for free gatherings of all sorts. This community-house, the playgrounds and tennis courts are used daily by young and old.

The building of the new club-house had been coincident with the beginning of the World War. It was dedicated January 4th, 1915. By this time the whole world was deeply exercised over the war in Europe. Drives of every kind were in the air. Everyone responded individually and collectively. Our club was the avenue through which the women of La Jolla could work as a unit. Sections for knitting sweaters, sewing for Belgian children, making hospital supplies and furnishing entertainments were formed. I recall one especially fine entertainment, a cafe dinner lasting several hours, which realized a large sum of money for Belgian relief. The young waitresses wore Belgian costumes and an entertainment of Belgian songs and dances was given during the dinner which was followed by a splendid lecture. This is but one example of our drives.

It has never been my privilege to work with a finer group of women. The contributions of that club to community interests and to war needs were simply stupendous considering its size. As the United States entered the war about the time my term of office expired, I was simply forced to serve another two years even though the by-laws had to be changed to permit it. Thus for four years, from 1914 to 1918, my local public service was mostly through this club. However, I was still on the State Federation Board as Chairman of Public Health. My work in this line became my special contribution to war work.

Before entering into the long story of my war work I must refer to another ply in the makeup of our home-life; the social side, which appeals strongly to my nature. During all my years of housekeeping there were nearly always some guests in our home. At the Biological Station this was not limited to friends but included visitors to the Institution from all over the world.

The village of La Jolla did not then possess a real hotel, though the growing town is over-rich with them now. So the visiting scientists were usually our house guests.

To illustrate whence they came, I will note an interesting coincidence. Two scientists from afar came at the same time to visit the Institution, each in pursuit of his individual line of work. Otto Sverdrup, the Norwegian arctic explorer who had been Captain of Nansen's steamer, the *Fram*, had just made the passage through the Arctic ice from Greenland to Alaska. He was interested in the migration of whales from arctic to semi-tropical regions. Professor Willy Kuykenthal of the University of Prague was the world's greatest authority on the embryology of whales. These two men had known each other's work but had never met, though they greatly desired to do so, and their native habitats in Northwestern Europe were but a few hundred miles apart. The first time they came face to face was in the huge living-room of our laboratory-home, on the opposite side of the world.

Another pleasurable memory among many was the visit of Professor Caullery of the University of Paris.

What a place that living-room of ours was for receptions! It combined all the facilities of a private home and a public assembly-room. Very large functions were not frequent, but a few are memorable.

Once established in our residence, I often said that all we needed to do was to put out a sign, "RITTER INN—Entertainment Free." Officials from the University—president, comptroller, surveyor—as well as scientists from all over the world were our house guests, to say nothing of the friends and acquaintances who kindly dropped in, in the course of their tours.

In looking through my book of house guests this first day of May, 1933, I am impressed with the array of names of people from different parts of the world that are inscribed on its pages. Aside from the round-the-world scientists, another group brought there from time to time by Mr. Scripps include such names as Clarence Darrow, Max Eastman, and Lincoln Steffens; also John Burroughs, an ofttimes guest of Miss Scripps.

More impressive still is the large number of names of persons in that book who have passed into the beyond. One cannot but question why so many friends have been called across the Rubicon of death and we be left. Both Mr. Ritter and I had descended into the Valley of Death, yet had been permitted to return.

Another memory that book brings to me is of its giver. Of beautiful Roman leather-work binding, it was a Christmas gift from Phoebe A. Hearst, another dear friend who had crossed the deep river.

But the book also tells more joyous tales. As the colony increased, some sort of social life for the occupants, as well as a common meeting place was necessary. It naturally fell to the director's wife to provide these things. So weekly or bi-weekly "at homes" were held in our house, to which the women-folk brought their knitting or darning, and the men dropped in after work hours for a cup of tea. Beside these informal colony gatherings there were occasional teas and frequent dinners. And when war-time came we ran open house all the time. No wonder

I appreciated having a domestic scientist at the helm during those five hectic years.

It would seem from all this that I was strong and robust. Quite the contrary. Each day an indomitable will drove a body unequal to the tasks imposed. Never a year passed without one or more breakdowns. One of the home-talent entertainments for the club was to be my paper on our trip to Japan, illustrated by beautiful lantern slides. Before the evening came I was so ill I could scarcely sit up, but tickets to fill the house to overflowing had been sold, and I must go through with it. I did, though at times I thought I should faint. Then home and to bed, which I did not leave for three months because of a recurrence of the cardiac dilatation, a condition of which I was never unaware.

At the Biological Institution the years of 1915 and 1916 were years of rapid growth and development. By 1915 all of the original twelve cottages were occupied. The laboratory was overcrowded so a larger building called the library was erected. But this building contained not only the library but the business manager's offices, the museum and some workrooms. The two buildings were connected by a two-story passage-way which necessitated planting the new building in the middle of the flower garden over which I had labored so hard. A sea-wall was necessary to protect these buildings from the erosion of very high tides.

The sea-work necessitated a wharf for the docking of large boats and a place from which to make temperature tests and other tests of the ocean water. A thousand-foot reinforced concrete pier was therefore built, reaching out to a depth of thirty feet at low tide. A small building on the terminal served as apparatus and work-room. Collections and temperatures were taken every two hours day and night to study diurnal variations in both the temperature of the water and plankton migrations.

A new power boat, named the *Ellen Browning* for Miss Scripps, was constructed in San Pedro. This greatly facilitated ocean-work in the immediate vicinity where the *Agassiz* was not needed.

The actual construction began early in 1916. And what a beginning year that was! January was a month of almost continual rain. All railroad bridges as well as traffic highway bridges between Los Angeles and San Diego were washed away, and on January twenty-ninth the Otay Dam went out, causing a disastrous flood back of San Diego. So flood-sufferers were added to the community burden. Even the heavy cranes used in building our pier were taken to help stem the flood of the usually dry San Diego River.

In the summer eleven more cottages were added to the colony, making twenty-six residences for staff, employees, and visiting scientists who came for extended periods of work. A larger cottage, called "The Commons," consisting of an assembly-room and kitchen, and a bedroom for a caretaker, was also built. Here many good times took place as the years went by—colony suppers, Christmas trees, song-fests, and other entertainments.

During most of this time, in addition to the directorship of the Biological Institution, Mr. Ritter's personal labors were devoted to the writing of books on philosophico-biological subjects. The prevailing spirit of the time urged him to make an effort toward contributing a helpful point of view in his book *War Science and Civilization*, published in 1917. This book seems to have been a prognostication of what is now occurring—the "new deal" fostered by our own government as well as by the World Court and the League of Nations: the attempt to settle differences by studying the other person's or nation's point of view.

Our entry into the war in April, 1917, brought with it a change in attitude toward life, both as to individuals and organizations. The dominating principle was the winning of the war, to do which all personal interests must be subjugated. The effect upon our household was probably typical; home duties were made secondary to the general good.

As one looks back on those hectic years, one can but wonder about their effect both on individuals and world conditions. Though it fostered a more unselfish spirit for the time and speeded up activities, many questions now rise in one's mind as to the ultimate results of these activities. Are the huge surpluses in farm and industrial products which seem to have clogged the machinery of the world due to this speeding-up process?

My own work dealt with moral issues to be described later. One can only hope that some lasting impression on those who listened to my talks has influenced their character at least to a small degree. Crumbs from the bread I cast on the waters have come back to me in the passing years, making me feel that perhaps my effort was not altogether wasted.

The biological staff was depleted by the enlistment of the younger men and the donated service of the specialists in various lines. Mr. Ritter and Mr. Crandall were soon drafted into line with the Federal Government in its effort to increase the world's food supply. The immediate avenues through which they worked were the Federal Bureau of Fisheries and the State Game and Fish Commission. Their field of work was the Pacific Ocean with its littoral border. All fishermen and fish canneries were brought under the jurisdiction of this Food Committee. As much of the richest fishing was done in the warmer waters along the coast of Lower California, which is Mexican territory, they had at once an international problem to meet. The connection with Mexico was particularly close and delicate and resulted in the visit of an embassy from the Mexican government to San Diego and to our Institution.

As I re-read Mr. Ritter's diary I see that it connotes what seems like a story of commuting to San Francisco and Los Angeles, combined with the narration of the visits of a stream of federal fish-commission officials who were often our house-guests. Mr. Crandall was appointed superintendent of the fishing industries which kept him from home most of the time. His time and services, as well as Mr. Ritter's, were donated by the Biological Institution. Another service was arranging courses of lectures for educating the public in the deeper meanings underlying the world upheaval.

So these long weary months of war passed, Mr. Ritter continually making trips on the food-production commission, and I, for lectures; with occasional intermissions for both of us on account of illness from overwork.

Mr. Scripps had hurried off to Washington to be near the source of "Ideas" that were governing our country's attitude, having a supply of his own to offer. Who had not? The added strain impaired his health and he was obliged to spend the winter cruising in his yacht in Floridian waters.

Meanwhile our home was open to war-workers of every sort—government officials, university specialists in the psychology of aviation or tropical disease, ministers in the Young Men's Christian Association work, soldiers, sailors, aviators.

Can one but wonder what this mad whirl amounted to when it all ended so suddenly? While we ate corn that our wheat might be sent to Europe (where they thought corn was only fodder), and sweetened our coffee with beet-sugar that the cane-sugar might go abroad, it seemed as if the millenium of brotherly love was just around the corner, and that the lesson in unselfishness could never be forgotten. But in the mad scramble of the 1920s, it has been difficult to find any trace of such benefits.

Yet there has been a League of Nations—fifty-five nations of all creeds and colors endeavoring to understand each other's points of view; there have been endless international conferences for the purpose of set-tling problems about which peoples have hitherto rushed to war; and there now seems to be a general acceptance of the idea that war settles nothing and leaves only physical and financial depression, if not ruin, in its wake. Perhaps by the end of a century the beneficial results of the World War will be evident.

* * * * * * *

But love and romance flourish even in war-time, perhaps to an unusual degree. At any rate Eros struck our house harder than Mars had done. One of our frequent week-end guests offered our trained home-maker a life position which she accepted.

So the year 1918 ended for us to the strains of a wedding march (more like a funeral dirge to me) and the third and last marriage of assis-tants in our home was consummated.

I afterward employed older, married women.

CHAPTER 15

My War Work

MY PERSONAL WAR WORK WAS SO DIFFERENT FROM THAT ALREADY related that I treat it separately. Beside my share in the local service rendered through our club those early years of the war, I was chairman of Public Health in the California Federation of Women's Clubs, which required correspondence with the officials of the Federation districts over the state. As I had always been in social service work of some kind, from the days of the beginning of Traveler's Aid in the late '80s, my conception of Public Health included social welfare. To help a northern district rid itself of mosquitos and thus remove the malarial menace, or to urge investigation of water and milk supplies in an inland county as a source of a typhoid epidemic, were no more public problems than were the social evils, those insidious foes not only to those originally infected but to innocent wives and unborn children. Thus my concept of public weal included healthy minds and ideals as well as bodies.

In one of my annual reports to the Federation I stressed the need of cooperation between the allied departments of Household Economics, Child Welfare, and Legislation with Public Health, that the great desiderata of community education and betterment of community conditions might be effected. This view of public health meant that food and sanitation and medical knowledge of prevention and cure of disease were not enough. There must be proper legislation to put necessary changes into effect, and behind all this there must be social hygiene or a recognition that sound morals are essential to community well-being.

Along this line I had been working for years before a world war was conceivable. But the war came, and with it the harbor of San Diego became a strategic point. The women of the vicinity soon realized that there was need of special protection and conservation of girls, as well as a need to help the soldier and sailor boys.

The results of the enlistment examinations were a startling confirmation of the doctrine that for years I had been voicing together with a large group of thinking women working along similar lines all over the country.

With the coming of hundreds and thousands of sailor boys on training ships to the naval and marine bases on Point Loma, the Government also established a large army camp on the mesa half-way between La Jolla and Miramar. The aviation headquarters on Coronado Point also grew by leaps and bounds.

My work as State Federation Chairman of Public Health likewise grew by leaps and bounds. I was called upon by schools and colleges to give talks to the girls. Women's clubs and civic centers in many localities sent for me. My field of work was the entire state but my physical activities were limited to the region between San Francisco Bay and San Diego, zigzagging east and west from the Sierras to the coast.

Many of my lectures were in Young Women's Christian Association groups. Here there was a double tie as I had been for years a member of the Pacific Coast Branch of the National Board. Hence my work as State Chairman of the Federation of Women's Clubs and local board member of the National Young Women's Christian Association was reported by the California Y. W. C. A. secretaries to the National Headquarters in New York.

So it came about that after our country entered the war, the National Board of the Young Women's Christian Association determined to establish nation-wide work of similar nature through the Social Morality Department of their National War Work Council. I was one of a hundred and fifty women physicians asked to meet in New York for the purpose of establishing a lecture bureau for sex education and social hygiene for young women and girls; in other words to spread the gospel of conservation of youth over the entire country.

This call seemed like an answer to prayer, for the difficulty of financing the work I was engaged in was almost insurmountable, and the thought of being one of a large group of medical women who were doing similar work was an added inspiration. Besides, the social backing of such an organization as the National Board with its supporters would give much greater weight to this work in the eyes of army and naval officials. So my telegram of acceptance was among the first received at Headquarters, and in a few days I was en route to New York, in an upper berth for the first time in my life, no other accommodations being obtainable on such short notice.

That convention in New York was an unforgettable one. All were fired with the desire to do their bit toward "saving the world for democracy." Many of those present had been enthusiastic workers in the field of social hygiene and welcomed, as I did, this opportunity to do concerted and superintended work throughout the length and breadth of the country, but particularly in strategic points near camps or wherever enlisted men were grouped. I happened to be living in one of the favored sites for such grouping and training headquarters for Army, Navy, Marines, and Aviation.

Because of the need of working in sympathy with the army and navy officials, the name of the section under which we were to work was changed to the Commission of Training Camp Activities, with Dr. Katherine Bement Davis at its head. Under this Commission, a lecture bureau of over one hundred women physicians was organized.

I was appointed to the California field and delegated to give courses of lectures myself, as well as to recommend other women physicians to cover the entire coast from the Canadian to the Mexican borders. Some seven or eight California women were enlisted. At first I was head of the group but later a secretary was stationed in San Francisco who could devote all her time to scheduling the lectures. A course of five lectures was planned for each high school or college group, and as many as possible for industrial groups. When full courses could not be arranged, the speakers, often standing on a box or table, addressed a room full of factory girls during the noon hour, or a group of clerks, particularly those in the Five and Ten Cent stores, after closing hours.

The subjects to be covered, as planned by the Committee of the National Board, coincided so nearly with the courses I had been giving as State Chairman of Public Health and Social Hygiene that I continued to use the same outline in the war work. In a newspaper clipping I find an outline of the course as given:

Lecture 1. The meaning of the sex principle in all living nature. Its manifestation in various phases of animal and plant life, leading up to its highest development in the human race.

Lecture 2. The highest attributes which distinguish the human being from all other animals, i.e. man's intellectual, moral and religious faculties. How man has developed all civil, commercial and social institutions out of the two primitive instincts, (a) the preservation of the individual life, and (b) the preservation of the race.

Lecture 3. Nature's plan for the preservation of the human race. Adolescence and its relation to health. Being well born. Influence of heredity and environment on individual and race. Causes of mental and moral deficiency. True heredity and false heredity. Intramaternal and extra-maternal environment.

Lecture 4. Social hygiene. Venereal diseases and their relation to individual and community health. Contagiousness and heredity of same.

Lecture 5. Relation of the sexes. Courtship and marriage. Meaning of marriage. Family highest unit of civilization based on primitive instinct of preservation of race. Proper and improper conduct of girls with men.

The contract with the National Board required the lecturers to be on call at all times and ready to make tours of from one to six weeks, and to give two talks daily in different schools in the same town or in towns sufficiently near to make this possible. Courses in Young Women's Christian Associations and also among business groups were usually given in the evenings.

This official work was carried on during most of 1918 and 1919, but my lecture work under the State Federation had begun in 1916. Meanwhile the United States Government had decided to instigate similar work in all localities where enlisted men were stationed. Upon announcement of this plan, the National Board with rare generosity offered their entire "bureau" consisting of the personnel of one hundred and fifty lecturers and the large sum of money they had collected for the expenses of travel and maintenance. They felt it was unwise to duplicate the work, and that they had assembled some of the best material in the medical profession, and that none but medical women were equipped to give such lectures. These lecturers had already had months of experience in handling this form of moral education. It would be impossible for the Government to duplicate such a group of trained women without great loss of time, so the National Board offered the entire "equipment" of an organized, financed working group of lecturers to the Government. The generous gift was gladly accepted, so we were transferred to a Federal Commission made up of the Secretary of War, Secretary of the Navy, Secretary of the Treasury, and Head of the United States Department of Public Health, to be known as the Interdepartmental Board.

This Commission had its headquarters in Washington. The American Social Hygiene Association loaned its leading officer, Dr. Wm. F. Snow, to be chief of this Lecture Bureau, under this Interdepartmental Commission of the Federal Government.

As already stated, I had to be ready for these extended lecture trips at any time, and was often absent from home for one or two weeks at a time, and on a few occasions for a month or six weeks, according to the distance covered. One rude interruption occurred concerning which I quote from a San Diego newspaper.

Mrs. Wm. E. Ritter of La Jolla has returned from San Francisco because of the influenza epidemic. The quarantine prohibited all meetings, so that the educational work of the war department in which she is engaged had to be temporarily suspended.

Not only is this lecture work of the social hygiene division of the commission on training camp activities carried on in schools and clubs, but in factories, mills, department stores, and all sorts of indus-trial plants where women are employed. Both the management and the women employees are eager to have the message of the govern-ment brought directly to them, and the appeal of the government to the women and girls of the country to help win the war by making the world safe for the soldiers morally, meets at least an interested response.

At the time the work was interrupted, about twenty-five talks and lectures were being given each week in San Francisco, Oakland and Berkeley. Dr. Ritter will return to the work as soon as the epi-demic is over.

* * * * * * *

Another arduous and most interesting line of work developed in San Diego. Because of its large harbor and its mild climate this community was probably more heavily burdened with war atmosphere and men in training than any other of its size. Often there were five or six thousand men on the streets looking for entertainment of some sort during their "on leave" hours—a different group daily. Coming as they did from naval training ships, marine base, army camp, and aviation headquarters, they were of all ages. The youths of the training ships were most in the minds of the mothers of the land—thousands of boys still in their 'teens.

This situation resulted in the foremost women of the town resolving to do something about it. All of the churches, Young Women's Christian Association, and other organizations began establishing quarters to pro-vide wholesome entertainment and opportunities for letter-writing, and thus provide a home-like atmosphere for the boys. But these efforts were scattered and took no concerted cognizance of the conditions of pub-lic dance-halls and all the other attractions that were luring the boys to spend their dollars in ways not altogether for their good.

So as soon as the United States entered the war, a group of prominent women decided to form some sort of a Civic Federation of Women as it was first called, and later abbreviated to Civic Center. Its purpose was to make women an organized influence in civic affairs of all sorts and to work for the betterment of the city and community at large. This is still a strong organization, but my province is to tell only of its war work.

For this a Social Service department was formed and I was appointed chairman. At first it seemed impossible for me to undertake it. To use my own expression in refusal, "It seems physically and geographically impossible. To carry on such a work as it should be done is impossible from my home so far removed from the center of San Diego. The chairman of such an active committee should be close at hand to be called on at any time." But the spirit of sacrifice was in the hearts of everyone, and I was virtually drafted both by the Civic Center and by the Interdepartmental Commission in Washington. My heart was in the work, I wanted to serve my country in every way possible, so the die was cast for another avenue of hard work lasting until we left La Jolla five years later.

Dr. Charlotte Baker had been made vice-chairman of this committee, which seemed to me like putting the cart before the horse, as Dr. Charlotte and Dr. Fred Baker had been active and ardent philanthropic workers in that community for the forty years they had been practicing there. But she had retired because of broken health, so could not take the chairmanship but promised to serve during my many absences for lecture work and other causes. So we undertook the leadership of the Social Hygiene Committee of the Civic Center. Our committee was soon accredited by the Interdepartmental Social Hygiene Board at Washington as their local representative, and we were provided with a secretary and local headquarters, and later with two trained social workers. We were also endorsed by the State Board of Health.

This work in San Diego did not end with the end of the war; in fact it increased, for the Government decided upon that site for the location of a large Naval Training School, and adjoining this another almost equally large Marine Training Base. After some time Camp Kearny was abandoned, but the Aviation Headquarters and the two naval schools are permanent assets of San Diego.

Our province was to help make our community a safe and healthful place for our added war population as well as for our young people. We not only wanted the city cleaned up but kept clean and wholesome, and yet attractive to the hundreds of homeless boys on leave, roaming our streets each night. The dance-halls and other places of entertainment were under the constant supervision of the two social workers, with frequent reports to the Mayor and City Council, as well as to courts and the Chief of Police.

Our desire was to work with the city authorities and to induce them to work with us. And it was then that a big thought occurred to one of our prominent women members, Mrs. Lillian Pray Palmer, former State President of the California Federation of Women's Clubs. She suggested that instead of our working as a separate body, trying to wield a "big stick" over the heads of our city officials, that we ask them to work with us on one big civic committee doing emergency war work.

The idea took root and grew into a committee of about fifty members among which was a representative of every branch of the city and county government which had anything to do with youths. The federal officials in charge of the various military and naval groups were also asked to join with the citizen group. All were struck with the efficacy of the plan and ere long the Mayor, a member of the City Council, the Judge of the Juvenile Court, the district attorney, city attorney, chief of police, county sheriff, probation officer, city superintendent of schools, head of playgrounds commission, Young Men's and Young Women's Christian Association secretaries joined our Social Hygiene Committee. If I have omitted any official it is due to faulty memory. All responded with a will and with the spirit of duty that had been aroused by the war. Admiral Welles represented the navy and attended many meetings, or if absent sent a representative. The chief surgeon of the Naval Hospital was also a member. There were also members from the Aviation and Marine bases. Beside our Civic Center kernel of women, prominent interested citizens were added. Our effort was to have a thoroughly representative group of San Diego in the large, including our federal officials. I was chairman of this half-hundred committee as long as I lived there. It meant often staying in San Diego over nights as well as days, but the plan worked remarkably well.

The Federal Department at Washington had said, "If you will take care of the citizen side of the proposition including the girls, we will take care of the military and naval side of the double proposition."

By thus working together with everything open and above-board, all conditions and problems freely discussed, no political scheming, all considering together what could be done for the benefit of all parties concerned, the situations and the motives behind all propositions were clearly understood. Meetings were called only when some specific action was needed, and the response was most encouraging. As I recall our meetings, there were never less than thirty-five present. We did not achieve a millenium, but many alterations in handling court cases, in protecting youths, in regulating dance-halls and other public places of entertainment that would have been impossible or taken months or years to accomplish, were made with astonishing celerity.

One spectacular result was effected in connection with the Mexican border, an international problem. Tia Juana, our near neighbor, was in Mexican territory. As is well known, it was a racing and gambling center, with no restrictions on liquor, "red-light" district, or any other social menace.

The twelve-mile drive to the border was over a paved highway and the danger to traffic from drunken drivers returning from Tia Juana became so great that two police officers were stationed at the border to intercept them. The San Diego probation officer soon learned that large numbers of high school students were making excursions to the Mexican town in the evenings, causing several very unfortunate affairs, and he determined to investigate the situation. From 6:00 p.m. to midnight during several week-ends he stationed himself with the other officers at the border and turned back all youths attempting to cross the line after taking their names, addresses and auto numbers.

His investigations revealed such an astonishing number of young people visiting the racing and gambling center, usually without their parents' knowledge, that our small committee decided there should be an officer on duty at the border all the time to prevent juveniles from crossing.

A meeting of the large committee was called to consider the matter and the probation officer presented his astonishing statistics. All agreed that preventive measures were necessary. The city and county officials who would have to deal with the unprecedented situation were present, making it possible to discuss the pros and cons of the constitutionality of the project and the financing of it. The first constitutional objection raised was that there was no such official position to be filled. Why not create a new official position to fit a new emergency? There was no precedent for creating such an office. Why not create the precedent? There was no money in the present budget for such an officer. A leading banker rose and said that our young people were of more importance than budget regulations. The city had an emergency fund which could be called upon for this.

Finally it was unanimously voted that it was the wish of the organization that such a position be created and filled at once. As all of the officials concerned, from Mayor to District Attorney, were present and agreed, it looked hopeful. The chairman was appointed to attend to the working out of the plan, with such help as she desired. I, the chairman, replied that we were leaving for Berkeley two days later so I could not take the matter in charge. It should be accomplished in two days, came the response, and we desire the chairman to head the committee.

Mrs. Haman, the president of the Civic Center, served with me. We consulted the District Attorney, Sheriff, and Chief of Police early the next morning. And then when all other obstacles were cleared away came the objection, "We have no one to fill such an office."

On our side, we replied that our Civic Center committee had canvassed this matter and had a candidate to recommend. We did so, and within forty-eight hours after the meeting the new officer was installed and began his work. This was lightning civic activity but shows what a community can do if it works as a unit. Would that more communities would cooperate in some such way.

The border problem was later taken to Congress, as no passports were required in crossing this international border. In passing, let me say that our correspondence with President Obregon of Mexico brought forth more sympathetic responses than we received from President Harding's cabinet. Our local Congressman, Mr. Phil D. Swing, was active in our behalf, and later the Congress passed an act closing the border from six o'clock in the evening to six in the morning. This act was in force until a few years ago.

As a result of this interest in Social Service, the Civic Center sponsored a plan formulated by Dr. Charlotte Baker, and in 1920 started a so-called Girls' Vocational Home in order to have a place where delinquent girls could be cared for without going to jail, the only place provided by the municipality for youth over fifteen years of age. A Detention Home cared for children under fifteen, but for unfortunate adolescents there was no suitable place.

The City Council and Chief of Police agreed to allow young girls picked up by the police or by the social workers to be placed in the Home under the care of a matron. This Home is now known as the Municipal Relief Home but is under the charge of a committee of the Civic Center, with Dr. Charlotte Baker as chairman. It cares for all friendless expectant mothers, most of whom are the deserted wives or sweethearts of the floating population brought to San Diego by the exigencies of the war. The girls were cared for during the necessary period and until work could be found for them or they could be restored to their homes. The Home could care for about fifteen girls at a time, and it was a constantly changing family.

Although later taken over by the city, this work was at first financed by citizens. An old residence was purchased and furnished by interested people on what amounted to a gentleman's agreement with the City Council. In the agreement between "gentlemen" however, it was a woman who figured as the largest financial sponsor, Mrs. Templeton Johnson advancing the money to pay for the property. But the City Government kept its promise as soon as it could legally do so.

Work of this civic and community nature kept me busy until we left San Diego County in 1923, at which time I perforce retired from this committee and the City Playgrounds Commission. Dr. Charlotte Baker succeeded me temporarily as chairman of the Civic Committee.

Meanwhile the Interdepartmental Social Hygiene Board at Washington had maintained our two Social Service workers as long as that committee existed. It then recommended that local communities where service men were permanently stationed should assume the financial support of the Social Service workers. Our Community Chest and municipality did so, but San Diego was the only city that continued this work. It was our belief that it was due to our all-inclusive committee, with citizens and officials working together not only harmoniously but understandingly, that this continuance of the work was made possible for several years.

With the passing of the spirit of post-war service the conditions and atmosphere have gradually changed, but that has been since my time.

CHAPTER 16

The Turning of a Long Lane

WHEN WE MIGRATED FROM THE ACTIVE CITY OF BERKELEY TO THE quiet village of La Jolla, I, with many of our friends, felt that we were to be isolated and lonely. There was something of that atmosphere for the first few years, but for the major portion of our residence there, I wonder, as I reread our diaries, if we ever had a quiet day. Very few are recorded except when one or both were "laid up for repairs." And even then in Mr. Ritter's case his meetings and conferences were only transferred from his office to his sleeping-porch or study; and I have been known to hold board-meetings in my bedroom.

I have already noted the constant flow of guests in and out of our home, some scientific strangers, and many official visitors including three university presidents: Benjamin Ide Wheeler several times, David P. Barrows twice; and once there were two holding that office, at our home at the same time, President Barrows just going out, and W. W. Campbell on the eve of his incumbency. These were usually overnight guests who were sometimes accompanied by their wives.

As to my family, instead of being separated from them, I saw them more than when we lived in Berkeley. My sister for frequent extended visits, and nieces and nephews were often our guests. After the cottages were built, the latter with their families came to the Colony for their summer vacations to escape the heat of Fresno. Having each of the boys of the younger generation with us as "chauffeurs" for several summers was a particular joy. Conrad Warner, a lad of thirteen years, came first in 1913 while we were still living in the laboratory. Beginning with the summer of 1916 he was employed by the Institution during his lengthy vacations. Will Warner Cockrill being younger, came later, his first summer overlapping Conrad's stay with us. The joy of having this young life about us is a lasting one.

But as to work: Mr. Ritter's scientific and institutional interests continually called him to various places. His diary is one succession of "offs": "Off for Berkeley," (almost every month), "Off for Los Angeles, Pasadena, Riverside," or some other place for lectures or scientific meetings. "Off for Cuyamaca" in the mountains back of San Diego, was a frequent entry. He was carrying on field-studies of woodpeckers in that region, making several trips a year. There were many camping excursions for a few days until highways and automobiles made it possible to make one-day trips.

On one such birding trip in the summer of 1919 both boys were with us, and fishing was added to the studies of animal life. Conrad caught a twenty-six inch trout in Cuyamaca Lake, much to his delight and Will Warner's chagrin. Baked, it made a feast for the family party upon our arrival at home the next evening.

These interruptions were sufficient to vary any monotony or feeling of isolation, and the constant flow of guests made a quiet life impossible.

And then the trips east at least once a year, and often there were two or three wearisome journeys across the continent. The growth of the institution made it necessary for Mr. Ritter to keep in close contact with eastern scientists through the great scientific organizations. He interviewed publishers and delivered many addresses. For several years he was away from home at Christmas time, attending meetings of the American Association for the Advancement of Science which convened during the holiday vacation week, requiring scientists from California to leave home before the holidays.

The meeting of this association in Minneapolis in the winter of 1917 was a notable occasion because of a blizzard that raged during that holiday week. It was almost summer weather when Mr. Ritter left San Diego on December twenty-second. Storms were sweeping over the Mississippi Valley when he reached there, and at Minneapolis he found a temperature of nearly forty degrees below zero. The university where the meetings were held was some miles from the hotel headquarters, and taxis were not always available. One late afternoon after being exposed to the extreme cold, Mr. Ritter became thoroughly chilled, and after unsuccessful attempts to get warm in his hotel room, he took two pairs of blankets off the bed, wrapped one around his legs and sat down on the floor with his back against the radiator and pulled the other blanket over the radiator and himself to try to thaw out. Needless to say a disagreeable bronchitis followed, but he was fortunate to have relatives in the city to care for him.

As I reread our chronicles of these years I am amazed at our activities. How fortunate it is that we can live but one day at a time, as reliving ten years in two weeks, as I have done in perusing these diaries, so overcomes me with the complexity of our lives that it seems impossible to untangle the varied interests sufficiently to make a consecutive story.

Mr. Ritter's routine was something like this: always a book under way, many lectures to be prepared, scientific articles to be written, staff meetings to be held, and constantly the future of the Biological Institution to be cared for. To these duties were added the frequent calls hither and yon, these outside calls increasing with the passing years as the building of State highways made rapid transit possible.

Of the early days when dirt roads were the rule, many amusing yet irritating tales could be told. It was not uncommon in wet weather to see autos mired along the highway. At one time forty were counted within a few miles, and a dozen were stuck in a swale between our home and the La Jolla grade a mile distant.

That evening several of the Colony women wanted to go to a church entertainment and the Institution chauffeur consented to drive us over in the Station bus, which was warranted to be able to jump all mudholes. We reached our destination safely but on our ten o'clock homeward trip the number of swamped autos having increased to two long lines on the narrow roadway, our chauffeur was forced to attempt to get around them. There was a ditch on either side, and our bus went down over the hubs. We had to climb out in the darkness, and down we too went "over the hubs," if human knees can be thus anatomically likened to wheels. A weary walk home, dragging first one foot and then the other out of the gripping mud finished not only the evening but our shoes and some of our best clothes.

As the years rolled by we became more and more San Diegans rather than just La Jollans. Our church and civic affiliations were largely transferred to San Diego, and after the roads were paved we traversed those eighteen miles back and forth several times a week.

In 1918 I was appointed on the Playgrounds Commission of the city, making it necessary for me to spend at least one more day a week in San Diego in addition to Civic Center day and those required for the meetings of my committee on Public Health and Social Hygiene.

The post-war work during the years of readjustment to normal life was especially active and Mr. Ritter's time was called upon heavily in various ways, especially in courses of lectures to help the world into a reconstruction on a firmer and more scientific basis. The formation of the League of Nations was paramount in every mind and I note many trips to San Francisco for meetings on this subject. The question of the world's food supply held so much interest that out of many long conferences with Mr. Scripps and others, there grew up a plan of an educational program for the Institution and for the San Diego public.

So it came about that in the summer of 1919 a Symposium was held for twelve days, with three meetings a day, on the general subject of "Population and Territory," or the economics of the world population and food supply. For this, authorities on various aspects of these questions from different universities were invited to take part, Mr. Scripps assuming all expenses.

At this Symposium, Johns Hopkins, Princeton, Harvard, and the University of California were represented, with Mr. Ritter as leader. Seminars were held daily at one o'clock at the Institution, with a lecture at four in the afternoon in San Diego and another in the evening. Great interest was manifested by the public and the whole perplexing subject was clarified in the minds of the participants.

This experiment was so successful that it was repeated in the summer of 1920, but without the arduous three sessions a day, added to the extra tax upon strength and time common to a gathering of social human beings. As an aftermath to the strenuous fortnight, some of the eastern professors sought rest at certain resorts, and I also remember that two days later Mr. Ritter was in bed on account of his only physical weakness, a lame back. When a slim lad of thirteen, in play, he had injured a vertebra, which was partially displaced. He had suffered all his life from occasional attacks which rendered him helpless for a few days or weeks. This summer was one of the troublesome periods, but work went on as usual, the writing, the staff meetings, the personal interviews, even though all must be transacted at home.

One important conference held while the director was confined to his couch was the first of many similar ones which led to a culmination greatly influencing our later lives. This conference, including some of the remaining participants in the Symposium, with the addition of Dr. D. T. McDougal of the Carnegie Institution, Mr. Scripps and his son, Robert P. Scripps, concerned the topic, "The Dissemination of Science through the Press."

The Symposium had been a result of the almost daily discussions between Mr. Scripps and Mr. Ritter. One important discussion concerned the lack of reliable scientific articles in the daily newspapers. A favorite post-war dictum of Mr. Scripps was, "If we must have a democracy we must make it more intelligent, and for this science must be relied upon." But how to get scientific advance and mode of thought over to the rank and file that make up a democracy was a difficult problem. Mr. Scripps rightly felt that it could be done only through the newspapers, the sole avenue into the homes of the masses. He often said, "Starting a new magazine would do no good as it would be read by only the few who have acquired the magazine habit."

For months, yes, years, this subject was mulled over from time to time until finally a definite formula, "The Dissemination of Science through the Press" took firm root in the mind of each. The more they talked of it, the more important though more involved it became. So it came about that the first of a long series of conferences with scientific and newspaper men was held in Mr. Ritter's study at five o'clock, August the eleventh, 1919.

A staff meeting was held in the same room the next evening after an entry, "up part of the day." And the next day the entry read: "General matters, preparatory to leaving for Berkeley tomorrow."

The summer sessions in Berkeley were always times of refreshment of spirits and delightful reunions with the dear old friends of the university circle as well as others.

One of the distressing features in writing this chronicle is the necessity of omitting the names of our many, many delightful friends, but once I began, my simple tale would broaden into a "Who's Who," in the hearts and lives of the Ritters. So I must confine myself to the few who really affected the course of our lives rather than attempt to include the many who added happiness to them.

After a month with the dear Berkeley friends we were off again for our southern home and another group of more recent but very close friends and associates. On this trip we took with us a new member of our family circle. Attending the university was the grand-daughter of my mother's brother, John Noble, who had migrated to Oregon in early youth. This girl, Bernadine Hobbs, had overworked to earn money to attend the university, and in consequence, broke down soon after she entered. So Bernadine came with us to our balmy southern climate for a winter of rest, and became a factor in my life.

Two months of the usual varied and hectic activities followed for both Mr. Ritter and me, during which time it was decided that Mr. Ritter should make an extended tour of the East to discuss the project of the dissemination of scientific news with scientists and editors. This was the first of several zig-zag journeys over the United States for the preliminary work of the foundation of a new enterprise.

We left home November twentieth, 1919, and though Mr. Ritter had a very troublesome back, he held conferences with groups, or discussions with individuals in fifteen cities. In Detroit there was an "Interprofessional Conference" in which he took part; in Boston an address before the Academy of Arts and Sciences; and another address at the Naturalists' meeting; another conference at Columbia University, New York; lectures at the Universities of Illinois and Princeton; the annual meeting of the American Association for the Advancement of Science in Washington, D.C., during Christmas week; a conference in Chicago ten days later, and another at Madison. These, with discussions with groups of scientific and newspaper men in several other cities, made up Mr. Ritter's itinerary.

Unfortunately it was interspersed with "laid up" periods, but in Boston he found a specialist who diagnosed his life-long trouble with his back as postural, and gave him great relief by a brace and special exercises.

Meanwhile many pleasures came to me in visiting our dear friend Mrs. W. F. Dummer in Chicago while Mr. Ritter made side trips, and through her seeing Jane Addams in her Hull House work, and Mary McDowell in her Stock Yards "Home." Another happy memory is that of being rescued from our hotel quarters by our good friends Dr. and Mrs. G. H. Parker and taken to their lovely Cambridge home. They were frequent temporary residents in our Biological Colony, as Dr. Parker carried on vacation work there for several years.

The memory of this journey is especially vivid because of its severity and wondrous beauty. It was the whitest winter I had ever experienced. We left La Jolla in November and made our first stop at Mr. Ritter's old home in Wisconsin where there was a family reunion for Thanksgiving. It began to snow and freeze so that the world was white. Back to Chicago, even that sooty city was beautiful in its heavy coating of snow. Ice was piled up in banks along the Lake shore as the stormy winds drove the freezing edges of the water into embankments. New England was a dream of beauty. Rivers were frozen over and even Long Island Sound was encroached upon by ice. Boston was beautiful, but oh, so cold! New York had a regiment of street cleaners struggling to keep the snow and slush under control. Christmas in frigid New York, then to Washington for the American Association for the Advancement of Science meeting, which convened in the national capital that year. The Susquehanna was frozen over; inlets of Chesapeake Bay were ice covered, and all Washington was skating on the Potomac—at least two or three thousand of the younger generations took advantage of this unusual opportunity. Such a beautiful white world! Certain memories of its frigidity and of our shiverings are not so pleasant, but those do not press to the fore; it is the beauty that remains. But the warmth of La Jolla in January was a welcome change.

Mr. Ritter's first duty upon reaching home was to write a report classifying the various sorts of responses to the idea of popularizing science through the newspapers. As a result of this, after conferences in Berkeley and at Miramar, a conclave of scientists including Dr. McDougal of Washington, Drs. Milliken and Noyes of the Institute of Technology in Pasadena, Dr. W. W. Campbell of Mt. Hamilton and Dr. George W.

Hale, director of Mt. Wilson Observatory, were called to Miramar for a week-end discussion with the promoters of the scheme.

At another time Mr. Scripps summoned several of his own editors from various eastern cities for a discussion of the project from their points of view, holding that newspapers must pay for the scientific material furnished them, and that scientists must be paid for their time and effort in providing the material. Both of these ideas were entirely novel and seemingly impossible of accomplishment, but they have materialized and Mr. Scripps' belief that such an enterprise could be made self-supporting seems likely to become an accomplished fact.

During these discussions, the slogan, "Dissemination of Science through the Press," was boiled down to, "Science News Service," and finally to its present official title, "Science Service," the name of an incorporated organization in Washington, D.C. The purpose of this corporate body with its staff of writers is to prepare bona fide scientific news for subscribing newspapers, and a weekly journal for distribution in schools and for interested subscribers.

Following the discussion at Miramar, Mr. Ritter was off for another trip east in April for further conferences, and again in June. During his peregrinations I occupied myself with another break-down and convalescence at Pine Hills in the mountains.

In July, after a repetition of the Miramar conferences, Dr. Edwin E. Slosson of New York was chosen as director of the first organized effort to make it possible for the public at large to have access to scientific news while it was news. Scientific discoveries, if not spectacular, were usually printed in brochures and distributed by the writer to university libraries and to his private exchange list of scientists, thus never reaching the public at large. Dr. Slosson was summoned for a conference at Miramar and the die was cast which was to materially change the course of our lives a little later.

In August the second summer symposium was held at the Biological Institution, and in San Diego, with only two daily sessions. The basic topic was the same as the year before, "Population and World Food Supply," with special emphasis on Oriental and Occidental relations from this viewpoint; the Japanese, in need of larger territory, having become a much discussed subject.

The speakers came from Columbia University, New York, Cornell, Harvard, Washington, D.C., and two from the University of California, each chosen for particular studies he had carried on. There were also two speakers who had been many years in educational institutions in China. Mr. Ritter was the only participant who had taken part the year before, he being the leader and with Mr. Scripps, the promoter of the plan.

These discussions during the two summers greatly impressed Mr. Scripps with the limitations of the world's knowledge on these subjects. Each so-called expert in his particular field was doing his work alone, unassociated with others working along allied lines, and was as a rule carrying on his studies as an aside to his university work.

After pondering this situation for some time, Mr. Scripps decided to endow a research foundation in some institution where men could devote their entire time to the solution of some of these all-important problems. This he did, but the account of it belongs to a later period.

The Symposium in the summer of 1920 left Mr. Ritter in a better physical condition than the preceding one, but even so he felt he had earned a vacation. Vacation! Yes, a real one, but taking his writing along as usual. The many business trips he made, which included scientific meetings, were not vacations but variations of work. Whatever writing he was engaged upon always went with him, and the oft repeated, broken journeys were tiresome in themselves. But even though the outing this time was for genuine relaxation it would not be interesting were there not something to be studied, to be learned.

This real vacation was made possible by Dr. Edgar Hewitt, Director of the Museum of Archeology in Santa Fe, New Mexico, and of a similar one in San Diego. Dr. Hewitt was to make an expedition into Chaco Canyon, New Mexico, where excavations were being made of the wonderful ruins of Bonita, especially Chetroketl, and the remnants of some prehistoric Indian race, possibly Aztec. This expedition afforded an opportunity to see much of the Navajos in their wandering mode of life.

After four weeks of out-door life, Mr. Ritter makes this entry in his diary: "Most wonderful vacation of my experience except the Harriman expedition to Alaska!" Immediately upon his return he was plunged into an orgy of work and travel including another wearying journey throughout the East.

The Christmas meeting of the American Association for the Advancement of Science was held in Chicago, where also he held conferences on Science News Service. After attending those, Mr. Ritter was off to Washington where the long gestation of Science News Service was to give birth to the infant, Science Service.

This fateful trip from Chicago to Washington was made the night of December 31st, 1920. A memorandum in his diary written that night reads: "And so another year! What has been done? But more important still, what is ahead? The possibilities for good in our Science Service are incalculable. Shall we be able to realize them, and what part in this effort am I to play?"

A fitting query to be written on the last night of a taxing year and the eve of a dawning New Year. The unknowableness of the future was startlingly answered that same night. Three scientists apparently in good health had left Chicago that evening. All went to bed in good spirits. In the morning one failed to arise, and after allowing time for late sleep, his friend called him. No answer. Examination showed that he had journeyed into that bourne from whence no traveler returns. So it was that Mr. Ritter and Dr. Vernon Kellogg reached Washington with the body of their fellow scientist sleeping in his berth the sleep that knows no waking.

For a year the Grim Reaper had crossed our paths all too often, and at that moment was swinging his scythe over two more near and dear ones. Two tragic deaths had occurred in our colony. A young woman had drowned while bathing in the surf, and one of the younger scientists had been suddenly snatched away from his little family. Two deaths had occurred in my own family. Maude Warner, Frank's wife, had succumbed to tuberculosis after a long battle, and beautiful sixteen-year-old Laura Cockrill, Edna's only daughter, had been taken after a brief and baffling illness. And before ten days of the New Year passed, twice more did the Grim Reaper strike.

On the seventh of January, Mr. Scripps' oldest son, James, was taken, and as I was on my way to his funeral a telegram came announcing that my nephew Frank Warner had been stricken with a fatal pneumonia when taking his little motherless daughter Jane back to her boarding school after the Christmas vacation. A wire from Mr. Crandall announcing this double tragedy, added to the fact that I was ill, brought Mr. Ritter hurrying home.

Meanwhile during the ten days in Washington, the infant project, Science Service, had been born; Dr. Slosson had been installed in an office, a business manager had been engaged, and the assembling of a writing staff and the securing of newspaper subscribers was in the air, making it essential that Mr. Ritter should be in Washington for some time to help guard the infant in its early puling days.

So it was that he came home only to make arrangements for a prolonged stay in Washington.

In February we set off for a six months' absence. Our good friends Professor and Mrs. C. M. Child of the University of Chicago took our house, a fortunate arrangement for both of us. Dr. Child had often come to the Biological Institution to carry on his scientific investigations during his periods of freedom from university work.

Aside from his work with Science Service, Mr. Ritter was writing a book for which he required extensive library facilities, so we located in a hotel on Capitol Hill near the National Library of Congress. We were only a block from the Capitol grounds and across the street from the office building of the House of Representatives and two blocks from the Library of Congress. While Mr. Ritter delved among the tomes at one end of Pennsylvania Avenue or racked his brain in the office of Science Service at the other, I began my intimate acquaintance with the Halls of the Congress, an acquaintance which was to continue for several years.

Aside from thus contributing to the mental pabulum of the Ritters, the restaurants of the Senate and the Library of Congress provided sustenance for the inner man, flavoring the physical food with the spicy conversation of the law-makers of our land as they too partook of the lowly meat and drink of the ordinary individual.

Luncheon was the only meal served in the Congressional cafes, so we usually dined at the Library restaurant, situated on the top floor of the building and overlooking all of the beautiful city and the lovely wooded hills of Maryland and Virginia. Arlington with its illustrious dead lay on the slope of one hill, with Lee's old home in its center near the beautiful new memorial mausoleum.

Mt. Vernon was beyond the range of the physical eye but not of mental vision. Evening after evening we dined on the balcony or by a window, drinking in the mixed elixir of Nature's beauty, the wonder of man's handiwork in the capital city with its increasing architectural memorials, and the historical interest of the makers of our nation. The Washington Monument and the Lincoln Memorial Building were directly in line as our eyes roved farther to the limits of Arlington.

Our interest in our country's history was inevitably stimulated, and our proximity to historic sites resulted in several short but memorable trips. The first was from Philadelphia to Valley Forge, where we tried to relive in imagination the perilous winter spent by Washington and his half-starved, half-naked troops during the darkest period of the war for our national independence.

Later in the spring, with our good friends Dr. and Mrs. Slosson, we celebrated our double wedding anniversaries by a two-day trip through battle-fields of the War of the Rebellion. Our distal point was Gettysburg, where we spent the night. The following day a guide showed us over the miles of battle-fields, outlining the position in those momentous battles. But more than the graves of the dead, the monuments to gallant officers, and the cannon that had helped to win the victory, the figure of the lonely abused Lincoln as he delivered that simple but undying Gettysburg address impressed itself upon me. Lincoln at Gettysburg, and Washington at Valley Forge had passed through a Gethsemane that our nation might live and be free.

One great pleasure in this first Washington experience was the finding of many old friends and the making of new ones. Among the latter there ranked first the director of the infant Science Service, Edwin E. Slosson, and his talented wife, May Preston Slosson, a friendship that has enriched our lives.

The trip to Valley Forge had been made during a visit to an old-time friend in Cynwyd, Philadelphia. While I remained there Mr. Ritter went to Ithaca, New York, to interview Dr. W. S. Thompson of Cornell University, one of the members of the preceding summer Symposium. Because of his studies and writings on population problems, Dr. Thompson was the tentative choice for the proposed research position Mr. Scripps was planning to endow.

For this interview, this viewing of the new problem from all sides, both as to the worth-whileness of the project and the change in the life of Dr. Thompson and his family, the two men went off on a three-day auto excursion through the lake region of central New York which was the district where Dr. Thompson had pursued his most intimate investigations, and chanced to be the homeland of Mr. Ritter's grandparents and the birthplace of both of his parents. Here he found distant cousins of two or three generations whom he had never met, which added interest to the excursion.

When the interview was over, Mr. Ritter went up into the Adirondacks for a long-wished-for opportunity for nature study, or the study of certain animals in their native habitat. His purpose was to watch the building habits of the beavers. These animals were protected by the State in this region, so were unusually numerous.

And here I feel inclined to loiter in my story, as Mr. Ritter was doing by the Adirondack streams, to explain the underlying stratum or "ply" in his seemingly futile interest in watching certain animals.

In writing his two-volume philosophico-biological treatise on the *Unity of the Organism,* that is, the life history of an organism, be it beast or man, from its germ-cells to its highest intellectual development, the problem of the part intellect or reason plays in the life of any animate creature became increasingly complex. He realized that no highly developed organ, as the human eye or heart for example, could be understood without so-called comparative studies, that is, comparing the development of that organ from its simplest manifestation in the lowliest animals up through more complex forms to its highest manifestation in mankind.

So he decided to study the activities of the human brain or so-called intellect in the same comparative way. In each great division of animal groups he chose a certain kind that seemed from its known habits to be especially intelligent. Among the insects he chose the harvester ants with their familiar nest-building and food-carrying habits and their communal life. For years at La Jolla his daily exercise was walking over the hills and watching certain ant colonies with their busy but often wastefully busy activities.

In the bird kingdom he selected the California woodpecker because of its conspicuous habit of acorn-storing in trees, fence-posts or telegraph-poles, and their small non-migrating colonies. To this day, not a week goes by without some hours of observation of these feathered friends.

About the most highly domestic traits among the more lowly mammals are the dam-building and the tree-cutting activities of the beavers. And here was Mr. Ritter's opportunity to observe them along the densely wooded streams of the Adirondacks.

For the higher vertebrates, the primates, his chance to study them came when we later lived in Washington, opposite beautiful Rock Creek Park in which extensive domain the National Zoo is located. These creatures acting so much like small children, led to the next step, the study of the human infant from its birth to about four years of age. On this fact rests the deep interest of this philosopher-naturalist in babies, and especially in the value of the nursery school for the directing of the "head-and-hand" activities of tiny tots, the developing of useful instead of useless, wasteful tendencies.

But the similarities of innate traits or "instincts" is not limited to four-year-olds. Whenever Mr. Ritter talks, either publicly or privately about these animals, their acquisitive habits, the useless gathering of far more food and building material, or even pieces of bright glass or stones than they can possibly use, he is invariably interrupted with the exclamation, "Why, that is just what human beings do!" So be it! I must return to my story.

My interest in Congress, in the Senate to be exact, was not that of a mere listener. Fortunately I found congenial work. By great good fortune Mrs. Maude Wood Park, President of the National League of Women Voters, lived in our hotel. She kindly included me in the meetings of the League's Council, a group of prominent women of whom only Mrs. Park and Mrs. Gifford Pinchot made an indelible impression. Another member, Mrs. Basil Manley, I already knew. I was not invited to be an ornament nor a useless inspector. The League of Women Voters was then actively engaged in trying to get the famous Maternity-Infancy Bill, known technically as the Sheppard-Towner Bill, through Congress, making it necessary to interview every member of both the Senate and the House. I, being the only Californian in the group, was delegated to visit all California representatives and senators. Mrs. Manley who had been born and reared in Oregon, was given that state together with its northern neighbor. So we teamed our work.

Did any of my readers ever traverse the halls of the Representative Office Building in search of twenty-five elusive, nearly-always-out congressmen? The senators were easy as there were but two to a state, and appointments to see them had to be made through their secretaries. Not so the congressmen! They had to be found, and found unoccupied with other visitors. To find a congressman reminded me of futile efforts to put one's finger on an elusive flea. How many miles of corridors there are in the several stories of the Representatives' Building, I have forgotten. The building covers a large city block built around a huge patio, two rows of offices with a corridor between on all sides of each floor. Fortunately there are elevators on each corner, but even so the weary miles we trudged during those hot months of April, May and June! And then the effort to make legislators understand the aim of the bill: that it was quite as important to have legislation to protect babies as to protect cattle and hogs; that the death-rate of mothers and babies in the United States was abnormally high, and that trained county nurses could do much in rural districts to prevent such a catastrophe by teaching expectant mothers how to care for themselves; and that mid-wives who attend most of the cases in remote districts, should have a standard training.

Then came days of trying and exasperating debate in the Senate Committee, in a hot stuffy basement room crowded to the limit of standing room. Such arguments as were advanced by the opposition, and such stalwart evidence as was given by the small but invincible leader, Julia Lathrop, Mrs. Park and other women, as well as by interested medical men!

The bill passed the House, but in the Senate it met great opposition and one of those exasperating filibusters. After numerous and trying delays, the bill had precedence for first place on a certain day just before the Fourth of July recess. The Senate gallery was packed by a crowd of us, led by Julia Lathrop and Maude Wood Park.

No sooner had the gavel sounded the call to order than a senator from West Virginia was on his feet to lengthily discuss the coal strike in that state. Talking himself out, before he took his seat a New Jersey member was on his feet to discuss the tariff situation; and ere he ended, another senator took the floor to talk, simply talk about some other subject far remote from the welfare of mothers and babies. The so-called ethics of the senate prohibits the interruption of any lordly member unless he graciously gives way to another speaker, as did these filibusterers, evidently by pre-arrangement.

So the day was lost without the bill securing a fair hearing. These tactics were continued until Congress adjourned for its Fourth of July vacation, but the senator who had it in charge succeeded in securing another exact date for the debate after the holiday. The bill was finally passed after a hard-fought battle.

This was my first and only experience at lobbying, but the result of the Senate contest made me a more interested listener in the Senate gallery during our later years of residence in Washington.

As the weather was insufferably hot I preceded Mr. Ritter in starting westward, and spent a week on Lake Chatauqua with friends from the University of Chicago. Meeting in Pittsburg, we came to Berkeley for a months' stay as the Western Division of the American Association for the Advancement of Science, of which Mr. Ritter was president, was to hold its annual session there early in August.

The autumn and winter of 1921 were similar to preceding ones in the number and variety of activities, yet different as to incidents. A new element had entered into our outlook of the future.

Mr. Ritter had made up his mind to retire from the directorship of the Biological Institution as soon as a satisfactory successor could be found. And so we came to the turning of the long lane of our life in La Jolla.

CHAPTER 17

Last Years in La Jolla

ALTHOUGH THE CORNER HAD BEEN TURNED IN THE LONG LANE OF building up a scientific institution, and all that that involved as to place of residence and mode of life, there was still a longer stretch of road ahead than had been anticipated.

Mr. Ritter's determination to retire involved many factors. First there was the future of the Research Institution to the creation of which he had given thirty years of thought and work. It had attained recognition in the scientific world and attracted scientific investigators from both Occident and Orient. Facing as it does the broad Pacific Ocean whose waters lap the Orient on its eastern side and the shores of many other lands to the south, and containing in its depths so many vexing problems, the seer who had first conceived the idea of such an institution, could now foresee a much broader and somewhat different future for it.

He was convinced that the research centered in this Institution should include every form of study that could be carried on in the ocean in its fullest scope. He felt that the Institution should establish reciprocal relations with every agency of oceanic study carried on by the Federal Government such as the Coast and Geodetic Survey, and the Bureau of Biological Survey as well as the marine observations and soundings of the United States Navy, and the Federal Weather Bureau. To a certain extent such relations had already existed to the advantage of both parties. The Institution had established subsidiary hydrographic stations on various coastal points, to correlate weather and ocean temperatures.

This policy would require strenuous effort for years to come and include many activities beside the biological, hydrographic and ocean-chemistry already being carried on. The institution he contemplated should be oceanographic in the sense of all that constitutes the ocean, namely, of the vast body of water with its mineral, gaseous and biological constituents. He spent months formulating such a policy to be presented to the President of the University, and with it appended the recommendation that the name be changed from the Scripps Biological Research Institution of the University of California to the Scripps Institution of Oceanography. This was done with the approval of the financial donors, who with the State of California were now supporting the Institution.

Facing the fact that in a few years he would have reached the age of compulsory retirement, and realizing that this policy outlined work for an indefinite period, Mr. Ritter felt that his successor should have the privilege of carrying out the modified policy according to his own ideas. He therefore asked to be relieved of the directorship as soon as a satisfactory successor could be found.

President Barrows accepted Mr. Ritter's recommendations with the proviso that he remain as director until the desired successor was secured, and empowered him to select and recommend the proper man to carry out the new policy.

Another reason for Mr. Ritter's desire to turn the Institution over to a younger man was that new and pressing demands were crowding upon him. In a sense he was realizing the fruits of his life work while still living, and the carrying out of other plans would demand all the time he could spare from his writings for the next few years.

As the result of the many years of discussion between Mr. Ritter and Mr. Scripps, both contributing ideas concerning world problems, sometimes agreeing, sometimes not, it had been decided that two definite efforts should be made to put these ideas into working form.

One of these plans was the development of Science Service for the dissemination of scientific news through the press. The first year of this work has already been dealt with. The other plan was the proposed Research Foundation for the study of the world population and food supply. This was still in the future.

The business side of Science Service was planned by Mr. Scripps. One principle of his economic philosophy was: "Two of the greatest economic sins are trying to get something for nothing, and being willing to give something for nothing." So he insisted that all writers for Science Service must be paid, and all newspapers must pay for the material they use.

Another bit of his economic policy was that the governing board should be dominated by scientific men, though newspaper men and his estate should be represented. Aside from these general principles he took no part in the organization, saying, "This is a matter for you scientists to carry out."

While he expected Science Service to become self-supporting, he set aside five hundred thousand dollars of his estate as a capital investment for the enterprise, the income of which at six per cent should be available annually. Often had he said, "Ritter, I will supply the money and help with the general outline of plans but it is up to you to see that they are carried out."

In the various conferences that had been held it had been decided that the Board of Directors should represent five groups of three each. Three of these groups should be from scientific societies, the National Research Council, the American Association for the Advancement of Science, and the National Academy of Sciences, which organizations should elect their own representatives. The fourth group should be newspaper men; and the fifth group, representatives of the Scripps estate, of which Mr. Scripps was one.

Mr. Ritter was president of this Board. This made it desirable that he should live in the East for some years that he might be in touch with both projects as they developed.

Mr. Scripps chose for his Population Research Foundation a university in Ohio. The headquarters of his business had always been in that state and he retained his legal residence there although he lived for the most part in California. Another reason for his choice was his preference for a small college with a far-seeing president; so it fell to Miami University, Oxford, Ohio, with R. M. Hughes as president.

The immediate outcome of the situation was another trip east for Mr. Ritter in search of a successor for the La Jolla Institution, and for lengthy conferences with President Hughes.

Mr. Scripps was at the time cruising on the coast of Florida in his yacht, the *Kemah*, and desired Mr. Ritter to join him for unmolested discussion on the carrying out of the plans, when his preliminary investigations were concluded.

After ten days with President Hughes in March, 1922, and a trip to Boston to interview the Harvard professor who was his first choice as his successor at La Jolla, Mr. Ritter joined his friend on his yacht. Dr. Thompson, the man selected for the Population Foundation also joined the party.

Meanwhile the year of 1922 was punctuated with accidents which brought both suffering and lasting results in their train. The winter was another of those recurrent wet ones. In January, while Miss Scripps was trying to protect her sleeping-porch bed from an oncoming storm she slipped and fell, fracturing her hip-bone into several fragments. At eighty-five years of age this was a serious matter. She had already built a hospital for La Jolla and to this she was carried and there spent many weary months. This was the first illness of her long life, her first personal experience with hospitals, physicians and nurses. The months of close association and her inside view of an invalid's needs aroused a keener interest in the progress of medical science, and out of this experience came the endowment for the Scripps Metabolic Clinic, the second institution of the kind in the United States. It was to this clinic or hospital with its most up-to-date facilities that I owe a prolongation of my activities.

February came in with a dreadful storm in which Bert Warner, his wife and six-year-old daughter Alice arrived to visit us. One morning little Alice came down stairs in a pretty new cotton-flannel dressing-gown to warm herself by the dining-room fire before her parents were ready for breakfast. Mr. Ritter sat reading by the fire while Alice stood in front of it, warming her back. Suddenly he noticed a flame creeping up the child's shoulders, and in an instant the inflammable fabric of her dressing-gown was a mass of flames. In his efforts to rescue her, Mr. Ritter was more badly burned than Alice, though at first she did not understand the rough handling he had given her.

The philosophical-biologist wrote his sensations and ideas concerning the incident before the acute remembrance could be effaced. Later Dr. George M. Stratton, Professor of Psychology in the University of

California, used these notes in an article on how a mind works under excitement.

The following summer I essayed to jump another precipice, this time in an automobile, with results similar to my previous attempt. The psychological effects of this are such that to this day I cannot bear to think of it and have always avoided discussing the subject, but it forms an essential part of this chronicle of events.

The spring and summer had found me exceedingly busy with Social Service post-war work, necessitating driving into San Diego at least twice a week and often staying overnight at a hotel in case of an evening meeting.

After Mr. Ritter's return from the East in May, colony affairs were humming more lively than ever. An unusually large number of investigators with their families were assembling for the summer's work, and others were coming for the college vacation period. At the Biological Institution there was no vacation period. Individuals took vacations but the scientific work never stopped.

To celebrate the thirty-first anniversary of our life together I had planned a holiday in the mountains combined with Mr. Ritter's regular field work. I had specified a comfortable trip with nights in hotels, but our good friends, the Bailey family, had come down for the summer and wanted to go with us. So instead of going and coming our usual way we made a round trip to other localities and returned by a different route. Alas, the road was closed for reconstruction and we had to make a detour of many miles over the worst road I ever traveled. I remarked to Mr. Ritter, "How any machine can stand such a racking as this without loosening every screw and bolt I cannot see!" A fatal bolt was loosened, though we reached home safely.

But I was the first one to drive the auto after the terrible racking it had received, as I was due in San Diego a day or two later. Fortunately I went alone. Some good angel prevented one of the young mothers with two babies going with me that morning.

As I was driving down a grade on a steep hillside, something which later proved to be the nut fastening the steering-wheel to the shaft struck my foot. I glanced down and so failed to see a trench across the street where a gas or water connection had been made. I struck it and evidently my foot slipped from the foot-brake onto the accelerator. At any rate the car shot forward like a demon, and jumping onto the sidewalk struck a telephone pole with such force that it cut it off at the bottom and swung it out on the car-track. The force of this blow was transmitted to my ribs by the steering-wheel and the concussion turned the car toward the protecting railing beyond the sidewalk. Through it the car plunged, and as it leaped into the air my head struck the top and the steering-wheel came off in my hands.

I was told later that there was a sheer precipice of eight feet before there was any ground for the car to light on. The car plunged downward about two hundred feet before it turned over. Oh, what a blessed relief was that turning over, and the stopping of the wild careening of the runaway car!

The crash of the car with the telephone pole and through the railing was heard for blocks, and soon I was surrounded by residents and passing motorists. Before I could be dragged out from the wreck the police had arrived and the police ambulance came clanging up the street. No one expected to find me alive. Fortunately one of the passing motorists was Miss Scripps' faithful chauffeur, Mr. Higgins. He and two policemen helped me to Miss Scripps' car. I thought I was not badly hurt. Legs and arms were intact, and I was too stunned at first to feel pain.

I had an important appointment at the Mayor's office so asked to be taken there. The Mayor remarked, "I think you would better be taken home at once." By this time there was a severe pain in my chest.

"I think I'll have an X-ray picture taken first," was my reply.

Higgins took me to a physician's office, and after the doctor had examined the radiograph he exclaimed, "I never saw a finer picture of fractured ribs; several of them are really bent inward!"

"Let me see it," I said, and after inspecting it I moaned, "That's the wrong side. That accident occurred many years ago."

The long drive home was excruciating, and by the time we arrived I could not move, and could only gasp words. I was carried into the house and to my bed where I remained many weary weeks with the mental suffering as bad as the physical. A severe pleuritis caused terrible pain, but that was no worse than the agony I endured every time I closed my eyes and made again that awful plunge down, down, down. Sleeping or waking my brain repeated that experience. The thought of ever riding in an automobile again seemed impossible. But I recalled severely criticizing a friend for yielding to that terror and determined I would not.

It was six weeks before I could sit up for an hour. I told the nurse to phone Mr. Crandall to come up to see me. When he came I said, "When the nurse gets me ready to sit up I want you to bring up one of the men, back my car (its broken ribs had been repaired more speedily than mine) around to the front door, and carry me to it and drive me up the Biological Grade," as a steep grade on our property was called.

"Can you do it?" he asked, startled at the suggestion.

"I must," I half groaned. "I have to get over this horror! But do not tell Mr. Ritter," I added.

"Very well, Mrs. Ritter; I will do it if you say so," he replied.

He was no sooner out of the room than I broke into a reeking perspiration from terror and weakness—a repetition of my frequent night-sweats. But my determination did not waver. I had to overcome that psychological condition of the terror of falling, and I decided the sooner I conquered it the better. In my own mind this act required the greatest amount of courage I ever displayed.

All went well in the twenty-minute drive, and it was repeated each day for a week, when I could ride for an hour or more.

Two months after the accident, Mr. Ritter had to go to Berkeley for his annual duties. I could not bear to stay at home, so our good friend Mrs. Templeton Johnson arranged to take me to my Mecca for recoveries, the Pine Hills Tavern in the Cuyamaca Mountains. By this time I could walk about the house with a cane.

The Johnsons had a fine big car in which I could be bolstered up with pillows. They took Mr. Ritter and me to their house for the night, thus breaking the journey and helping to get an early start for the sixty-five mile mountain drive.

Going over that narrow dirt road along those precipitous grades was another psychological experience, but I forced myself to look down into the depths, hundreds of feet below.

Arriving safely, they left me at Pine Hills during Mr. Ritter's absence. Here I drank in the soft mountain air and the fragrant odor of the pines and aromatic shrubs, and gained strength. But another test still faced me—to overcome the dread of driving a car.

When Mr. Ritter came for me after his return from Berkeley, he drove the fateful car in which the accident had occurred. He was to remain three days to accomplish his field work.

The drive to Cuyamaca Lake was about twelve miles over very high and narrow grades on dirt roads. I said I would go with him. He was surprised, but I went—with a purpose to still further overcome my dread of grades, and perhaps . . .

After we had crossed the bad grades we came down onto a mountain meadow as we approached the lake.

"Now I will drive," I said.

"Do you think you can?"

"I want to; I must!" was my only reply as I slid over under the wheel.

I drove three or four miles until I felt both confident and weary. That was accomplished!

But after reaching home again, I note that for more than a month someone drove for me as I took up my San Diego duties again. I was not strong enough to drive. It was just four months after my fateful drive that Mr. Ritter notes in his diary, "Mary drove to San Diego alone for the first time!"

* * * * * * *

We had anticipated that Mr. Ritter's retirement would occur that summer, but the Harvard professor whom he had chosen as his successor and who had personally favored the opportunity for research work for himself at La Jolla, found that for family reasons he was forced to decline. The University President insisted that Mr. Ritter remain another year and again empowered him to find a man who could carry out the new oceanographic program.

This, together with the constant call from Science Service, meant another hard trip East, which was more than I could undertake. So I settled myself in a hotel in San Diego during Mr. Ritter's absence, to be near the scene of my labors which were particularly arduous at that time, especially with regard to the menace of the Mexican border and Tia Juana in luring high school boys and girls into its gambling-dens.

But by this time another element had entered into the eastern journey. During his war work some years before, Mr. Scripps had had a slight "stroke" and his physician had advised a winter on his yacht, with as much time as possible spent each year quietly at sea. His yacht, *Kemah*, not being large enough for long trips, he had built the *Ohio*, a much larger boat which was to make its maiden voyage among the islands outlining the Caribbean Sea and along the northern coast of South America, through the Canal and up the Mexican coast to San Diego. He invited us for the trip, being especially anxious that Mr. Ritter should accompany him. Though Mr. Ritter felt he could not spare the time he finally accepted, as it seemed the only means of obtaining necessary conferences with Mr. Scripps concerning their mutual projects.

By the time he had decided on the voyage, and I was ready to start with Mrs. Scripps on the overland trip to Florida to join the yachting party, a telegram came saying that my place had been filled by Mr. Gilson Gardiner of Washington, D.C., for many years a writer on the Scripps newspapers. My great disappointment in missing so unique a cruise was but partially assuaged by the pressure of my social service work in San Diego.

The cruise included visits to the Greater and Lesser Antilles and many stops and excursions along the northern coast of South America. They made a leisurely trip through the Canal region, stopping days at a time in some places. Coming up the coast of Mexico, Mr. Ritter's most acute memory is of an ulcerated tooth. As he was suffering greatly, the boat was run into the nearest port, Manzanillo, to secure the services of a dentist. Alas, there was none, though it was announced with pride that there had once been a dentist there but he had left. But this did not relieve the throbbing pain though Mr. Ritter writes in his diary: "Much touched by solicitude of whole party, particularly Bob Scripps' effort to radio the United States Consul at Mazatlan to have a dentist in readiness when the *Ohio* anchored next day."

This was accomplished and after two sessions with the dentist, the offending member and the pain were extracted—in large part. At least his diary notes laconically four days after reaching home that "Dr. Post finished tooth-pulling left over from Mazatlan."

Each day's summary of experiences on the trip begins with "Worked on ..." (Some chapter in the book he was writing) before his other entries. I quote the memoranda for January 30, 1923, the day after the tooth was extracted. "Pleasant day's sail—much cooler. Good progress on 'Self Injury of Animals.' Very important talks with E. W. on heredity, Institution affairs, and consciousness." Some variety of topics! Then he adds, "Bob received wireless of Campbell's acceptance of presidency of the University of California. This may mean much for our oceanographic plans." The next day at Magdalena he notes:—"Got off message of congratulation to Campbell ... Fine day's run.... Good talk with E. W.... Decision to cut out Guadalupe and Ensenada and make directly for San Diego, arriving Saturday morning!"

The yacht docked in San Diego harbor February 3, 1923, having left New York on November 18, 1922. Mr. Crandall and I went aboard with the Customs officer.

While in Washington, Mr. Ritter and President Barrows had interviewed Dr. T. Wayland Vaughan of the United States Geological Survey concerning his assuming the position of director of the Scripps Institution of Oceanography of the University of California. This new name of our Biological Institution did not imply a change of personality or of purpose but a linking up with a broader purpose. It was in fact a wedding of two purposes, where the bride changes her name but continues to be very much herself. In this linking up, the biological staff remained intact while new men and departments were added. Dr. Vaughan's work had been oceanographic, particularly on coral reefs and bottom deposits. Through his work in Washington he was in close touch with the divisions of Federal scientific work which Mr. Ritter had hoped would cooperate with the Biological Institution in converting it into the broader Institution of Oceanography.

Thus it was decided that we should leave La Jolla in June, 1923. Meanwhile Mr. Ritter had been delegated as one of the representatives of the United States Government at the Pacific Science Congress, convening in Australia in July. Dr. Vaughan was also a delegate.

As this decision was reached soon after the termination of the yachting trip in February, there came the confusion of winding up all of our civic and social activities, writing reports, and getting the Institution affairs into proper shape to hand over to a successor.

This was a complicated time. It was at this time that the two presidents of the University of California, David Barrows retiring, and President-elect Campbell, with his wife, came for an overnight conference about the future of the Institution and a survey of the entire situation. This was Dr. Campbell's first visit to the Institution.

In April came the recurrent necessity of a trip to Berkeley and the East, and again Mr. Ritter was "off for a month." Although spending most of the time in Washington at Science Service headquarters there were various side trips to be made to interview prospective members of the Science Service Board of Directors, and a trip to New York to see the publishers of his forthcoming book.

When Mr. Ritter returned in May he found me up to my eyes in work, sorting our belongings for indefinite storage of furniture and an indefinite residence in trunks, beside preparing for a tour of the southern half of the world.

In the midst of this diversified packing, I had the great joy of the first visit to the Pacific Coast of my Connecticut cousins Mr. and Mrs. J. A. Macdonell (Loraine Beeman) of New York. On June the second, they with my twin cousins Edmond Bennett of Los Angeles and his sister Alice Campbell of San Francisco, came for a brief visit. It was the first time we four cousins had ever been together. Three of us, Edmond, Loraine and I, were born the same year; Alice was considerably younger. Joyous as was this reunion, it was of necessity a short one because of the upset condition due to moving. The rest of the visit was postponed by arranging that I should leave La Jolla a week earlier than was necessary to catch the steamer for Australia, and visit with them at the Beverly Hills Hotel in Los Angeles.

Scarcely had they departed when Dr. Vaughan arrived to inspect the Institution and the scene of his future home and scientific activities. He was our house-guest for four days, and then Mr. Ritter needed to go with him to Berkeley to make certain required arrangements with the University authorities.

Mr. Ritter's diary reads: "Home June 12th. June 14th, packing begins in earnest. June 19th, Mary's last day in San Diego."

Added to the internal confusion were the external "lasts" and farewells,—last meetings; last club luncheon with us as guests of honor; last Colony party as a farewell to us; farewell receptions and dinners hither and yon; all pleasant occasions, with the overtones of friendship and gaiety, and the dull undertone of sadness at the severing of connections which had meant comradeship for the past fifteen years. All in all, leaving La Jolla and San Diego proved quite as severe a heart-wrenching for me as had the departure from Berkeley a decade and a half before, to begin this new life.

I had engaged vans and a furniture packer from San Diego, and expected the man to come for a full week's work. Alas, in spite of frantic telephoning, instead of one man for seven days to pack books and dishes and crate furniture carefully while I labeled each box and barrel as to contents, not until the day before my departure did a train of three huge vans and seven men come to do all the packing and moving in a few hours.

It was accomplished, but when eight barrels of dishes and kitchen utensils stood in the dining-room, I had no idea which was cut-glass, fine china, or pots and pans! Such a mess! Books, pictures, bric-a-brac, and all sorts of things were likewise lost in boxes and cases with no indication of their contents. I was simply frantic, but what could one woman do with or against seven expert packers, bent on speed, and the "boss" away off in San Diego leaving me with no court of appeal. Is it any wonder that the precious box containing my personal lecture notes and diaries has never come to light?

The day ended, the house was empty, and we went to Miss Scripps' home for the night, where Mr. Ritter made his headquarters until he followed me a week later.

I was off the next morning for Beverly Hills to join my cousins and enjoy the visit and much-needed rest. This was a never-to-be-forgotten week of loving kinship, a factor in my adult life which had been all too infrequent, as I had left home and kindred so early.

A spicy flavor was added by this first and only proximity to the Hollywood world. Many movie fans lived in this quiet hostelry. Theda Bara, the first soulless vamp of screen life, at whose wicked smiles I had often shuddered, sat demurely at the next table to our gay group. No couple passed in and out of the dining room more quietly and unostentatiously than she and her tall, lank husband, and no conversation in the room was more subdued than theirs. In appearance she was "every inch a lady," even in her downcast eyes and modest demeanor. I was surprised!

One evening Jim Tully had a showing of his first scenario in the hotel theatre, with a crowd of movie notables there to criticize it. If I remember correctly, it was a failure. What a jumble life is!

The week sped by. Mr. Ritter joined me at the station, en route to Berkeley and our Australian steamer.

A grateful interlude was this six-months' trip after the busy, hectic first half of the year and the heart-strain of closing another chapter in our lives.

The entries in Mr. Ritter's diary during the last three days as director of the Institution he had created and tended throughout its years of adolescence until it attained its majority, contain the following: "June 23rd. Drove from Miss Scripps to the Institution. Ate my cold lunch in yard of our home, alone, with many stirring thoughts. Our empty home ... very empty. Our thirty-second wedding anniversary ... Long letter from Mary." "Tuesday, June 24th. Beautiful day ... Last conferences with staff, devoted to last touches of getting ready to leave tomorrow ... Luncheon at Spindrift, guest of Crandalls ... Feelings such as never experienced before at last leave-taking of house at 5:30 ... Last dinner with the Harpers." "June 25th. Last breakfast with Miss Scripps ... off for San Diego via Dr. Baker's for farewells to Dr. Charlotte and Dr. Fred ... latter to train with me ... Reach Los Angeles on time and catch 'Lark' for San Francisco for World Conference on Education" (where he gave a paper).

Then "All aboard" for Australia! What a host of friends boarded the good old English ship *Tahiti* to see us off on our journey to the other half of the world.

CHAPTER 18

The Other Side of the World

FAREWELLS ARE APT TO BE MORE OR LESS SAD, ESPECIALLY WHEN one sets out to sea. The ocean seems a barrier as one leaves the homeland, and one's native shores become dimmer and dimmer. We stayed on deck until the Bay shores had receded, the Golden Gate closed behind us and our good but fated ship *Tahiti* began to climb the swells on the bar. Descending into our stateroom we were greeted with an array of flowers that made me catch my breath, but when we saw the glorious box of fruits and sweets sent by the La Jolla Colony, all my pent-up emotions burst the bonds of self-control and I indulged in a good cry. What a relief tears are! Even Mr. Ritter's eyes were moist as we half cried, half laughed with the mixture of sadness and happiness.

Leaving the temperate zone in midsummer, cut off from every person we had ever known, we found ourselves in a tiny floating world, sailing for four weeks over unknown seas, first into the northern tropics, then through equatorial heat, through the southern tropics, on, on southward through the Pacific until we crossed the fortieth parallel of latitude which forms the unmarked border line between Pacific and Antarctic oceans. Those names denote the changes we experienced, from equatorial heat to antarctic frigidity.

During the first weeks we sailed on placid seas, getting warmer and warmer as we entered the tropics. Passing through the zone of calms, or the Doldrums, so disastrous to old-time sailing ships, we crossed the Equator and saw the Southern Cross in the heavens for the first time, as our familiar constellations receded. Still another thousand miles before our first sight of land at Tahiti.

All these two weeks and those to follow, Mr. Ritter was working on his addresses for the Pan Pacific Conference in Australia. There had not been time to put these into shape before leaving home.

In sixteen thousand miles of sailing on the high seas we never once sighted another vessel (except near ports) until between Honolulu and San Francisco on the homeward journey. On the other hand, though usually from ten to twelve hundred miles from land, it was never so far but that birds—albatross, the stormy petrel or Mother Cary's chickens—followed in our wake, traveling so much faster than our boat that they could circle round and round our ship. The graceful flying fish and schools of dolphin also raced and played about day after day and week after week.

Only two islands were touched on the southward voyage, Tahiti in the Society group, and Raratonga, one of the Cook Islands, and a two days' stop at Wellington, New Zealand.

The praises of Tahiti have been sung too often for me to repeat them. The beauty of her mountains and flowering forests cannot be exaggerated.

Her natives, with their sunny, kindly natures, are attractive but so sophisticated that they have lost most of their original charm.

We drove around the rim of the island (the interior being jagged volcanic peaks) to visit the spot where Captain Cook, the famous explorer, took the first observations of a transit of Venus in 1769.

Our vehicle was a good trusty Dodge which seemed to withstand the wear and tear of nature's roads, largely of Volcanic rock. But passing as we were through a bower of waving cocoanut fronds, mangoes, breadfruit, bananas, wild oranges, and all sorts of tropical bloom, we could not find fault with stones and ruts underneath. Mixed with the ever-present green foliage and vivid colored blossoms were glimpses of the blue, blue sea, breaking in spray on the white coral reefs.

But autos are not the rule. The native chariot is a two-wheeled cart drawn by a diminutive pony, usually a rack of bones, which looked as if it might be a left-over of the tiny three-toed horse of prehistoric ages.

On our drive we saw one such outfit, in which was a native of huge size, clad as were most natives, in a white cotton undershirt and white cotton trousers. His shoulders were as broad as the seat of the cart. He lolled far back to make room for his bay-window front and enormous legs. We were told later he weighed three hundred and fifty pounds. He looked it. We began to laugh at the comical scene when our native chauffeur solemnly announced: "The King, the native King." Sure enough, it was his majesty, Pomare VI. Such was the royal personage, the royal robes, the royal equipage! We later passed the royal palace, an ordinary small one-story cottage, on stilts, as all houses are, to avoid ants and other insects (there are no snakes) and to provide shelter beneath for the domestic stock, horses, cows, dogs and chickens.

In the most tropic climes a two-hour rest from all business is taken at mid-day. Everyone indulges in a siesta. To illustrate the effect of white influence on the native character: while shopping we passed a stout Tahitan lady arrayed in a light blue voile dress embroidered in white, conspicuously a ready-made American product, and a white sailor hat with a pink veil around it, while her rugged brown feet were guiltless of shoes or stockings. Strolling back down the street after the shops were closed for the noon rest, we saw the same lady lying on the sidewalk in front of one of the largest European stores, sound asleep, her head pillowed on the bundle she had been carrying. No one appeared to notice her, and she was far from being the only one taking the mid-day siesta wherever the sleepy hour overtook them.

Creeping out of the beautiful but dangerous harbor at midnight, with the jagged coral reefs flouting us on either side, we turned our prow southwestward, headed for the Cook Islands.

Here our first storm overtook us. It delayed us three days, as these Polynesians who live in the water half the time would not unload the cargo in the rain!

We had to anchor outside the coral reef there being no entrance through it, and run out to sea each night. This island of Raratonga is small but wondrously beautiful with its jagged peaks, the usual tropical forest and tropical fruits and flowers.

Again turning southward, in two days the balmy breezes lost their balminess, the tropic sun lost its heat. Crossing the tropic of Capricorn was like plunging into a cold swimming pool after a hot bath. Leaving Wellington, the Tasman Sea lived up to its reputation for storms, rough sea, and chilly winds. But the inclement weather only delayed our good ship one day, and as the fourth week waned we found our-selves entering beautiful Sydney Harbor, the fascinating door-way to "lonely Australia."

In its remoteness and its individuality, Australia is well named "The Lonely Continent." It is lone, unique. Nothing is like things called by the same name in other lands. No indigenous plant or animal is like any plant or animal found elsewhere in the world. The native Bushman is considered one of the lowliest types of humanity.

Australian hospitality is well known, and it deserves its reputation. Both individually and nationally the Australians make the stranger within their gates feel their welcome.

We went there to attend the Pacific Science Congress, and scientists from all the countries surrounding the Pacific Ocean were in attendance. Congresses of all kinds are familiar enough, but never had we experienced anything approaching the extent of entertainment and travel that was accorded the overseas delegates in Melbourne and Sydney. I do not think it would be possible under our laws to duplicate their program of hospi-tality. The Commonwealth government and the several states contributed largely as hosts, and they own the railroads.

About the size of the United States, Australia has a white popula-tion somewhat less than New York City; hence at a glance one can see that the problems of transportation and everything else are numerous and formidable.

Apparently the pioneers who entered this new continent had a restricted vocabulary, and coming to a land where everything was strange, they named things from external resemblances, regardless of the vast dif-ferences there might be in the real nature of plants, animals, or even the earth's structure itself. So Australia is a land of contradictions, the veri-table land where "things are not what they seem."

Nothing is what it is commonly called. The wild rose is not a rose; bears are not bears; oaks are not oaks, and with one exception even moun-tains are not mountains geologically speaking. Instead of so-called moun-tains being elevated above the sea by gigantic earth-convulsions, their ranges are remnants of a great plateau in which have been eroded enor-mous canyons, cutting their way down to sea level.

Riding through the dense primeval forests which clothe these rugged ranges, one is shown ash, pine, beech, birch, mountain laurel, and many other familiar species; but when one comments on their strangeness, the reply is, "Oh, they are all forms of Eucalyptus,—we have fifteen hundred varieties and they resemble almost every other tree." Next to the Eucalyptus in number come the Banksias or bottle brush trees, and the Acacias, which likewise are bewildering in their diversity and resemblances.

The only large animal is the kangaroo, of which there are many species. Evidently it sets the style for all the other mammals, for one and all are marsupials and carry their young around in their apron pockets. Mice and rats, foxes, opossums, bears—none are true to their nicknames, for all are of the apron-pocket type, a very primitive type, indicative of what the animals of other parts of the world may have been some millions of years ago.

So one's bewilderment grows until one calmly accepts "oaks" with needles, "pines" with large leaves, and all other contradictions that fancy can picture. The wild flowers are beautiful beyond description, but utterly distinct from any other flora.

The Congress was divided between the two capitals of Victoria and New South Wales. Melbourne in the extreme south had the first half, so we were immediately transported thither. Going south in that other half of the world means going farther from equatorial warmth to more and more antarctic cold. We arrived at Melbourne, the Paris of the southern world, in a driving storm as it was midwinter there.

One great discomfort which our genial hosts could not remove was the different gauged railroads. No two adjoining States use the same width of track so it is impossible to run "through" sleeping cars. The trip from Sydney in New South Wales to Melbourne in Victoria is about like going from San Francisco to Los Angeles, an all night trip. But alas, about midway all passengers have to disembark from a broad gauge train and transfer to a narrow gauge; not a very comfortable experience at midnight in a frigid, driving storm. The warmth of the reception for the delegates made up in large measure but did not prevent severe colds.

The Congress was extremely interesting, representing all nationalities bordering on the Pacific, even including the "mother country," England.

In fact the English delegates especially contributed to our pleasure, then and since. Outstanding papers and discussions by outstanding men from all around the Pacific Ocean made the Congress an outstanding event in our lives. But the sudden plunge into midwinter storms took hard toll on several delegates, two of whom were from the University of California. Mr. Ritter contracted a severe cold ere reaching Melbourne but was able to fulfill his part in the program there.

The return trip to Sydney on another cold, rainy night with another midnight change of cars increased its severity. On the day of our return we attended the Lord Mayor's reception, followed by a luncheon and general opening exercises of the Sydney Conference, with the result that Mr. Ritter went to bed with a temperature of one hundred and two degrees. He was to make the response to the Governor General's address of welcome at the opening session next morning. About two in the morning he called me and I found him having a severe chill! Pneumonia was my first thought and through the rest of that night I relived the La Jolla experiences with that fell disease.

Fortunately Dr. Vaughan was in the same hotel. I called him early and asked him to get the best physician in Sydney and to arrange for a substitute for Mr. Ritter at the Conference. In getting Dr. Smith, a brother of the famous London archeologist, Elliot Smith, I am sure we had the best doctor in Sydney. The illness proved to be not the dread pneumonia but a severe bronchial influenza from which he recovered sufficiently in a few days to carry out his part of the conference program.

At the conclusion of the three weeks session most of the delegates sailed for home, but Mr. Ritter accepted an invitation from the Government of Queensland to make a tour of investigation, with a few others, along the two thousand miles of coral reefs known as the Great Barrier Reef. They were guests of the Governor of that northern State of Queensland, Sir Matthew Nathan, who accompanied them on the voyage of exploration. As only small vessels can negotiate that dangerous conglomeration of sunken reefs, a "tug" was used for the three weeks' trip. There being no sleeping accommodations except the skipper's cabin, which was given to the Governor, rolls of blankets were provided the guests, most of whom slept on deck, but Mr. Ritter and two knighted

Englishmen monopolized the benches in the small mess room. The exploration of this unique portion of the oceanic-world was a never-to-be-forgotten opportunity.

Meantime I too was having wonderful experiences in sightseeing and hospitality. Thanks to some influential women I was permitted to live at the Queen's Club, an exclusive women's club of Sydney. The days were for the most part kept busy by my new-made friends. Even so, seeing all of our American friends off for home left a hollow feeling, and three catastrophic occurrences had filled the air with gloom. The first was the terrible earthquake in Japan with the devastating fires in Yokohama and Tokyo. The distress of the large delegation of Japanese over the probable loss of families and friends cast a gloom over the entire Congress. The leading seismologist not only of Japan, but of the world, died from the effects of this strain added to an attack of the prevailing influenza and his advanced age.

A few days later, Sir Walter Davidson, the Governor General was stricken and died suddenly. Less than three weeks from the time Mr. Ritter was to have replied to his address of welcome, the whole country was draped in mourning for their leading statesman.

While the Governor's body lay in state, and I was acutely feeling my aloneness, half-way round the world from home, with my husband two thousand miles away in a small boat exploring very dangerous reefs, one of the most famous graveyards of ocean-going traffic, my eye espied a two-line cablegram in the *Sydney Morning Herald*. It ran: "Berkeley, seat of the University of California, destroyed by fire. Three hundred students killed." Can you imagine my distress and the many questions that filled my mind? Was all of Berkeley destroyed, including the University? Were my young grandnephews who had been with us so often in La Jolla among those killed? Was this and that friend homeless? No further information could be obtained. A code cablegram had brought this item. When I inquired about cabling to Berkeley I learned why the news was so brief. Cables to and from the Antipodes are prohibitive in expense. No letters could reach us before sailing. Mr. Ritter was beyond any communication with the outside world. There was nothing to do but wait, wait. How keenly I sympathized with the poor Japanese, and recalled our other waiting experience in Japan at the time of the San Francisco earthquake and fire! Six long weeks I had to wait until I found some San Francisco newspapers in Samoa. And these had been brought there by the Captain of a lumber schooner who left San Francisco two days after the Berkeley fire. Every newspaper is treasured in the Antipodes and passed around from hand to hand for news of the outside world. Thus these had been given to the steamship agent in Samoa. I had been searching for papers at every possible port, and so traced these down finally, to my great relief.

The interesting excursions in Australia I cannot relate, though they were many. The wintry July and August had passed through the budding September spring, and then into the beauty of full-fledged spring in October, when we left a dock from which many new-made friends waved us adieu, as we sailed out of the wonderful Sydney Harbor, with our arms and our stateroom filled with flowers with familiar names but strange faces.

Out of that peaceful harbor we again plunged into the stormy Tasman Sea, to another new but totally different land—New Zealand.

Here our stay was all too short, but full of weird interest, for we hied us away to those mountainous regions where "the world is in the making." The famous Rotorua and Wahrakie geyser-lands are bordered by volcanoes which in recent years, in one titanic explosion, blew up a whole mountain and changed the contour of the earth for many miles. Old lakes were sunk, new lakes formed. We rowed across one small lake that was boiling on one side and cold on the other, so that fish could be caught in one part of the lake and cooked in another, almost with one swing of the fishline.

Walking over this bubbling, splashing earth, where one never knows what may be underneath one's feet, and where geysers may break forth any moment, gives one a genuine thrill; yet the tattooed Maoris live complacently in these steaming lands, use the steam to heat their houses, and cook in the potholes nearest their domicile. If one pothole blows up, they calmly choose another. Yet fatalities occur frequently enough to add zest to the picture.

The steam from the boiling cauldrons is often so dense that one must watch his steps most carefully, as a misstep would mean fatal scalding.

And every few minutes there are eruptions from one or another of the larger cauldrons.

New Zealand is a land of varied scenery, agricultural in the north, Alpine mountains in the south. I was surprised to find that three-fourths of it lies in the Antarctic Ocean. It is totally distinct from Australia in its fauna, flora and geological construction. Apparently in the unknown past there has been a land connection with South America, possibly through the Antarctic continent.

Leaving New Zealand, we set sail for the South Sea Islands in the tropics.

CHAPTER 19

The South Sea Isles

OUR FIRST STOP ON THE HOMEWARD TRIP WAS AT THE PORT OF SUVA, capital of the Fiji Islands. Of all the groups of islands in Oceanica, this is to me the most beautiful. Its mountains are jagged and colorful, and it is all mountain peaks with tortuous inlets of the sea between the rugged isles.

Here we disembarked from our trans-Pacific liner as I was determined to visit several groups of the South Sea Islands while we were in their midst. Mr. Ritter felt he could not spend the time for a leisurely cruise of two weeks, so we established ourselves at the Grand Pacific Hotel where he could devote himself to his writing. I had arranged to meet a French woman, a fellow-traveler on the *Tahiti*, at this hotel, for the inter-island trip.

As an illustration of the smallness of the world, we had scarcely entered the hotel lobby when we met a friend, Dr. Casey Wood, a noted oculist, formerly of Chicago. Dr. Wood had long been making a comparative study of bird's eyes with their highly-developed, far-sighted retinal cells. This study he was then pursuing among tropical birds.

Two days later my traveling companion, Mrs. de Nivernais and I were aboard the *Tofua*, the relatively small inter-island steamer. I felt a sinking of the heart when I saw one hundred and fifty black Fijians with their scant attire and the frowzled huge kinky pompadours just as pictured in my childhood geographies file into the hold of our vessel. I thought of them as I had seen them pictured, as cannibals, but later learned that they were preferred as longshoremen, because they were more dependable and more energetic than the brown-skinned Polynesians.

The first group visited was the Tongan Islands. Captain Cook named the Tongan group the Friendly Islands, because the natives treated him well. But they were a warlike people, making constant raids upon the neighboring island tribes. Especially menacing were they to the Fijians, many of whose islands they conquered before both groups were taken under English protectorate. The Tongans are a proud and haughty race, considering themselves not only superior to their Polynesian and Melanesian neighbors, but looking with contempt on the colorless whites as well. They had a native queen, twenty-two years of age, who lived in a large wooden house which seemed like a palace in contrast to the native thatched cottages. She was quite Europeanized, but if calls were made by the English officials during siesta hours, she had been known to grant them audience in Mother Hubbard gown and bare feet.

The Tongans have worked out a fairly efficient form of government, but one we could not very well copy. For instance, over the jail door is a sign which reads: "Any prisoner who does not return before six o'clock will be locked out." It works. The prisoners who are allowed leave on various pretexts, scurry to get back to evening meal and shelter before the prescribed hour.

We visited several of the flat Tongan Islands, all formed by elevated coral reefs. Such elevations are still occurring. Stops were also made at other small groups, as the *Tofua* is their only means of getting mail and supplies.

While the *Tofua* seemed small as compared with the great ocean liners, she seemed alarmingly huge when we were winding between the hundreds of coral reef islands, especially through one tortuous channel so narrow and crooked that the boat could scarcely pass through. The jagged reefs could almost be touched on either side. But our young captain had been familiar with those channels all his life.

Samoa, the land of Stevenson, came next. His residence is now the home of the English governor, having been rebuilt by the Germans before war times.

Have any of you essayed the climb to Stevenson's tomb? If so, imagine attempting that precipitous ascent through the dense tropical jungle just after a heavy rain, when the clayey soil was wet and slippery. Suffice it to say, we slipped and skidded until I abandoned the attempt and sat down in despair. Long may he lie in his hallowed grave on the hill-top! He will never be disturbed by me.

The Samoans appear to be a high type of Polynesians, but even so they adhere to a primitive mode of life which we would find impossible. Their houses are communal, with several families under one roof. And it is only a roof, a thatched roof supported on slender poles; no side walls, no partitions. The only pretense at partitions is about a six-inch board laid lengthwise on edge on the rubble floor. The floor is made of cobble-stones varying in size from that of an egg to an orange. For beds, a straw mat is laid down on the cobble-stone floor. In the house we visited, four families lived under the same roof, divided into four sections by the six-inch boards, their main purpose to limit the excursions of the creeping babies.

We visited one boys' school considered of high rank, the teacher of which was a native but a Harvard graduate. The building was of the same wall-less type, though larger than the houses, that is, the roof was larger. As our guide led us in we found only the teacher and one pupil, both ill with malaria. The college-bred man lay on the cobble floor with only a straw mat between his aching bones and the orange-sized stones, and a make-shift pillow, too ill even to talk. Those woven straw mats, very beautiful in design but very thin, are slight protection from the round stones on which we found it difficult to walk.

Tattooing is a favorite method of body decoration and before the days of the white man was the only dress except a clout. It is still practiced, though against the white man's law. Our driver and guide, who had been schooled in America, was tattooed over almost his entire body, the patterns being most elaborate. As he was little more than a youth, this adornment, desired even at the price of torture, must have been recently acquired.

Circling round among these tropic isles, we crossed that exasperating 180th meridian four times, and dropped days and picked them up again in a bewildering manner. One week would have two Wednesdays; the next one no Saturday; until it was impossible to keep one's dates by any calendar. Likewise the seasons. Here we were basking in a late November Spring which gave us foretastes of what a tropic December Summer had in store. In these southern climes Christmas is apt to be the hottest day of the year. One could be comfortable only in a minimum of clothing, while depending on the constant trade winds for the breath of life.

We returned southward to the two hundred and fifty emeralds dotting the South Pacific, the peerless Fijian Islands. And here most unexpectedly we found the gem of all our experiences in the southern world. For the story of our month in the Fijis, I append descriptive letters written while on the ground.

Suva, Fiji, November 11, 1923.

Dearest Family:

Next Sunday morning we will be "on the rolling deep" again, and will have left this most idyllic spot. I was never more loath to leave any place! It is almost perfect.

The only "fly in the ointment" is the measley little mosquito which poisons me, giving Mr. Ritter hope that I will be willing to leave here; but mosquitos and all, how I should love to stay here quietly for another month, to drink in the beauty, and rest. The view from our windows defies description. The climate is perfect, neither hot nor cold, but warm and balmy both night and day. This hotel is a joy, with its sixteen-foot veranda extending all around two "storeys." It is built for the climate, the cool trade winds or balmy breezes blowing through the house constantly.

Being in the tropics, everybody sleeps with open doors. We do not close them even when we go out, though the servants are the so-called light-fingered Hindoos. I am growing fond of these good-looking, brown-faced, barefooted, white-robed and turbaned men. As always with that nation, each man will do but one thing. It takes three to "do up" the bedroom, three more for table service, two for office, two to escort one to a taxi, and all of them to carry in or out one's luggage.

For the bedroom work, the chief upstairs man makes the bed in the morning and opens it and spreads your mosquito net at night. He wears a "sash" to his turban, to distinguish his rank. Next comes a light brown smile with a small man attached, to brush the floor, not sweep it. Down on his knees he goes to brush the rug or fibre mat with a hand brush the size and shape of a large clothes brush. Then he wipes up the concrete floor and the smile vanishes to the next room. Then comes a wavy-haired black man to empty the washbowl and slop-jar. (Are there such things as faucets and stationary bowls in bedrooms?) This man comes three times a day—in the morning, again before time to dress for dinner, and before bed time.

At table we have our regular waiter beside the water-boy who purveys all fluids, for which one has to pay, even for water. There is also the chief steward in his green turban with two sashes, who takes orders and repeats them to subordinates; and at your last few meals, fully half a dozen wait upon you obsequiously. You may imagine this retinue keeps one tipping until one feels tipsy, but they are so smiling and good-natured that one cannot resist. Tips in this country are not small, by the way.

This is the fifth Armistice Day, and in ten minutes we start by taxi for the Government Buildings to see the Colonial observance of the day; then to the Fijian church to hear the wonderful singing in a language so musical that it is almost like listening to a chant. We heard a most remarkable choir last Sunday at Bau, and thereby hangs a tale of the crowning experience of all this varied trip.

To begin with, Bau is the ancient Fijian capital situated on a tiny island just large enough to hold a little straggling village, crowned by a hill used as the chiefs' cemetery, and the missionaries' home.

The titular King of the Fijis, Tui Viti, still lives there, and likewise a resident member of each tribe subject to him. It was here that the Fiji Islands were ceded to England nearly fifty years ago, with the understanding that their tribal relations and tribal government should not be interfered with, and that the Colonial Parliament should consist of both races, a contract that is being carried out in good faith by both parties, as far as practicable.

It so happened that this month the English Governor and his staff were making a last round of the various districts, before his departure at the close of his four years' tenure of office. The culmination was to be a Council of Chiefs at Bau, lasting a full week. This affair was to be the most conspicuous conclave that had occurred there in forty-four years, and the great ceremonials were to take place on Saturday, November the third. Naturally we Americans wanted to go, but it seemed impossible until the day before, when we succeeded in chartering a large launch for the two days' trip. Boats of considerable size can only make the trip at high tide, owing to the miles upon miles of coral reefs and sand bars, so we had to stay over night and sleep (?) on the wooden seats of the launch. But the sights were worth almost any sacrifice of physical comfort. One can recover from and forget fatigue, but one never forgets such ceremonies as we witnessed—the held-over barbaric ceremonials of ancient Fiji. The old feature of cannibalism was left out, but scores of entire hogs roasted to a crisp in the old cannibal ovens, were there as substitutes.

About twenty tribal high chiefs, with between two and three thousand of their subjects, were present. As a present to the Governor each district is ordered to bring so much of such and such foods amounting to tons and tons of cocoanuts, yams, bananas, pineapples, taro, and puddings made of pineapple, cocoanut, taro and sugarcane tied up in banana leaves. There were also about thirty huge turtles and the above-mentioned roast hogs, some of which were prize boars weighing three hundred pounds or more, imported for the occasion from New Zealand. The chief of the fishermen, with scores of his underlings, brought several tons of fish strung on poles, each pole laden to the capacity of two men to carry on their shoulders. All this and unlimited quantities of yangona roots and stems to make the native liquor, kava. After being presented with an elaborate ceremony of kava-making, and drinking by all out of the same cocoanut-shell cup, this food is then distributed by the Governor to the tribes, and after the day is over they hold one glorious feast or "gorge." The pile of food presented was twenty-five feet high and about seventy-five feet long by six or eight feet thick, held in place by a bamboo frame or fence built up higher and higher as the food accumulated.

In the afternoon three tribes gave their war-dances, each vying with the other in the intricacy and ferocity of their dancing, and attacks with war clubs, as well as in the brilliancy and number of decorations on their war costumes. The costumes were composed of garlands of flowers around the neck, shoulders, wrists and ankles, and a skirt made of flowers and grasses, under which was a clout or sulu, their only garment.

The skirt consisted of a wide wreath of flowers or colored grasses, or tapa sashes around the loins, with strands of the same forming a skirt to the knees. The gorgeousness of color beggars description. The inner bark of certain trees had been dried and split into ribbons as thin as tissue ribbon, brilliantly dyed, and varying from a half inch to three or four inches wide. Most of these were then crinkled or "fluted" by hand, until they stood out like the finest ballet costume, and rattled delightfully. Some had lovely skirts of a fresh green marsh-grass, one-eighth of an inch wide and two feet long. Others had skirts of pendulous twigs of flowering shrubs. The costumes were beautiful over their bronze skin oiled and polished till it shone like satin.

One tribe adorned their huge mops of frizzled hair with wreaths, and another with huge colored rosettes or bows and curious ornaments fastened somehow to the very top of the upstanding pompadour, from three to five or six inches high before adornment. Others had bull's horns on their foreheads; others the sacred whale's teeth, (their diamonds and pearls) around their necks; or large breast-pieces of mother-of-pearl.

To make themselves look ferocious in these fascinating decorations, their faces were painted in all sorts of designs, with red and black paint. One had a broad red band down the middle of his face, another a black band. Similar bands stretched across the eyes, like a domino; one had his face half red, half black; others had all sorts of curious splotches of paint. It was said each design had some significance. It did make them look weird and ferocious—oh my!

It was altogether the most gorgeous spectacle of its kind any of us had ever witnessed. The rhythm and beauty of their concerted movements were wonderful. They were arranged in solid squares with two hundred or more men in each, moving like one giant body. No Queen's Guard was ever better trained.

Each group had its human band sitting on the ground singing the war songs and beating time with hands or feet or hollow bamboo rods which produced musical tones. Everything was in perfect rhythm. Tiny children, not in the band, beat time correctly with sticks or anything they could get. They are a musical people through and through. And such voices! The bassos are like great organ tones, so powerful yet so melodious. The tenors, sopranos and altos are likewise exquisite. Even little children sing in parts, like our negroes. Harmony is a part of their nature.

At church the next morning we heard a choir that was simply wonderful! They have no instrumental accompaniment but the organ tones are all there. Any artificial accompaniment would be entirely superfluous.

Later:

We have just returned from the Armistice Day services, beginning and ending with a drill and parade of the native constabulary and band. Five hundred people were in the church, and not a shoe or hat except on the few Americans and white officers on the platform with the minister, but the bronze legs and feet are charming. The soldier's uniform is attractive and fitting for the climate, consisting of a khaki shirt waist with plenty of brass buttons. The officers have their waists piped with red. Then a sulu of white cloth, the bottom edge of which is in deep Van Dyke points. These points reach to the knee. The sulu is a piece of cloth three-quarters of a yard wide and two yards long, wound round the hips as tightly as possible, making a one-legged trouser. The end of the sulu is tucked in the belt on the left side, leaving ample room for freedom of movement in walking, as the two ends overlap in front. A leather belt completes and stabilizes the uniform.

White is the usual color for men. The highest chiefs wear the same nether garment, the sulu, but only soldiers and police may have the lower edge pointed. Some chiefs and dudes dress like white men from the waist up, wearing shirts, collars, neckties and tailored or custom-made coats, but are bare from the knees down. Some even have the sulu of the same goods as the coat, but this is the height of swelldom or foppery. Even the king himself wears no hat or shoes. The chiefs are very handsome in physique, and some in face.

Tuesday morning, November 13, 1923.

9:15 a.m.

Sunday afternoon we went for our last long drive, winding along the shore and in and out of the mountain gorges. The roadway is dotted with thatched villages—Hindoo and native. There are about sixty-five thousand Hindoos here (introduced long ago by the English for labor in the sugar and cotton plantations) to eighty-five thousand natives—about three to four, or more than that about Suva where the Indians cluster, while the pure-blood Fijians remain in their mountain and coastal villages. The Fijians do not take kindly to city life: those living here are not true Fijians.

It is complained that the early white planters imported Hindoo laborers accustomed to agricultural pursuits, because the Fijians will not till the soil. This is not sheer laziness as they will work about boats, and they are great fishermen. They will also work in large numbers for village needs, being intensely communal and having a prejudice against working alone. We took ninety Fijians on our boat to handle the cargo at the Polynesian ports because the Tongans and Samoans cannot be relied upon to do that kind of work.

When one looks at the problem from the Fijian standpoint, why should they do the white man's hard work to get something they neither need nor care for? They do not value money as such, and exchange it at once for something they do care for. Whales' teeth or tambria are infinitely preferred to gold or silver. Nature supplies all their needs; they wear only such clothes as the whites force upon them. Tapa and other vegetable fibres supply all the covering they need for decency or warmth, and the whites have not yet induced them to contract bills for either shoes or hats. As for shelter, the forests provide the thatch, poles, and rope (braided fibres of a vine or cocoanut palm) that they use for binding and decoration. The construction of their walls, being woven in diverse patterns, is artistic and decorative. The ridge poles are decorated in lovely designs of these colored vegetable fibres, very beautiful in their finer houses and temples. Not a nail is used in construction.

They do not need to work for food. In the lower ranges of mountains through which we passed on our Sunday drive, within seven miles of Suva were forests of breadfruit, mangoes, bananas, papaias, fern-trees (used as a vegetable) with taro, yams, sugar-cane, wild pineapples, and yangona growing beneath. True, they have times of stringency, but so do the cultivated areas all over the world. What is more common than failure of crops? In this country droughts are almost unknown and the shortage of food is usually due to the effect of hurricanes on the fruit crops, but even so, there are many tubers and small plants they can resort to, and they have unlimited quantities of fish and turtles on the endless coral reefs, in streams and in deep water. These foods, most of them luxuries to us, furnish them all the necessities of life. But they like meat, and these islands produce no animals suitable for food. Fortunately the white man has introduced the hog and poultry which fill this need. But alas, before this occurred and for some time afterward, the upright biped was their chief source of animal food.

Cannibalism was rife everywhere among these meatless south-sea islands, but the Fijians, Papuans, and Marquesans were the most voracious, but ably seconded by the Australian Bushmen and the New Zealand Maoris (the last, Polynesians). The Fijians and Bushmen are blacks or Melanesians.

Until fifty years ago the roasting oven for human flesh was seldom cold in Bau, where we were last week. All prisoners of war were eaten after they were fattened, and as tribal wars were incessant, the supply seldom ran out. If it did, the chiefs proscribed that certain families should be set apart to supply a victim as occasion required. Horrible? Yes, but a custom that has existed for thousands of years in various part of the world. Cruel? Yes, unspeakably, but equaled many times in European history.

Look the world over and you will scarcely find a finer-looking group of men than those twenty chiefs assembled in Bau last week; splendid physiques and many handsome physiognomies. Chiefs are inbred and "to the manner born." They must excel not only in physique and personality, but in athletic prowess. They must be able not only to outrun their subjects, to throw the spear farther and wield the war-club better, but they must also be better fishermen, house-builders, tree-fellers and so on. They must truly be looked up to, in order to retain prestige. The present king of Bau is a handsome and very able man, and, I take it, would be a gentleman anywhere. He is a grandson of old King Thakombou, the greatest chief Fiji has produced. It is said that all families from which chiefs descend have an admixture of Tongan blood. It was to prevent being conquered by these warlike Tongans that King Thakombou finally made overtures to the English Government in 1860. The islands were not definitely accepted until 1874, fourteen years later.

In his legendary and historic greatness, King Thakombou is almost an "Arthur of the Round Table." A Swedish sailor ship-wrecked on this island years before had been protected by him because he possessed and used a gun. The guns, rescued from the wreck, reversed Fijian history, making Thakombou king instead of only a tribal chief.

King Thakombou was a terrible cannibal until he was converted by the missionaries, after which he issued an edict abolishing can-nibalism in all the tribes he had conquered. Yet around his resi-dence today is a palisade of upright stones, each stone representing a human victim eaten under his hospitable roof. Every little way a second stone uplifts its head like our fence posts, signifying an enemy chief who "has adorned the festal board." We stood on the stone on the temple (Bure) steps where the victims' heads were laid to be clubbed. Wicked whites dub it the "Nut-cracker." Atrocious slang, is it not? The upright stone used to brain little children who furnished the piece de resistance of a feast (a la suckling pigs) is now the baptismal font in the Wesleyan church, and today every house-hold in Bau has family prayers each morning.

We were told to be at the church early if we wished a seat. We followed the advice and were placed up in front. As the congrega-tion strolled in, every person knelt in prayer, huge chieftain, vir-ile youth, giggling girls, little children and their staid mothers; all except one foreign clad dude in the choir who did not want to soil his white trousers.

It is the change in one generation that amazes me so. Only one missionary, a Dr. Baker, was actually eaten, though many lost their lives. Dr. Baker was unnecessarily rash in his stubborn determination to "carry the Bible clear across Fiji." The shore-tribes begged him to turn back, but he would not; then he stupidly committed a terrible breach of etiquette and greatly insulted the cannibalistic chief who had entertained him over night. To be sure, the chief had offended his etiquette by sticking the missionary's comb in his own unsanitary hair, at which the missionary snatched it out, thereby defiling the sacred head of the chief, for which he lost his own. At Bau I saw an inoffensive-looking old man who as a boy had partaken of the feast supplied by the missionary. At another village we saw a fine stone church, the Baker Memorial, which had been erected to the memory of the martyred missionary by the children and grandchildren of those who had eaten him—surely a remarkable transformation in one generation.

Although dangerous cannibals in the past, the Fijians were never murderers or thieves as we use the terms. With their extreme communal system, where everything belonged to everybody for the asking, burglary was unnecessary. In forty years from 1870 to 1910 as Resident Magistrate among the more remote hill tribes, A. L. Brewster, an English official, tried only one case of murder. In a suicide pact, the girl had succeeded in killing herself while the man had not. He was convicted and sentenced to be hanged. The sentence was remitted to ten years in prison. After his release he was elevated by his tribe to the highest honor in their power to bestow, because "after such long residence abroad he would be the man best fitted to deal with and understand the customs of the white man."

Since abolishing cannibalism, they are singularly free from vice, in fact their record places them almost if not quite at the head of all law-abiding people.

Their family life before the days of the missionaries was peculiar. All were polygamous, having three or four wives. The men did not sleep at home, but in public houses, going home in the morning to breakfast and for the day. This was partly that they might be ready for possible attack by other tribes. All family relations were absolutely private, in the woods or in remote cottages. After a child was born, the mother was set aside religiously for four or five years, it being considered indecent for a woman to bear a child oftener than once in that length of time. If she did, her relations raised an insurrection, beating the husband severely and jumping on him until he was sometimes seriously injured. The civilized monogamous marriage has increased the number of sex offenses as well as increasing the hardship of woman kind among the Fijians. Any married man who strays from the straight and narrow path is sent to jail.

Of all the criminals and insane or dependents of any sort in the Fiji Islands, ninety-five per cent are Hindoos and whites. The five per cent of Fijians who go to jail are sent either for sex offenses or minor infractions of English law such as failing to pay taxes, especially a dog tax, or some other trivial ordinance they do not understand. In one inland district of six thousand natives, there were not enough men sent to prison to keep the grounds clean. They are remarkably peaceable and do not quarrel among themselves.

The Hindoo population has adopted the Fijian thatched house, making it impossible to tell a Fijian from a Hindoo village except by the people themselves. The men are clothed similarly to Fijian men. The women and little girls wear long, much beruffled skirts, fully seven yards round, the girls' dresses relatively as long as their mothers', with tight-fitting waists. Their heads are covered with veils wound round their necks and reaching at least to their knees. And oh, such colors! The brilliant yellows and orange seem the favorites, but pinks, blues and terra cottas follow closely. And then, such adornment! Everyone has a filigree gold breast-pin in the left side of her nose, and if the family can afford it, a large gold ring through the septum of the nose, reaching down over the mouth, often with filigree pendants falling below the chin. Then to paraphrase Mother Hubbard, they have "rings on their fingers and rings on their toes; rings on their ankles, wrists, neck and nose." The more silver or glass bracelets and anklets and necklaces, the better, and if the purse will permit, each toe has as many silver rings as it can carry.

Thursday, November 15, 1923.

The second to the last day in Fiji is waning, but it is a day to be remembered. This forenoon at high tide, we took a launch and went over a small part of the coral reef which extends almost around the Islands. It goes without saying that coral reefs are beautiful. Color does so love tropical climes! Even the fish in the reefs are brilliantly colored. The corals build only as high as low water, so are covered most of the time. The entrance to this reef, like nearly all we have seen, has the tip of a wrecked vessel protruding sufficiently to add danger as well as give a significant warning. Corals cannot live in fresh or even brackish water, and as most of the islands have streams, the partly freshened water opposite the mouth of the stream prevents the coral growing there, allowing a narrow passage through which vessels can enter.

After leaving the reef this morning, our boatman took us through lagoons to the mountains that we so dearly love. He approached nearer and nearer the precipitous cliff until once we stuck on the reef and broke the propeller. We could see no break in the rugged hillsides, but he turned a point, and lo! we were in a little river with the mountains on both sides, and these indescribable jungles covering their steep slopes. Naturally nearly all the trees and plants are strange to us except such things as we cultivate, such as hibiscus, bougainvilla, oleanders and so forth. But even the huge forest trees blossom. Many have brilliant red blossoms; others have pink, terra cotta, yellow, blue, white—blossoms of all colors, and such fragrance! The frangi pangi tree is everywhere and its bloom is most odorous. Stephanotis and other familiar perfumes bear their waxy blossoms in these jungles. Then there are orchids on the ground and growing as parasites on the trees. I wish I could take home the lavender orchids we picked last Sunday on our drive, which are still fresh and blooming anew. Tree-ferns and the tall cocoanut palms wave their graceful fronds everywhere, and banyan trees are omnipresent. I am wondering how Honolulu will stand the contrast. Honolulu is very lovely but less primitive, and the natives here are far more dominant and natural. The only thing I leave without a pang is the pesky, poisonous mosquito.

But it would be sad indeed to find an unalloyed paradise and have to leave it.

Through the tropics again, recrossing the equator to the Hawaiian Islands which are about as far north of the equatorial line as the Fiji Islands are south of it.

Honolulu, with its mountainous background and beautiful shore line, stood the comparison with its southern rival well, but it is a cosmopolitan city.

Our stay was brief but our friends were all the more active in their hospitality on this our third visit to the charming place.

Another week and we were homeward bound—weary and worn. As if to welcome us, other vessels passed us for the first time, in this last lap of the more than sixteen thousand mile voyage. But this is a much traveled path across the ocean deeps while all the rest of the journey had been off the beaten track.

CHAPTER 20

Retirement

HOME AGAIN IN DECEMBER AFTER AN INCONGRUOUS YEAR OF TWO winters and two springs, and only half a summer—winter and spring in La Jolla, and a bit of summer in Berkeley; winter and spring in the southern half of the world, reaching San Francisco in December, to jump from tropical heat into a California winter.

I said "home again" but we had no definite home save that California is always the homeland. What awaited us? A series of interrogation points as far as I could see. We had reached that fabled happy position of retirement, where one has no compulsory duties.

Retirement from active life while one is still able to continue his activities leaves a gap that tells heavily on both the physical and mental well-being. For that reason, when Mr. Ritter retired from the directorship of the Scripps Institution, it was a matter of choice and was only to undertake two or three other jobs quite as time-consuming. But for myself, when I had to retire from my active work in San Diego, I felt that the time I had always dreaded had come—a serious climacteric in my mature life-history. I realized that the necessarily unsettled residence of the next few years would not give time for me to strike root deeply enough to become a working force in any community.

My sympathy goes out sincerely to anyone compelled to retire from any congenial active work because of the force of circumstances.

Mr. Ritter, fortunate man, had before him an amount of writing laid out that has from that time to this kept him wondering how he would ever accomplish it. This served as a *vis a tergo* for him, and to a certain extent to me, inasmuch as I always worked his manuscripts over again and again for the elision of errors. He had also the building up of two new institutions as incentives for the future. Science Service was a year old but was calling to him for advice all the time. The new foundation of World Population and Food Supply, waiting to be founded, was also calling him. Both of these pressing interests made it seem imperative for him to be in Washington. Should we go there at once?

In opposition to this call from the East was the necessity of his remaining near his own library and vast collection of notes for a book (later divided into three) which he was writing. He also desired the assistance of a co-worker, Dr. Edna Watson Bailey, now a university professor in the department of education. Her biological teaching had been applied to human beings and she had become an authority on health education.

So our lot was cast in Berkeley for the year 1924. Before settling down we went to Fresno for a family reunion at Christmas-tide. After New Year's I proceeded to San Diego to arrange for the final removal of our household "lares" to Berkeley. During this siege I resolved that our household goods should no longer be my household gods. I determined to dispel the "tyranny of things." Hereafter, things necessary to comfort must serve as a means to that end, not as something for which I must be a slave in caring for them. This beneficent philosophy was engendered during the rearranging and shipping of a carload of furniture from storage in San Diego to storage in Berkeley, when it was evident that for the next few years, if ever, there would be no settled home in which these goods and gods could tyrannize over me.

In San Diego, amid the confusion and assortment of that medley of unmarked boxes and barrels and crates of furniture, I renewed the old associations with my co-workers in San Diego and La Jolla. It was a happy two weeks, with committee meetings and club functions in which I was an honored guest. My headquarters were with my beloved friend, Miss Scripps, and all the friendly overtures revived both the happiness of the past and the sadness of a final parting. We were tearing up the last roots of our eighteen years in our southern home. Mr. Ritter joined me later and we started back to Berkeley in our faithful Dodge laden to the limit with some of those "lares."

In Berkeley we were domiciled at the Whitecotton Hotel for that year. Hotel life has the advantage of readiness at all times for extra guests at table, and of these my diary recounts an endless number, with an equally endless number of entries of dining out with the Strattons, the Kofoids, the Riebers, the Freemans, the Nobles, the Baileys, and many other friends. These added an overtone of pleasure to cover the deep undertone of the unhappiest period of my life.

I had lost my life work. There were no definite duties awaiting me each day; no civic responsibilities for which I must muster all my energies. There were not even household cares which I must oversee. So I felt a sense of groping, of a lost personality, or however that dire complex resulting from retirement may be defined. Whatever it may be called, it induced a restless, unhappy state of mind that lasted several years, until I found myself anew and assumed a more quiescent and acquiescent personality.

It was not that I was not busy. How I kept going at the rate my diary connotes, I do not know. But the busy-ness was not soul- nor self-satisfying.

To begin with, as soon as the carload of furniture arrived, there was a siege of unpacking to find the things we needed, repacking, selling off the excess from a large house, giving away much that I could not sell, segregating all of the books and cases of notes that Mr. Ritter needed in his study in the University Library building, kindly assigned for his use; also all of the things we could use to make a hotel suite homelike, or would need in Washington. The remainder was stored for four years. It was during this final siege that I completely renounced the tyranny of things.

This transitory job completed, and even while it was going on, I devoted some hours each day in correcting the penciled grist from the mill of my husband's brain. In editing these manuscripts Dr. Bailey afterward said she had the "hardest task of her life," for out of the vast amount she finally segregated three books instead of one. The omniverous scholar had not been content to leave out anything pertaining to his main theme, so someone else had to classify and sift out the subsidiary from the main topics. Three years more of work resulted in a volume, *Natural History of Our Conduct*. This title sounds very simple, but viewed in its entirety would include all animal activities, even the over-productivity of the writer. Is not the tendency to over-produce among human beings the same as that of ants and wood-peckers and all the other animals he had studied regarding their so-called intelligence? In the quarter of a century during which I have worked with Mr. Ritter on his manuscripts, I have learned full well that books do not just grow. While the list of his published books seems a goodly output, the number of articles in scientific journals would equal it, and a third portion fully as large if not larger, is still in manuscript. Mr. Ritter often humorously alludes to his "five-foot shelf" of unprinted books.

By this time I had resumed club affiliations old and new. In addition to the Charter Club in Berkeley, the Town and Gown, I was deeply interested in a new organization, the League of Women Voters, which the advance of women had created. This organization kindly put me to work as Vice President, a real kindness which helped to assuage that lost feeling due to laying down my former activities.

Unfortunately ill health was telling on me more and more. During these tiresome months of mental and physical distress, one of my college girl patients became my good angel and faithful physician, Dr. May H. Sampson. Much of the year I spent in bed. But that rarely means idleness to me. Unless too ill to use my brains, my mind and hands find something to do, and correcting or writing manuscript is to me a bed habit.

Travel too had its share of this retired year. Twice Mr. Ritter was called East for scientific congresses. The plans which he and Mr. Scripps were formulating for the developing activities also made inroads on his time.

After the Caribbean trip Mr. Scripps set off in his yacht for the Orient and was away many months. In March Mr. Ritter received a message stating that the *Ohio* was in San Diego harbor and asking him to join Mr. Scripps to talk things over.

In April Mr. Ritter went East for the annual meeting of Science Service and other business. I took advantage of his four weeks' absence to go to Pasadena to the sanitarium of my good friend, Dr. Josephine Jackson, for dietary treatment and general inspiration such as she can give in a unique manner. My return to Berkeley was timed to meet Mr. Ritter's train. Unfortunately he arrived with a cold which I promptly acquired, and was down again with my arch enemy, "Flu." Later this resulted in a happy convalescence with my niece, Ruth Cody, in Palo Alto, while Mr. Ritter was attending a Scientific Congress at Stanford.

The happiness of this year was largely contributed by my family and the association with the old-time friends. My poor paralyzed sister was established in Alameda with her nurse and a housekeeper. Bi-weekly visits were paid to her when I was able. Her son, Bert Warner, and her daughter, Edna Cockrill, made frequent trips from Fresno to see her. Both had children in college, so there was a double lode-stone. These several opportunities to be with my loved ones were sources of deep joy and satisfaction.

Commencement week was a time for the gathering of the clan. Elizabeth, Bert's daughter, completed her college course, and to add a note of excitement, there was a suitor in the offing. My diary brings to mind a dinner party for Elizabeth and Floyd Hammond, who later became another nephew.

In July another message from Mr. Scripps announced the arrival of the *Ohio* in New York harbor. He requested Mr. Ritter to come on for further arrangements about his new endowments, joining him and Mrs. Scripps on a cruise to the Marine Biological Stations of Woods Hole and Bermuda.

This being the only means of discussions with Mr. Scripps of his plans for the development of the "Ritter ideas," the request was complied with. Out of this conference came the decision that Mr. Ritter should go to Washington for an indefinite period. This month of Mr. Ritter's absence I spent in the summer home of my niece, Edna Cockrill, located on Huntington Lake in the high Sierras. I had always looked to the hills as the source of strength, and this fine mountain air renewed my strength of mind, body, and soul. The visit with the two generations of nieces and nephews was also exhilarating, as Edna's two sons, Warner and Robert, and Frank's orphaned daughter, Jane, were there. During this visit the problem of Warner's continuing at college was discussed and settled, and Robert and Jane became real entities to me instead of almost unknown children. This stimulus to my affection for them resulted in their introduction to the joys and sorrows of travel.

At the time of the "Big Game," the Cockrill family came to Berkeley to see the game and to visit with Warner and Edna's mother. While driving over to see my sister, I said to Robert, "You will graduate from high school next June, will you not?"

"No, I finish in January at mid-year."

Instantly an idea popped into my head. Why not take Robert to Washington for six months to serve as my chauffeur? It was becoming more and more apparent that unless I was to be house-bound in Washington I should need such a helper. I said nothing at the time, waiting to discuss it with his mother and Mr. Ritter. Both assented when I mentioned it to them, so the next day when the recent presidential election was under discussion, I said, "How would you like to see the inauguration, Robert?"

"What inauguration?"

"Coolidge's, of course."

"What are you giving me?" he inquired with school-boy slang.

"A trip to Washington," I replied. "Would you like to go with me in January and be my chauffeur until we return for the summer in July?"

"Try me and see!" was his enthusiastic response. And thus Robert's love of travel was inaugurated, and in January, 1925, we again pulled up the plants of renewed Berkeley friendships, to see if the roots were sprouting. They were.

And right here let us look at some of those roots that have never died regardless of numerous transplantings. A few of our many close friendships have already been noted, but most of them have not been mentioned. Life without them would not have been the same, so I must incorporate a few more in this narrative. Mr. Ritter had three friends in his class of 1888, who were particularly congenial. They were George Stratton, Henry Rieber and Theodore Palmer. The last named was the most constant companion in undergraduate days because of their similar work, but he went to Washington soon afterward and was awaiting a renewal of friendship when we came there to live. The other two continued graduate study in the University of California as did Mr. Ritter, and after their advanced degrees in Harvard and Germany, all three became professors in their Alma Mater. A life-long friendship has continued which includes their respective life mates. Berkeley would not be Berkeley without George and Alice Stratton; and although the Riebers have followed the University to its southern half, the intimate friendship has not been broken.

An added bond in this case came through Winifred Rieber's art as a portrait painter. She has transferred Will Ritter's lineaments three times to canvas, and one of the greatest joys of the year in Berkeley was her sojourn of two months at our hotel while she was painting his portrait as well as that of President Campbell and Dr. Hosmer, the aged writer of hymns. The portrait of Mr. Ritter, begun here and completed in La Jolla, was later presented by Miss Scripps to the Biological Institution he had created. How much our lives have been enriched by these friendships it is impossible to estimate.

Other very close associations for a third of a century have been with the Torreys and the Baileys. Dr. Torrey like Dr. Esterly and Mr. Crandall had married a university girl of my particular choice, though my advice was not asked. Grace Crabbe Torrey's brilliant mind and charming personality have during these later years been among the brightest beads—scintillating, opalescent beads—on my rosary of precious friendships.

And then the Baileys. In a sense Edna Watson Bailey and her children have been more nearly a part of the Ritter family than any others. As student and research assistant, Edna Watson was very closely associated with us before her marriage. The friendship continued unbroken when she married Dr. Ellsworth Bailey, who was another of the biological students forming the summer groups. When upon his death Edna was left with two little girls, Mr. Ritter, in a grandfatherly sense adopted the children, participating as a naturalist in their formal and religious education. That interest continues now in their college life and has done much to open up the out-door world to their inquiring minds.

The roots of friendship had deepened with the years, but with the beginning of 1925 we must again be transplanted to Washington, D.C. As we planned to return to California each summer it was evident that we could not strike root deeply there.

So the first year of freedom from regular duties came to an end. Again I assert that the happy part of retirement is largely a myth.

CHAPTER 21

Washington Days

WHEN WE TRANSFERRED OUR PLACE OF ABODE TO WASHINGTON IN January, 1925, the trip was difficult, due to my ill health. We went first to La Jolla for a farewell visit to Miss Scripps, and to give Mrs. Rieber the opportunity to finish Mr. Ritter's portrait with the La Jolla shore as a background. The Scripps Metabolic Clinic, named for its donor, had just been opened, and as I was lying on her couch one day, Miss Scripps suggested that I go there for a thorough examination. To please her I did so, and an endocrinal disturbance was found which contributed largely to my unhealth. It was urged that I spend a few days in this hospital. The few days were prolonged to two weeks ere I could continue our journey, but without doubt that two weeks and later sojourns under the same treatment prolonged my life by some years.

Robert joined us in La Jolla for the eastward trip. I had planned to go by the southernmost route via New Orleans and through the Gulf States to Washington. This was a new route to me, and would give Robert a glimpse of the Southland and of the Mardi Gras. Mr. Ritter was to leave us at New Orleans to interview President Hughes of Miami College. I was glad to rest two days and give Robert the opportunity to prowl about this quaint old city and witness the annual Mardi Gras carnival.

A new automobile had been ordered from the factory in Detroit to be forwarded to Washington. It reached there the day Robert and I arrived. Thanks to a good friend, Adrienne Conybeare, who had found us an apartment-hotel, we settled in Cathedral Mansions opposite the entrance to beautiful Rock Creek Park where I loved to drive daily, and

Mr. Ritter had a fine opportunity to study the intelligence of apes and monkeys in the National Zoo. The location was ideal, and Robert a great acquisition to our household.

Almost at once I began "listening in" on the Senate discussions, and also joined a weekly Current Events lecture course in which things of local and world interest were reviewed. My impressions of senators and senatorial discussions were various.

As an addendum to my experience three years earlier, one filibuster struck me as especially exasperating and an unnecessary waste of the people's money. The final signature to the Isle of Pines Treaty was before the Senate—and had been for twelve years. The treaty was only a matter of business justice to the people of a Caribbean Island which had been decided in their favor twelve years before, but certain New York interests objected to it and had succeeded in preventing its validation all those years. Approval of the bill's passage was almost unanimous, the only objection coming from a New York senator. When ready for final passage this man gained the floor. On his desk was a pile of books more than a foot high, and he announced that he would keep the floor all night unless the Senate would adjourn without passing the bill. He began reading a passage from one book, utterly irrelevant to the subject, and talked on that as long as he could find anything to say. Then he took another book, read a passage on a totally different subject and talked on it as long as he could. Another book, another subject, another discussion. This he repeated until the afternoon waned, adjournment hour had passed, and dinner time was so close that the listeners began to file out. As I was leaving, the speaker hoarsely addressed the president of the senate, saying, "My voice is giving out, but I shall keep on until the Senate adjourns." He won his point that day, but later the bill was passed and long-delayed justice was granted. This was an unusually clear instance of what filibustering means, and how it can be accomplished.

My opinion of that Senator and of the powers by which he was dominated was not enhanced. On the contrary my conviction increased that the Senate rule that the dignity of a member of that body was so great that he could not be interrupted, no matter how badly he abused that privilege, should be abolished.

February had been a month of snow and wintry winds, but early March indulged in a deceptive spring-like warmth which succeeded in deceiving the young Californian who had never experienced the extreme changes in temperature which often occur in these less pacific climes. The day after the filibustering experience was uncomfortably warm and muggy. Robert, who was going to dinner with a boy friend and to the theatre later, could not be persuaded to take an overcoat. In the evening a sharp thunderstorm came up, and after sitting three hours in a heated theatre, he emerged into a sleety rainstorm which had caused the temperature to drop forty degrees. He faced a three mile ride home in his friend's open car. Result—pneumonia, with ten days of great anxiety, and daily telegrams to his parents.

By the first of April he was ready for drives through the beautiful spring blossoms to places of interest within easy reach of Washington. One notable trip was our visit to the quaint old city of Annapolis and the Naval Academy. We went to Baltimore several times, visiting Johns Hopkins University and historic points. Mount Vernon, the home and burial place of George Washington, and Arlington, the National Cemetery in which stands General Lee's old home, were points of interest to which we often took friends who chanced to visit us.

My desire was that Robert should see as much of the country, of historical places, and of universities as possible: in other words to make this pre-college half-year an educational one. Naturally we visited every nook and cranny about Washington again and again, and April brought an opportunity to explore a section of our country which was as new to me as to Robert.

The National Convention of the League of Women Voters, to which I was a delegate from the Berkeley Chapter, was to be held in Richmond, Virginia. Every mile of the over seven hundred mile round trip was crammed with historic interest. The first day we lunched at Fredericksburg and visited the homes of George Washington's mother where he lived as a child, and that of his sister, an unusually fine colonial mansion restored by the women of the South. By evening we were housed in the quaint old Jefferson Hotel in the capital of the one-time Confederacy.

The convention was notable, but it is of Robert's historic trip that I am thinking. Richmond, so beautiful, so full of interests old and new, caused memories to tumble over each other. From the confederate days we leaped back to colonial times as we sat in the pew in which Patrick Henry arose and made his undying speech, sat and listened to the sexton of the small but venerable church as he feebly imitated Patrick Henry's fiery pronouncement, "Give me liberty or give me death!"

One had to rapidly adjust one's historical sequence as we were taken down the James River to Jamestown to view the tower of the first church erected in what is now the United States, and also the statues of John Smith and Pocahontas. While dreaming of Indian scalpings, we were hustled into a modern bus and taken to Yorktown, to jump over the centuries as we read the inscription about Cornwallis' surrender. Then to Williamsburg to dine in the refectory of William and Mary College, still in active use by young men and women of today.

After a week of ardent conference on political issues affecting modern women and children, we crossed the Valley of Virginia as we toured from the hotel named for Jefferson to the site of the University he founded and largely built, the University of Virginia.

I had written Mr. Ritter to join us at Charlottesville for the homeward journey. Although we had visited the University of Virginia previously, the architectural genius of Jefferson impressed me more this time. What a monument he has left both in the great educational institution and the beautiful quadrangle and buildings in which he housed it. Monticello, the mansion he planned and built for his bride, the ingenious devices he invented, the beautiful landed estate on the sloping foothills of the Blue Ridge Mountains, and the family cemetery, are impressive indeed.

We were loath to leave the Dolly Madison Inn to cross the Blue Ridge to the famous Luray Caves. I left the exploration of these miles of caverns to the two men, but next day at Shenandoah Cavern I descended in an elevator to glimpse the beauties of the bluish stalagmites and stalactites in their weird formations.

We traveled up through the Shenandoah Valley where northern and southern troops chased each other back and forth until Winchester, in its center, had been captured nearly a hundred times. It is said that the residents had to look out each morning to see which flag was flying in order to know which army was their captor.

As we were driving through the country where Sheridan made his famous ride, the sky became so dark that we had to turn on the auto lights at three o'clock. A huge menacing black cloud swept toward us with such thunder and lightning as I had never experienced, and the rain came down in a deluge. I was sure that one bolt of lightning struck our radiator, and that the top of the car was crushed in as the simultaneous thunderbolt deafeningly hammered on our heads. To my surprise we still lived, but two or three miles ahead we were stopped because an auto was on fire and the gasoline flames spread the width of the highway despite the torrents of water falling on it. All traffic was stopped until the gasoline fuel was exhausted. Winchester in mid-afternoon had its street lights burning and all places of business illuminated. By these lights I could note that the rivers rushing down the streets flowed over the rims of the auto wheels. The deluge continued during the fifty mile drive to Harper's Ferry where we spent the night at Hill Top Inn. Again our minds were simply gorged with historic events from John Brown's raid and tragic execution, to, a little later, the town, the house, the window where Barbara Frietschie is supposed to have waved her flag of defiance at the invading troops. Was there a Barbara Frietschie?

Beside the interesting places we saw on this trip, another source of great pleasure was the southern spring with its budding flowers and trees, the fertile grain fields, blossoming orchards, dogwood and red-buds. The awakening of nature after a dormant winter is a thrilling sight to Californians who have never known what the dead of winter really means.

Washington was just as prolific as the open country with its vernal display. Rock Creek Park is an improved bit of natural woods on rolling hills with a beautiful stream dashing through, deserving of its name. Much of the flora of eastern woods was native in the park, which was our "front door yard" all the time we were in Washington.

Another favorite spot in the national capital was the Tidal Basin with its border of Japanese cherry trees. This year they were wondrously beautiful and almost daily we circled the Basin while waiting for Mr. Ritter in the late afternoon. This was convenient as the Science Service headquarters were in the beautiful new National Academy of Science building opposite the Lincoln Memorial. Was there ever so fitting a memorial as that stately Greek temple with its portico of forty-eight huge Corinthian columns, one given by each state in the Union? And within, the colossal figure of the martyred president sitting there in deep contemplation with the destiny of the nation on his bowed head.

On either side, engraved on the marble wall, are two of his undying addresses to his fellow-countrymen. One day when I had taken a friend to see it, a young couple came in, a bridal pair. From their conversation it was evident that the bride was a northern girl wedded to a southern youth. She was all enthusiasm; he stood in sullen silence, keeping his hat on. The heads of the other men were bared. She whispered to him to remove his hat. "I will not take off my hat to that tyrant," replied the hereditarily sore-hearted southerner. A few moments later they stood before the engraving of the Gettysburg address, she reading, he looking out toward the Washington monument. "Please read it," she pleaded, "you will understand him better."

"I don't want to understand him."

"Then do it for my sake, if we are to be happy together," she begged. He turned toward the inscription and she read aloud in a low tone. Slowly his sullen expression changed, his face softened. When she was about half through, he slowly removed his hat. At the close, a moment of silence, then with a glimmer of moisture in his eyes, he took his bride's arm and said, "I did not know he ever said anything like that. I will understand your people better for this."

Again had Lincoln saved the union of the North and South—in marriage.

Between the monument park and the Tidal Basin was a municipal golf course where the army and navy teams practiced their polo games once a week. My life-long love of horsemanship and sport lured me there frequently on Wednesday afternoons. Thus with the beauties of architecture, the attractions of the Senate and Supreme Court, the Congressional Library, and our many friends, the days in Washington sped by. But Robert and I were soon to start on another motoring trip to follow up the springtime in the North.

All of these pleasures were interspersed with the usual correcting of Mr. Ritter's manuscripts, for that grist mill never stopped. His mornings were given to writing, then we all went to some interesting nook for luncheon, and left him at the Science Service offices where he worked with the staff until we called for him about five o'clock.

Just at this time occurred the most interesting convention I ever attended. It was the unique Quinquennial meeting of the International Council of Women. Women from forty-six nations took part, the Countess of Aberdeen presiding. Her broad Scotch accent and very deliberate speech were in striking contrast to the vivacious French officers, and the alert American hostesses. Almost every variety of accent and of racial color and physiognomy were depicted, while the presidents of the forty-six National Councils were extending their greetings. The diversity of topics considered covered everything from disarmament to women's status in their native countries. The warmest discussion next to disarmament was on the subject of equal morals for men and women. This convention had naturally drawn many acquaintances, from California to Australia, beside several from European countries, so Robert and I and the "Dodge" daily took what I finally dubbed the "forty-mile drive," showing these friends some of our favorite places in and about Washington.

For the double purpose of extending Robert's course in geography and history, and of realizing a day-dream of motoring through New England, we planned a month's trip northward to the Canadian border. Mr. Ritter decided to go to his beloved Cosmos Club during our absence, so we packed and stored our personal belongings and planned our itinerary to meet Mr. Ritter in New York on our return, as he was to make one of his frequent trips to that metropolis. I invited my friend Adrienne Conybeare to go with us, as she could be companion to both Robert and me, and substitute as driver if need be.

Colleges and universities stood near the top on our list of sights. Princeton came first, and after visiting twenty-four more or less famous institutions, this was Robert's favorite. After two days in Philadelphia for its many historical interests, plus its noted university buried in the heart of the city, we drove down the Palisades and crossed the Hudson on

Dyckman's Ferry at Two Hundredth Street and entered New York from Riverside Drive, thus avoiding the heaviest traffic.

Robert's first three days in New York were intensive and extensive as to sight-seeing. The first evening I insisted that he take a taxi to the theatre, a distance of some three miles, as I feared the country youth would lose his way or be held up by pick-pockets. He objected but finally yielded. Imagine my consternation next morning when he related his experiences, saying that he had taken a taxi down town in the early evening but had walked home after the theatre! I decided then and there not to restrict the young man again with older generation qualms.

To me New York holds the lure of a reunion with my cousin Loraine Beeman Macdonell. Through all the years since my girlhood visit in Connecticut, our friendship has been renewed by these frequent reunions on one side of the continent or the other.

As we left the metropolis behind us on the fourth morning I made a call on an old-time Berkeley friend, Chancellor Brown of New York University, while the young folk visited the college. Then we proceeded up the Hudson, calling on several younger generation cousins; then over Bear Mountain Bridge and Storm King Highway to West Point to watch a drill and to explore the grounds. Next day we went on through the Adirondacks where spring became less evident, up to Lake Placid. Truly we had left full-leafed spring behind us. Here in the cool Adirondacks the fruit trees were just beginning to bud.

Our indefinite itinerary was wherever the whim led us, stopping when night shadows fell. We traveled to the extreme north of New York, ferrying over Lake Champlain, on across the Green Mountains of Vermont and the White Mountains of New Hampshire, across Maine to its southeastern coast line, down the rocky coast to Boston, and finally back to New York via the ancestral home of the Bennett and Beeman families in New Preston, Connecticut.

The only member of the family now living thereabouts is my genial cousin Will Beeman of New Milford. Throughout all the years since my girlhood sojourn with them, I had returned many times to visit Aunt Mary and Aunt Ruth, the last members of the ancestral family. They were no more, and in all probability this was to be my last trip to the beautiful Lake Waramaug region.

In New York we met Mr. Ritter, who joined us on the two-day trip back to Washington.

Two more busy weeks in Washington and we were off for Chicago, homeward bound. Arriving there July first we found it so cold I got out my sealskin coat! The westward trip was made as extensive as possible for Robert's benefit and my own pleasure. Mr. Ritter was busy in Cincinnati and Oxford, Ohio, and visiting his sisters and brother in Wisconsin, while Robert and I loitered in Chicago and then in Minneapolis where we spent the "glorious Fourth" with another cousin, Edwin Beeman Jr. Mr. Ritter joined us here and we fulfilled a life-long desire to visit Yellowstone Park, where we vacationed for a week in viewing its wonders.

Robert's geography lesson would scarcely be complete without seeing something of the north Pacific Coast. Also that adopted cousin-niece, Bernadine Hobbs, was luring us to Seattle, so thither Robert and I went. Portland and the Columbia River Highway also halted us a few days. Altogether, Robert toured thirty-four states, visited twenty-four universities, and saw the sights of many cities in his six month's pre-college travel course. When, after his graduation from college he sailed on a freight steamer to work his way around South America, and the following year hiked through Europe, he wrote me, "You know you are responsible for lighting up my desire to see the world." I felt no sense of guilt. The "see your own country first" tour with Robert meant much to me in my battle with the doldrums of retirement.

A busy summer in Berkeley followed, Mr. Ritter being hard at work. August took me back to La Jolla for another session of treatment at the Metabolic Clinic and a visit with Miss Scripps. Then a fortnight at Huntington Lake with the Cockrills and Warners. Mr. Ritter joined us for a few days at the Lake ere we were to leave California for Washington once more.

Scarcely had we reached Berkeley when a cable came from Bermuda asking Mr. Ritter to join Mr. Scripps again on his yacht for further discussion of plans. This meant a hurried departure, leaving me to complete the business and packing prior to making the trip to Washington alone early in October.

If meeting interesting people, attending interesting lectures, theatres and conventions spelled happiness, surely the autumn in Washington should have been blissful. Mr. Ritter was constantly on the go to New York, to Chicago, Cincinnati or St. Louis, which meant lonely though active days for me. I retaliated by leaving him for a week of Convention in New York which Edna Bailey wired me to attend.

The Bailey family, consisting of Dr. Edna Bailey, Anita Laton and the two girls, were located in New York for the winter, the two teachers taking a sabbatical year at Columbia University. The need for cooperation on Mr. Ritter's book resulted in our going to New York before Christmas to remain six weeks, a hectic but doleful Yuletide. Telegrams brought word of my niece Edna Cockrill being suddenly subjected to a life or death surgical operation, and a cable brought news of the death of Mrs. Slosson's sister in San Nemo, on the Italian Riviera. Then, due to our removal from Washington, Santa Claus lost track of me, a trivial, laughable incident now, but the last straw then. When none of the California packages had arrived by mid-January, I set the whole Post-Office Department to tracing them. They were found carefully stored away on a closet shelf in our apartment in Washington. As our close friend Professor George Stratton was carrying on some work with the National Research Council, we had invited him to occupy our apartment during our absence. He was the only person I had not instructed about forwarding the Christmas packages, so he had carefully put them away!

January in New York, with its snowstorms, art galleries, operas, conventions, and hosts of friends, took all the strength I had to spare, while Mr. Ritter plodded faithfully on his work with Dr. Bailey. Such pleasures, such weariness, such unrest of spirit! While the diversions were interesting, educational, and thoroughly worthwhile, and the friendly intercourse was delightful, they did not dispel the sense of loss of work. I wanted a real personal task to accomplish, a feeling of being useful in the world. How can women live idle lives, filling in their days and much of their nights with bridge playing and social entertainments? I had not yet learned the lesson of being a mere looker-on at life.

The return to Washington was welcome as there I was playing at work on a welfare committee, which often took me to the court for wayward youth, and then there was always the Senate on which to fall back. In early December, soon after the opening of the Congress, I had heard the introduction of the famous bill to join the World Court, and had listened to several discussions of it. When we returned the last of January it was still under discussion. On January 27th, I find this entry in my diary, "Rushed off to Senate early in order to get a seat. Stood outside the door from 9:15 to 11 a.m., opening time, to hear final discussion on World Court admission, which was promised for one o'clock. Endless talk. The reservation proposed by Senator Moses was defeated; then the Reid obstruction amendment was defeated at 6 p.m. Final favorable vote taken on Protocol at 6:52, ending a discussion lasting three and a half years." A very lively skirmish occurred in the late afternoon. One would have thought it might end in blows, hair-pulling, or at least in broken knuckles, due to the vehement pounding on the desks by the angry debaters. But no blood was spilled, no hair lost, and apparently no knuckles broken.

Eight months later I was to hear this same measure discussed in Geneva by a committee of representatives of forty-five nations to determine if they could accept the fatal reservation which was slipped in at the last moment, to prevent a filibuster. It was the clause that the World Court could not act on any matter in which the United States "has or claims to have an interest." Oh, those fatal words, "or claims to have." But more of that later. Geneva is eight months distant.

Realizing that Mr. Ritter was becoming restless to be settled in Berkeley with his own books and copious notes (cases and cases of them), I decided that if we were ever to see Europe again it would be much simpler to do so while we were on the Atlantic coast. I therefore urged a trip to Europe that summer instead of to California. Little we dreamed of what the near future held in store.

During the winter Mr. Scripps had been touring the world in his yacht. A letter from the Cape of Good Hope announced that he expected to spend the summer in the Mediterranean. He asked Mr. Ritter to join him there to review the progress of Science Service and the new Foundation on Population in Miami University, and to make plans for their future, as well as for another project—another "Ritter idea." Mr. Ritter accepted this invitation which necessitated a change in my plans.

Late in March, two calamities struck us. One cold snowy evening we detected smoke coming up through our floor and could hear the crackling of flames beneath. A hurried fire alarm to the hotel office, and a scurrying to save our clothing, ended only in our being driven out by the dense smoke. Soon firemen filled our rooms, and floors and partitions succumbed to their axes. The building was saved but our apartment was a wreck, with thirty-four broken window panes to admit the sleety storm beside the holes chopped by the firemen.

The next day after our upheaval a cable arrived stating that Mr. Scripps had died on his yacht, of a cerebral hemorrhage. The *Ohio* was anchored off Liberia, western Africa, and the American consul and his wife were dining with Mr. Scripps when he was stricken. Ere they reached shore half an hour later, their dinner host was dead.

Anticipating such an occurrence Mr. Scripps had left instruction for a simple burial at sea. Wrapped in a tarpaulin, his body was lowered into the ocean he loved.

The loss to Mr. Ritter of the most intimate friend of his life-time was very severe. Beside his personal loss, there was the alteration in the future of their joint projects, as Mr. Scripps had awaited Mr. Ritter's report of the year's test before making adequate financial arrangements for their continuance.

CHAPTER 22

Europe Again

OWING TO THE CHANGE IN PLANS CAUSED BY MR. SCRIPPS' DEATH, Mr. Ritter decided not to go to Europe but to return to Berkeley for the summer, where he could have access to his own books and notes. I felt that for me it was now or never again to Europe and I was particularly desirous of spending some weeks in Geneva attending the League of Nations Convention.

Knowing that my grand-niece, Elizabeth Warner, and her friend, Florence Bradford, were anxious to go to Europe but that their parents would not permit them to go alone, I wrote them my plans for taking auto trips through some parts of Europe off the beaten track and asked if they would like to join me. They heartily agreed. These girls had finished their college courses and wanted to see Europe before they settled into domestic life. Another grand-niece, Jane Warner, just out of high school joined the party.

They arrived in Washington late in March for two weeks of sight-seeing in the Capital and in New York before sailing on the tenth of April. I had meanwhile met a San Diego friend, Mrs. Hazel Waterman, who was sailing about the same time. She gladly annexed herself to our party, which was a great advantage to me. We took an Italian liner direct to Palermo, Sicily, and slowly followed the Spring northward.

Sicily with its beauties of nature, its towns on hill tops, decorated carts and horses, its execrable roads, narrow streets, and primitive customs reminded me of Italy thirty years earlier. But its wonders of ancient art in the 12th century mosaics, said to be the finest in the world, its ruins telling of Greek, Arabic, and Norman conquests, and its picturesque but devastating volcano are individual.

In Palermo we found the delightful Hotel des Palmes. Good hotels do add so much to one's comfort in traveling!

After viewing the glorious mosaics we were taken to an interesting Albanian village, Piana dei Greci, in existence before Columbus discovered our unknown continent. It is hidden among the hills where the famous banditti were still numerous.

From Palermo we took an auto for a week's trip around Sicily. The first day surprised us with a freezing Sirocco and blinding dust storm. Our first stop was at Girgenti with its famous Greek temples of the sixth century B.C. Beautiful they were looking out upon them by moonlight. Upon closer inspection they were fine, but not quite equal to the temples of Paestum. Two days later we reached Siracusa where in the beautiful gardens of our hostelry, the Villa del Polito, are the devilish quarries where the conquered Athenians found a living tomb, being thrown into these great caverns and left to die. Now large trees grow therein and we could look down on them from the gardens. With my mind filled with these ancient atrocities which befell many of the intelligentsia of Athens, I finally fell asleep to be awakened by the bray of the omnipresent donkey and the whir of a modern aeroplane.

After two days in each of these interesting places we went on to Taormina the Beautiful, nestling at the foot of imperious Etna. We were bowling merrily along in mid-forenoon with Etna's majesty luring us onward when the auto engine suddenly stopped and no amount of coaxing from the chauffeur could start it. In despair he finally started to walk the nine miles to the next town, Catania, leaving us helpless in the middle of the road. We had a good chance to view Etna 'tis true, but with four long hours of waiting even Etna, smoking from various clefts, lost some of its charm.

We had taken our lunch with us and we ate it sitting on some "new mown hay" which proved to be a brilliantly-flowered pea-vine. As the peasants in their decorated carts, which we had passed so gaily earlier in the day, passed us one by one, it was now their turn for gaiety and much laughter and merriment at our predicament.

In the afternoon a carload of Sicilian gentlemen came along in an auto and seeing five lone foreign women sitting stranded in a car in the middle of the road, they gallantly insisted on rescuing us. Though their car was as full as ours they tried to induce us to go with them after failing to find a tow-rope. We tried our best with words and gesticulations to inform them that our chauffeur had gone to Catania for repairs and would return, but even that international word chauffeur, did not register. They gave us fruits and offered us wines, and finally one of them produced a piece of cord about the size of a lead pencil with which they were determined to tow us. In spite of our shaking heads they were working vigorously to fasten our car to theirs when an auto hove in sight, proving to be that of the mechanic who was bringing back our chauffeur and the repaired magneto. Surely those Sicilians were gallant—and persistent.

By nightfall we reached our hotel in an old Dominican monastery where we could watch Etna smoking first through a rent on one side and then on another while all the time spurting from its crater top.

The lovely drawn linens and laces of the Taormina nunneries were alluring to the girls but our chauffeur insisted on taking us to Messina where he left us to pass between Scylla and Charybdis as best we could on our passage to the shore of Italy. In this rugged mountainous heel of the Italian boot there are no passable roads, so we took a night train to Salerno whence we planned to go by auto along the wondrous shore drive to Sorrento.

An agent of Thomas Cook and Sons was at the depot and kindly conveyed us to a hotel for breakfast. I consulted him about an auto for the day's trip to Ravello, Amalfi and Sorrento. He offered to provide us one with a reliable chauffeur for twenty-four dollars of our money, but it sounded so large in Italian lira that the girls thought it too much and insisted on finding something cheaper. They started out to search and soon returned triumphant at having secured an auto for eight dollars. My heart sank and I asked, "Are you sure that the man understood he is to take us to Sorrento?"

"Oh, sure! We told him Ravello for lunch and then to Sorrento." The bargain had been made with a man who could not speak English.

I was fearful, and the Cook agent said to me, "You will never be taken to Sorrento for that sum." But the girls would not listen, and we set forth in an auto of ancient vintage.

All went well until we started up the steep, winding, and narrow grade to the hill-top town of Ravello. When nearing the top the chauffeur was having difficulty in steering the car. He could scarcely guide it around the sharp turns. The precipices below did not look alluring as we lurched along. When we finally reached the top, some Italian idlers shouted to the driver. We jumped out to see one front wheel at an angle of almost forty-five degrees. It was discovered that the axle was broken inside the hub. How we were spared going over that precipice I do not know!

Here we had to wait until another machine came to our rescue as we supposed, but alas, it was only to tow the broken car home. They took us down the hill to the main road below hill-top Amalfi where our driver stopped and took our luggage out, set it beside the road, and insisted that we get out. He had been engaged, he insisted, to take us to Ravello and no farther. The eight dollar bargain covered about one-third of the journey and the chauffeur would not take us to Sorrento even for extra pay. There we were dumped!

How Mrs. Waterman and I should have loved to spend the night in the old monastery hotel at the top of the Amalfi cliff where thirty years before Mr. Ritter and I had watched one of the most beautiful sunrises we ever saw from the windows of two of those monastery cells where we had spent the night. But the majority ruled that we should not even go up to Amalfi but proceed to Sorrento. A swarm of vettura drivers surrounded us. These tiny one-horse carriages looked romantic to the young folks, and choosing one of the better appearing horses, the three girls crowded into the little vehicle and started off in great glee over the adventure.

Mrs. Waterman and I followed less gleefully but I will admit that the views from that famed Amalfi-Sorrento cliff drive were so beautiful that we felt resigned to the slow jog trot as we drank in the beauty of the water-view and the terraced hillsides with orange trees growing over lattices, one row on each terrace. But as the afternoon waned and darkness dropped upon us with Sorrento still miles away, the joy of scenic beauty was replaced by the pangs of empty stomachs and aching backs.

I was amused to learn that the girls grew fearful that they were being kidnaped by banditti. It was the cold evening air and the weariness that troubled me.

Lights finally appeared and we reached the suburbs of straggling Sorrento. Our drivers stopped at a hostelry named El Paradiso and would go no farther. Here we spent a comfortless night, and if that is a sample of Paradise I do not want any more. The next day in a pouring rain we procured a taxi to take us some distance to El Tramontano, one of the better hotels in the real Sorrento.

It was the first of May during which month we slowly meandered through southern Italy, first to dear old Naples where Mr. Ritter had worked in the Marine Laboratory on our former trip. Naples connotes its wondrous environs, Capri, Pompeii, and Vesuvius. In Rome we joined our steamer friends, the central figure of which group was my little diphtheria patient of long, long ago, with her husband and half grown son.

Another auto journey through the famed hill-towns of Assisis, Perugia, and the rest took us to Florence. After two weeks of sight-seeing I decided to rest while the others went to Venice, and to rejoin them in Milan on the way to the Italian Lakes.

Mrs. Waterman and I remained at Bellagio on Lake Como while the girls made a rushing trip into the Alps, as it was their only opportunity.

The beauty of those Alpine lakes! After enjoying Como's circle of snow clad Alps for ten days we traversed three lakes to visit Locarno where the famous pact had been signed.

Reversing our northward trend we returned to Genoa. Mrs. Waterman and I motored along the lovely Italian and French Riviera to Nice where the girls met us, then to Monte Carlo where my chief interest lay in the Marine Aquarium of the late Prince of Monaco, who was an ardent collector of sea-life. The girls twirled the wheels of the gaming tables a few times for the thrill of the game of chance. Meanwhile we elders watched the look of desperation in the eyes of the old habitués who, bedraggled and worn, clung to the hope of sometime regaining their losses.

Some of the quaint towns in southern France, Avignon, Arles, and Nimes, yield memories of wonderful Roman ruins, and interesting tournaments of modern peasant games, from a street bull-fight to an athletic contest in the old Roman amphitheatre which has been in constant use for over 2,000 years.

On to Carcassonne, the wonderfully preserved medieval fortress crowning a hill-top at the foot of the Pyrenees. As we drove through the portcullis of Carcassonne's impregnable double walls with their fifty-four observation towers from which missiles could be thrown upon any attacking foe, I felt as if I had dropped back a thousand years—save for the auto. For streets there were narrow lanes of cobblestones worn by the tread of feet for over five centuries. With apparently no change in fashions the brightly clad boys and girls go marching on. One modern innovation we appreciated, a tourist hotel.

From Carcassonne over the Pyrenees, a two day trip to Lourdes, weird Lourdes. Beside the indescribable beauty of mountain scenery, much the same everywhere, yet always different, the only unique sight was the tiny republic of Andorra in the distance, and the picturesque peasant women working in the hay fields.

Pathetic Lourdes! and the still more pathetic faith of the devout. The time for healing is appointed for various regions. At this time the Bretons of northern France had brought their dying friends. In the evening a double procession a mile long marched around a great park, all carrying candles and singing their dolorous prayer, "Ave Ma—ri—a! Vita, Vita!"

To the mystic grotto hundreds were carrying their sick and dying in chairs or on stretchers. While we were watching, forty in chairs and twelve on stretchers were brought into the grotto to receive the miracle of healing, while hundreds of the faithful sang their doleful petition. No sign of healing was evident, but such faith! Poor deluded mortals!

We went on to Paris by a night train and I took a rest cure while the others saw some of the sights of the city.

This trip differed from any other foreign travel in that I had hitherto accompanied my husband or made the journey with others of my own age. Almost two generations stretched between the members of our party and tastes varied as much as age. I was more interested in things of the past, historic places, cathedrals and works of art. The present, with the activities of moderns, whether in palaces or at the Lido, attracted the younger ones.

I soon realized that in their estimation I was an inexperienced old lady fit only for a shelf of antiques. The lack of physical strength to keep up their pace I acknowledge. Fortunately our party could divide into two groups, two elders and three youths, in our expeditions either together or separately. This plan worked nicely until we reached Paris where Mrs. Waterman left us to join other friends from San Diego.

While the exigencies of travel are trying at the moment, time puts a softening haze over the memory pictures and the glaring vexations become humorous episodes. Doubtless the girls have many jokes to tell on me, but one or two incidents seem so ludicrous to me now that I am sure they will forgive me for relating one of them.

In Paris one minor incident showed me plainly my standing in their estimation. Although somewhat indignant at the time it gives me great amusement now whenever I think of it.

One day when driving in a taxi the girls were discussing the "Follies Bergere" which they had attended the previous evening. I exclaimed, "Oh, I wish you had told me you were going; it is a thing I have wanted to see."

It was not the exhibition in itself that I desired to see but I wanted to know what modern Paris was giving as entertainment. My interest was the outcome of my social-service-morality work of many years. So when the response came from one of the girls, "That wasn't a fit thing for you to see, Aunt Mary," I was as nearly bowled over as ever in my life.

Not fit for me to see! I who at their age was seeing the nudity and drabness of life while dissecting human cadavers alongside men students, witnessing with them the most trying of operations, treading the streets of San Francisco slums at all hours of the night with another student, to usher some poor waif into the world. Then nearly fifteen years of medical practice before they were born. I who had been active during all the years of their girlhood in social hygiene or morality work in the State Federation of Women's Clubs, and later during the war had carried on the same kind of work under a Federal Commission! I thought of the nights when with a trained social-service worker and guarded by a plain-clothes policeman, I had inspected the haunts in San Diego—haunts considered dubious for the sailors and soldiers to visit.

I think that I fully appreciated the feelings of Alice in Wonderland when after taking a magic potion she shrank and shrank and shrank. Yet mine was no unique experience. Probably all parents have had similar ones. It was the viewpoint of youth in that very serious period following "commencement" of independent life, as opposed to that of one of ripened years looking back upon completed tasks.

As I look into the merry sparkling eyes of the three- and four-year-old children of these same girls, I doubt not that some time they will better understand my consternation at their judgment concerning my attendance at the "Follies Bergere."

Paris is Paris; always the same, ever different. Of its environs, memories of the glorious opalescent windows of Chartres Cathedral stand out, and also quaint Barbizon in the forest of Fontainebleau, where we lunched one day outside the house where the artist Millet worked and almost starved, selling his pictures for the merest pittance that he might obtain food for his family. O, Life, Life! Why does it take so long to recognize talent?

I well remember when *The Man with a Hoe* was exhibited in San Francisco, and the newspapers flaunted the statement that nearly half a million dollars had recently been paid for this one picture of a cloddish peasant beaten almost dumb by his hard life. And the creator of that work of art had likewise been crushed to earth by his own hard life and the lack of appreciation.

The girls and I left Mrs. Waterman in Paris when we went to London. Part of our six weeks in the British Isles was spent there and the remainder was passed in an auto trip around England and Scotland, the two elder girls driving. This was to me the pleasantest part of our trip together. Their Mecca was St. Andrews and Gleneagles where they wished to play golf on the mother-links. It was the cathedrals from Salisbury to Durham and York, and the beauties of English and Scottish lakes and mountains and a bit of Wales that filled three weeks with joy for me. At Edinburgh and Cambridge Universities, reunions with friends made in Australia added enjoyment.

We then returned to London where Mrs. Waterman rejoined us for more sight-seeing. She had decided to turn her face homeward. The girls were soon to sail for home. It was hard to let them go; in fact I could not bring myself to see them off. So the morning before they were to sail I arose early and left for Paris before they were up.

Having arrived there I first attended to some dressmaking and then regardless of the prudent warning of my grand-nieces, I went directly to the "Follies Bergere" determined to despoil my character by the, for my age, improper display of beauty and nudity. The only thing that worried me was an apparent pickpocket beside me, who seemed interested in my hand-bag.

Geneva, the Mecca of my trip, followed. I planned to arrive there a week before the opening of the seventh annual convention of the League of Nations, that I might attend the lectures of the International Institute of Education, preparatory to the Convention's proceedings. Dr. Zimmerman, President of the Paris Institute, and other notables delivered daily courses of lectures.

During this week I learned that the World's Court Committee was discussing the reservations of the United States' application for admission to that Court. They were the same five reservations that I had heard discussed for weeks in the Senate at Washington, closing with that fiery debate which seemed likely to end in hair-pulling. Here in Geneva, a committee consisting of emissaries from forty-nine nations discussed the reservations for three days in morning and afternoon sessions, and while the discussions were animated there was never an impolite word nor a rude action. What a contrast! And it was not that they did not understand our country nor the meaning of that fifth reservation.

Four items were readily accepted, but that fatal clause in the fifth item, "in which the United States has or claims to have an interest" could not be agreed to, since it would undermine the power of the World Court.

The way in which Sir George Foster of Canada analyzed his neighbor country was eloquent and understanding but not entirely flattering. A prince from India made a clear statement of the situation; likewise delegates, usually premiers or other high officials of the countries represented, talked straight to the point, but there was never a raised voice nor an epithet that our Senate could resent. But of course they could not accept that phrase, "or claims to have."

This is past history, but it was most interesting in the making. Other history in the making at the convention gave me two of the greatest thrills of my life.

One was the election of Germany as a member of the League, and a permanent member of the Council as one of the six great nations. The meeting was solemn and impressive as all felt it to be one of the most advanced steps that the League had taken.

The German delegation arrived late the next afternoon. For a week, up to that hour, the weather had been inclement. There had been no sign of the Alps around the gray lake. But as the train bearing the German envoys entered the city, the clouds parted and Mt. Blanc seemed to come forward to greet them. It was looked upon as a good omen, and was so used in the addresses at the Assembly.

The next day I was fortunate in gaining entrance through the closely guarded doors to see the German Embassy enter from behind the official platform. Slowly they descended the steps, led by their Premier, Herr Stresemann, to occupy the front seats reserved for l'Allemand. The entire delegation was seated alphabetically according to the ruling French language, placing the Germans second on the list. Blonde Estonians sat next to black Ethiopians, and had the *Etats Unis* been a member of the League, her delegates would have sat on the other side.

The drop of a pin could have been heard while Herr Stresemann made his long speech of acceptance. Then Briand, the fiery orator of France, responded in the name of the League. Such eloquence! Sparks seemed to emanate from his finger-tips, since he talked as much with his hands as with his lips. Each time he uttered the dramatic words, "C'est fini!" tears filled his eyes. They rolled down Briand's cheeks while Stresemann wept openly. There was not a dry eye in the house. It seemed that the occasion marked a turning point in world affairs, and I can but believe it is true, even though only yesterday, at the fourteenth assembly, Hitler announced that Germany would withdraw from the League.

Even so, all that the *Societe des Nations* has done toward establishing a better understanding among the peoples of the earth cannot be wiped out. The effect of those fifty-five nations of all races and colors, striving to understand each others' problems, is a step toward the Brotherhood of Man that can never be entirely undone.

We are so apt to forget that the Commission of Peace, while doubtless the most pertinent at present, is only one of the six international commissions of the League striving to understand and remedy world conditions. The Commission for International Education, with its college open to students of every race in the world who aspire to diplomatic vocations, will alone create a far better understanding among nations.

The days in Geneva were filled to overflowing. At half past eight each morning, Dr. Zimmerman explained the proceedings of the previous day in the Assembly and gave an outline of what was to be done that day. Lectures were given all day and in the evenings for the benefit of those who were not fortunate enough to gain admittance to the assembly meetings. The meetings of each commission were also open to guests. Famous speakers were to be heard on every side.

Then there were the luncheons of the International Club which were followed with talks by noted men. The description by Nansen, the North Pole Explorer, of his experiences while lost for many months in the Arctic was the most thrilling. He was also one of the most prominent figures on the Assembly floor.

At the end of three weeks the never-to-be-forgotten conference came to an end. Friends from far and near had crossed my path and gone their various ways. What a place it was to meet friends old and new. Dr. Josephine Jackson from Pasadena came from Paris to join me for a few days, and a friend from Queensland, Australia, was one of the women delegates.

Two of the happiest events of the weeks in Geneva were due to the receipt of group letters from my dear girls, one sent from Cherbourg, their first port, and one from New York.

To leave Switzerland without a closer touch with the Alps was impossible. Two days at Montreux were spent en route.

A visit to the "Prison of Chillon" one afternoon made me realize that civilization had progressed a long, long way from Chillon to Geneva, since the days when the chains of the captive feudal lord wore grooves in the stone pillars of his neighboring lord's damp, cold cellar below the surface of the Lake which the chateau overhung. Immediately overhead the sounds of revelry and feasting wore even deeper grooves in the captive's heart.

From Montreux I went up to Wengern although the season was well advanced, too far advanced, as I found the village deserted of its summer residents. The inns were closed; it was nightfall and no more trains came or went. One kindly matron of a Swiss chalet, the "Silberhorn," took me in for the night. The moon was full and the clouds lifted over Jungfrau that she might say *gute nacht* and a rosy-tinted *guten morgen.*

The next day I reached the top of the Sheidigg on the funicular to bask in Jungfrau's beauty. The peak of my wanderings had been attained. I turned my face homeward.

Going down to Interlaken in the late afternoon I found all hotels either closed or closing. The host of the Villa del Polito in Syracuse, Sicily, kept a summer hotel there. He opened a room for me, facing the Jungfrau. The night was as clear as a bell and I watched the moonlight play on the snow-covered maiden until sleep shut out her silvery form. But awaking at half past two in the morning I was greeted by a sight which repaid me many-fold for this bit of wanderlust. The slender icy peak of the mountain was a glittering bluish tint in the clear moonlight. Ere long a rosy tint appeared, a pre-dawn glow. Then King Sol touched the Jungfrau with his golden wand and she seemed to come much nearer. Then the shadow of another peak intervened and she became a great white spirit, and then a phantom, so far did she seem to recede. Four times was this golden-hued advance made, followed by a loss of color and seeming recession into the dim distance before Old Sol had surmounted the intervening peaks and cast all of his glowing splendor upon the Jungfrau.

My plan had included a trip to Zermatt to visit the Matterhorn, but my hotel host dissuaded me, declaring it was too late in the season. Another desire that remained unfulfilled was a flight from Geneva to Paris over Mt. Blanc, as I feared to risk the altitude.

So I returned to Montreux and went by train to quaint old Dijon for a night, and from there to Paris to get my dresses which of course were not ready.

London drew me once more for a two weeks' visit to the Nursery Schools, of which London is the mother. The search for these led me through devious slums far beyond where taxis are to be picked up on the streets. Only the great busses penetrated those remote districts.

Mr. Ritter had requested me to learn all I could of these schools, especially those in the poorer regions which were more or less under the supervision of the City Government. It was an interesting and beneficial experience and one that I recall with especial pleasure.

But late October had come and my two months of roaming alone over Europe at my own sweet will had passed. The time of homecoming for both Mr. Ritter and me had arrived, he from California, and I from London. It was not au revoir but farewell to dear England when I sailed from Southampton to Cherbourg to pick up my various belongings that had been stored in travel—and Queen Marie.

CHAPTER 23

Sunset and Afterglow

THE LONE TRIP ACROSS THE ATLANTIC IN OCTOBER, 1926, WAS MADE on the *Leviathan,* which brought also Queen Marie and her party to America. Due to my royal escort misfortune befell me for we entered the New York harbor at four o'clock on a cold, rainy morning. The Mayor and other officials of New York had arranged the usual parade for the Queen and planned to take her off the steamer at ten o'clock. So we had anchored before daylight and the engines being idle there was no heat on the boat. After the great hullaballo of the Queen's escort of tugs and brass bands, the tide was too low for our *Leviathan* to enter the channel. There we lay until four o'clock in the afternoon, nearly frozen. It was dark by the time we had passed the customs officials, and New York was bitterly cold. Result—I too partook of the "cold."

As Mr. Ritter was to arrive in Washington from California two days later I took a train that would reach there shortly before his train was due. Alas! his train was delayed by a freight wreck and I waited in the cold depot until I was again chilled, then drove three miles to our former apartment to find it cold and dreary. I turned on the heat and went to bed.

When Mr. Ritter arrived late in the evening he found me with the usual high fever and aches of Flu. It was a severe attack, so thanks to walking the same deck with a queen I had a winter of illness ahead of me.

November 19th brought Mr. Ritter to that number of decades which in biblical times measured the life span of man. He was well and hearty, but he had always disliked time-consuming administrative duties. Science Service was well established and he felt that the strong Board of Trustees and the able Director and Business Manager could carry it along, so he decided to retire from the presidency the next year and return to Berkeley. Retirement was not his goal but his opportunity to carry on unmolested what he considered his major work, writings which he had in mind and in which Mr. Scripps had been deeply interested. He felt that he would be more nearly fulfilling the wishes of his friend by so doing than by remaining at the helm of a craft which could be guided as well by someone else.

To illuminate this statement I must deal further with the relations of these two friends. While a deep affection developed between them during the years of their intimate association, the basis of their relationship was that of minds rather than of hearts.

In the discussions of these two very dissimilar men, there was not only the world-wide interests of both to be taken into account, but the contrasting method of approach to problems that elicited each other's interest. Without holding any definite creed or philosophy, Mr. Scripps was by nature a humanist. Every topic discussed would almost inevitably bring out the question, "But of what use is all this to mankind?" Mr. Ritter, on the other hand, considered everything from the strictly scientific point of view, and while not a philosopher in the academic sense, he was so tinged with it by nature and so deeply dyed by years of reading, that the philosophical angle had always to be considered.

Mr. Scripps was an omniverous reader. In the center of his study stood a large library table for magazines. Arranged in piles thereon was the annual output of virtually every magazine in the English language from the *Westminster Review* to the *Black Cat*. He had formerly had French Journals as well, but preferring now to save his eyes by having Mrs. Scripps or a secretary read to him, he confined himself to English subscriptions.

Another illustration of his reading proclivities is shown by this incident. When in war-time his physician sent him for a winter's cruise off the coast of Florida, he told his secretary to write to Brentano and order every recent book on economics, psychology, ethics, sociology and philosophy.

Cases containing about four hundred volumes arrived on the yacht. Mr. Scripps scanned through every one of them and then had his secretaries read to him those of which he desired to know the contents. What powers of concentration and what a memory that man had! He could quote the gist of almost everything he ever read. Discussing world topics with a man of such a mind and of such wide reading was no child's play even for a highly trained academic man.

Both lives were deeply influenced by these years of intellectual clashing. Mr. Ritter's interests became more and more humanistic. Man as an animal—whole—his body, activities and intellect or "soul" became an object of years of study. This was due doubtless to Mr. Scripps' constant prodding with the question, "What is this damn human animal anyway? Ritter, you are a zoologist, a student of living things and you ought to help the rest of us to understand ourselves better."

When the war came and men rushed madly to the front to kill each other, and all those left behind were urged to sacrifice everything—lifework, homes, money, and even flour and sugar to provide for the fighters and their deserted families—his urgency on this point became a genuine prod. He was stirred to the depths of his being by these contradictions in human nature and turned to his friend for scientific help.

To quote from a disquisition on these two men: "It is hardly the ordinary thing to find a business man, a humanist and a philosopher of sorts turning to a biologist for information as to the ways of men. Something in Mr. Scripps' knowledge of men, admittedly extraordinary, led him to feel that this particular biologist could interpret us to ourselves with sanity, science and common sense, could he but be badgered into the undertaking. Mr. Scripps' line of reasoning seems to have been: if scientific knowledge is useful and indeed indispensable to the most efficient making of glass and steel and houses and newspapers, it will in all probability be found to be equally useful and perhaps indispensable to the most effective conduct of all human affairs. In these he included, not just those humble affairs of getting food and clothing and curing ailments, but those high affairs of love of God and man, faith and hope and loyalty."

Out of these questionings came, as I have said, the founding of Science Service and the studies on population at Miami College. But there was another side to these questions, that of the religious factor in man's nature and of the proper handling of the individual problem of reproduction.

On these points Mr. Ritter had some ideas that appealed to Mr. Scripps. They were that all mankind is religious whether it be a cave-man with his little stone idols or an ascetic devoting his life to meditation. Likewise mankind reproduces his species just as animals do with this difference, that in animals it is an instinct merely, while with man it is or should be connected with his highest faculties, not only of emotion but of intellect and reason. How to induce his highest faculty, reason, to dominate both of these natural instincts was one of the problems into which Mr. Ritter was delving. In some way the child should be taught to appreciate and think naturally upon both of these subjects from its earliest years. How to instruct them is one of the unsolved problems of child-education.

Mr. Scripps was deeply impressed with these ideas, and it was to this line of thought particularly that he referred when he said that his philanthropic bequests should be to endow the "Ritter Ideas." Neither of them felt that the study of human society could solve the knotty problem of what a single human being is, psychobiologically considered.

At once Mr. Scripps placed five thousand dollars in the hands of President Hughes for Mr. Ritter to draw upon for experimentation on these ideas. Meanwhile Mr. Scripps went off on his yacht for a world cruise. All of these projects, Science Service, the Miami Foundation and these indefinite plans for child education were to be fully discussed when he returned from his cruise. Hence the message from Cape Town for Mr. Ritter to meet him in the Mediterranean in the summer of 1926. Had the contemplated six weeks' of discussions been realized after each man had been thinking deeply about them for a year, what the outcome would have been will never be known.

Mr. Scripps left a large sum to be used at his son Robert's discretion for projects that his father was interested in, but there were no definite instructions, and the interested, ever-inquiring mind was not there to interpret.

The financial side of the dealings of E. W. and W. E., as the two men were dubbed, was peculiar. No money ever passed between them. Their collaboration was not on a financial plane. In the founding of Science Service, when Mr. Ritter was traveling almost constantly, a sum was deposited with the Board of Directors with which to refund his expenditures on his scientific trips. Likewise part of the Hughes fund was for refunds of Mr. Ritter's outlays for this purpose.

In the early years of their association at La Jolla, when the gifts to the University were made for the building of the library, pier, and sea-wall, Mr. Scripps stated in a letter to the Regents that he and his sister, Ellen Browning Scripps, were not making a gift to the University as such, nor to a Research Institution only, but rather they wished to endow the life-work of one man, William E. Ritter. All of Mr. Scripps' donations to Mr. Ritter's work were on this basis. There was never a direct gift during his lifetime nor in a bequest.

But to return to my story. It is difficult to evaluate the worth of one so near. If I overestimate or underestimate my life-companion, my excuse is that I have had but one husband so that I have no good basis of comparison. Is the pedestal of this household "lar" too high or too low? But laying aside joking, I will turn to others for certain estimates that parallel mine.

For that November anniversary a banquet was planned by the Science Service officials. It was held in the dear old Cosmos Club, the former home of Dolley Madison. The date of the banquet was delayed a week that I might be there. When it came it was a cold snowy night and although I was sitting up only part of the day after a month of Flu, I was determined to go, and was well repaid by the rich memories although it resulted in a prolonged relapse.

Messages came to Mr. Ritter from far and near as well as from those present. Later a brochure was published with a digest of the addresses and a sketch of the guest of honor. From this I shall quote a few extracts. One quotation I have already used.

The brochure begins with this statement regarding the change in thought between the old prophets and the present-day seers. "Seventy years is no longer regarded as the age of man: we think now of a septuagenarian only as of one who has begun his second maturity. Yet enough remains of the septuagesimal tradition that when a man reaches seventy we think it not inappropriate to pause and take stock of the things he has done to justify his length of days upon the earth."

A synopsis of the man and his work is given thus: "According to his own testimony this naturalist's motto is 'Neglect Nothing.' Applied to a creature of the complexity of an amoeba, this constitutes a sizable life-work. Applied to a human being, the task is staggering. It has called for delving with patience and precision into an enormous mass of material. Psychology, physiology, neurology, anthropology, sociology, with their many ramifications, have been explored and made to yield tribute. An onlooker at these tremendous labors is aware of a very good reason why biologists have not long since dealt thus with humans. The mass of facts and interpretations of facts to be synthesized is so great that we shall not often find a mentality able to cope with the task, or a temperament willing to tolerate its appalling exigencies. The mass of material demanding attention now is enormous compared to that available in Darwin's time. It is cause for genuine satisfaction that Professor Ritter has done certain fundamental thinking so thoroughly it need not be redone for some time. In the future, the humanist seeking sound scientific foundation for his concerns will find safe conduct through a great mass of irrelevant and fruitless theorizing, because one man with human sympathy and super-human patience has so faithfully 'neglected nothing.'"

As stated before, his studies of human conduct were by the comparative method, through ants, birds, beavers, apes, and babies. To study conduct in early childhood he found the nursery school was the best avenue. Convinced of this he used the fund Mr. Scripps had left with President Hughes for educational studies, in bringing from Boston on a two year contract, a trained nursery school director. The first year she spent in an experimental school in West Oakland. The second year she was loaned for a Berkeley experiment known as the Children's Community, now officered by the mothers themselves. This has proved a decided success.

Dr. Bailey who had general superintendence of the Oakland school, writes: "What glass-fronted aquarium tanks are to the observation of eels and starfish, nursery school play-spaces are to the study of the young animal, with the added advantage of freedom and 'everyday-ishness' quite impossible to the imprisoned sea creatures. There is no doubt that just this careful individual study through long stretches of growth will yield insight into adult conduct, exactly as honest and painstaking analysis of animal activities gave the clue to their significance for human activities."

In the spring of 1927 Mr. Ritter resigned from the presidency of Science Service and was succeeded by Dr. J. McKeen Cattell, a psychologist and editor of *Science* and other scientific journals.

Would it be fitting to call this resignation the setting of the sun of his official work? The afterglow is yet to be depicted.

In April we left Washington. Mr. Ritter hastened to Berkeley while I loitered on the way.

At first it was difficult for Mr. Ritter to find working quarters at the University as the great building which was to house all the life-sciences was in the early stages of erection, and the various departments were swarming in old wooden buildings that had been moved and fitted up for temporary quarters. Dr. Kofoid tried to make room for him by doubling up, but Dr. Joseph Grinnell could offer him a room to himself where he was comfortably located until the huge new building was completed. Here he now has a large airy room in which to delve for the remainder of his life among his beloved books and his endless cases of notes clipped from many sources through two-score years of reading.

And what is he doing? Going on with the same old studying and writing. Study to him does not mean the reading of books alone, but observing, and thinking as well.

Last evening I cornered him and said, "You must give me a summary of your work. Think it over and tell me as briefly as possible." This morning he said: "A bird's eye view of my professional career would reveal a double stream. One of them would be concerned with the theory of life and the other with the practice.

"The theoretical stream started in 1896 with a purely technical treatise on animal development. This led eventually to my conception of 'wholeness,' in the *Unity of the Organism,* and is focusing in the Problem of Human Wholeness on which I am now working.

"In other words my effort in the theory of life has been to help bridge the gap between psychology and biology. Psychology has been understood to be the science of the mind, and biology the science of the body, as if the two could be independent of each other. My theory of 'wholeness' includes both as part of one living organism.

"The practical stream was the organizing of the department of zoology in the University of California, the Scripps Institution at La Jolla, Science Service in Washington, and lastly my part in starting the Scripps' Foundation on Population in Miami University, Ohio, and the Nursery School in Oakland and the Children's Community in Berkeley."

Since our return, travel has been greatly lessened but in 1931 Mr. Ritter was invited to London to participate in the proceedings of the second International Congress of the History of Science. He was invited because his views on "wholeness" led him directly to the works of Aristotle who was the first adequately to grasp the conception of "complete reality." Mr. Ritter's contribution to the Congress was on this aspect of the history of science.

Apropos of his work in this line, at a meeting of scientific societies in Chicago this summer, massed there because of the Century of Progress Exposition, he was talking one day with a prominent psychologist on this subject of closing the centuries-old chasm between the theoretical views of mind and body, when the psychologist said, "Yes, the chasm is lessening, and you are surely doing your share, Ritter."

The special object of Mr. Ritter's trip to Chicago was to attend a meeting of Science Service, the purpose of which was to learn from scientists of other countries what they were doing for the dissemination of science. There is no other institution for this specific purpose though attempts are being made in various ways to spread scientific knowledge.

The afterglow of Mr. Ritter's life-work as evidenced by his interest in the instruction of children from their earliest months may best be expressed in the closing paragraphs of the Washington brochure:

"This latest phase of Professor Ritter's work is peculiar in that, while most of his life-work has been directed toward pure science, this enterprise is concerned also with practical applications. Because of his insight into the nature of human capacity for regulating conduct with regard to organismal welfare, the results of these present observations are bound to be of arresting importance for education. Perhaps it is not at present justifiable to speak of education as an applied science; but if the trail which

Professor Ritter is now blazing is carried through to its goal, there will be available psychobiological knowledge adequate to the creation of such a science.

"We are agreed without argument that 'the race moves forward on the feet of little children'; we are willing to spend free-heartedly to smooth the road before these feet. To bring the great learning, the keen powers of observation, the sure logical mind, the fruit of a lifetime's ripened scholarship into the service of children, not merely to smooth the old road, but to strike out a new and safer way to more abundant life—that seems a not unworthy climax to the life-work of a gentleman and a scholar who loves his fellowman."

What better afterglow to a long lifetime of study could a man ask than to return to his Alma Mater, be comfortably located in a permanent work-room near the great library, and at liberty to use his time as he pleases?

In these afterglow years there have been light scattering clouds, else the setting sun could not have reflected its coloring. But three points of radiance have been particularly bright. The first was that our dear friend, Ellen Browning Scripps, presented to the Institution of Oceanography for which she laid the foundation, a life-size portrait of Mr. Ritter painted by Winifred Rieber.

The second was the honor conferred when President Sproul and the Regents of the University named the latest and largest building at the Institution the William Emerson Ritter Hall.

And last but not least, at the last Charter Day commemoration of the University, his Alma Mater conferred upon him its highest honorary degree of Doctor of Laws.

* * * * * * *

Our last winter in Washington was one of semi-invalidism for me with variations of the genuine article. I was still rebelling against retirement and my determination to keep going only prolonged the resented state of affairs.

One lasting result was the first section of this book. For a long time it had been borne in upon me from outside as well as by my own sense of duty, that I should write an account of our pioneer ancestors, all of whom had passed into the Beyond, for the three generations of their descendants who had no record of them. So sitting up in bed, I spent the mornings writing the account of their lives and of my childhood days, as an illustration of the California of that time. This was laid aside with no intention of doing more than some day having it mimeographed for "the clan."

In April we returned to California via La Jolla to see Miss Scripps. I remained ten days while Mr. Ritter proceeded to Berkeley to search for an abiding place. While in La Jolla my friend, Dr. Jackson, drove down from Pasadena to urge me to come to her for another two weeks' rest. This I did, and en route paid a last visit to my dear cousin Edmond and his wife, little dreaming that they would precede me across the deep dark river.

From there I went to Fresno to visit my family and to await the wedding bells of my grand-niece, Elizabeth Warner, which rang on May 14th, when she became Mrs. Floyd Hammond. I was also greeted by the first member of the fourth generation, little Mary Warner, the daughter of Conrad and the great-granddaughter of my sister.

Again in Berkeley, this time to remain. We established ourselves in an apartment at Hotel Claremont as the best solution of our living problem.

The years have passed with ever-increasing speed. Reunion with the old friends has been a great joy. Travel for me has been confined to our own state, but that state I have learned better than ever before. For four summers, long auto trips, canvassing the range of the California woodpeckers, have taken us the length and breadth of the state through the great valleys and along the mountains at an elevation of from four to five thousand feet.

When Mr. Ritter went to London in 1931 I longed to see dear old England again but did not dare venture so arduous a trip. Instead I went to Fresno to visit my niece and nephew and their families. Then I induced them to go with me for a week's sojourn in Yosemite. I was eager to see it once more though all my sight-seeing must be on wheels. The freshened memories of the mountains and the falls are precious but the journey was too strenuous.

My motto has been, "I shall keep going until I drop." I virtually did so. While realizing that a rest was imperative, I was determined that Mr.

Ritter, who was due in a few days from England, should not find me in bed. He came on Thursday. Sunday was church day. Could I make it? I determined to go with him, and did. Home for lunch. That was too much. Dr. Torrey, who was with us at table, noted my distress and led me out of the dining room.

The dictum was, "Go to bed for a week." I did so, in fact stayed there for a year, deep in the valley of shadow. In the following year and a half of semi-invalidism I have found the brightest part of my afterglow.

The year of severe illness was brightened by the love and thoughtfulness of friends. There was never a day without flowers in my rooms and quantities of books to be read. But there were months when too weak to read, I could only ponder on what life is and what makes it worth while.

The rebellious spirit was quelled and contentment and gratitude took its place. Why are we so slow to learn? More than three thousand years ago a Sanskrit sage wrote:

> Look to this Day, for it is Life!
> Yesterday is but a dream
> And Tomorrow is only a vision,
> But Today well lived makes
> Every Yesterday a dream of happiness,
> And every Tomorrow a vision of hope.

I trust that I have now learned this lesson, but why should it take a lifetime to learn to make it a part of daily experience?

Only last Sunday a modern sage said to me in explanation of a part of his own life philosophy, "The present is not made up of years but of memories and experiences."

This same logician, by name Henry Rieber or Dr. C. H. Rieber, Dean of the College of Arts and Sciences in the University of California at Los Angeles, gave several definitions of the difference between a pessimist and an optimist. One illustration I took unto myself as well fitting my own life-history.

Two pails in a well had been going up and down, down and up, for lo, these many years. One day in passing, the full pail said to the empty pail,

"Isn't this a wretched life? I no sooner come up full with my heavy load than it is poured out and I have to go down empty."

"Oh," said the empty pail, "I was just going to remark, "Isn't this a fine life? Every time I go down empty, I come up full."

To myself I said, "Yes, I've been forced to go down into the depths of the well many times, empty of strength, but so far I have always come up full of courage and determination to forge onward."

So it has been this time. Though I am still confined save for an afternoon ride, in spite of the depth of the well into which I sank, I have come up filled to the brim with renewed faith in Nature's God, greater hope for world betterment, more love of humanity, and courage to face whatever comes, and determination that "Today shall be well lived."

Two tasks awaited me. One was what I call my bedside clinic, my bedside to be sure, where messages come by letter and by phone in addition to a continuous stream of stricken friends with woes, sorrows and calamities of all kinds. Ofttimes my nurses have been distracted and at times it has been hard on me—intensely wearying physically, but spiritually it has been a blessing. To feel that I am still of use, that many lean on me for strength and courage, and can go away with "healing in their wings," is a real comfort and uplift to me. May I not live until I can no longer be of use to anyone.

Then I have had leisure, enforced to be sure, to read, to listen to glorious symphony concerts from afar, and to write this resume of a lifetime of memories.

Formerly when confined to bed and pillows, I spent the mornings writing letters. This is one long, long letter to my family and friends, all of it written lying down or sitting up in bed. Whether it is worth the effort only you can tell, and your reactions will be various.

To me it has been the emptying out of my overflowing pail of innate energy. Like the woodpeckers, I have to peck holes and fill them with acorns, stolen almonds or stones as the case may be.

If this effort fills a purpose by recording the advance of California from the gold-seeking days of the pioneers; if it hints of the progress of our State University from its early years to its present rank as one of the largest and best in the Union; if my almost pioneer days as a woman physician form a background to the great advance of modern medicine; and if the pioneering of my life-comrade in his biological undertakings is a stimulus to others of his kind, I shall be content.

At any rate I am content, and deeply grateful for life and the comradeship of my life-mate.

In the words of Tennyson "we twain" bid you au revoir.

> And so these twain upon the skirts of time
> Sit side by side full-summed in all their powers,
> Dispensing harvest, sowing the 'to be,'
> Self-reverent each, and reverencing each,
> Distinct in individualities,
> Yet like each other even as those who love.

Berkeley, California,
October 17th, 1933.

AFTERWORD: AFTER FIVE YEARS
(INCLUDED IN THE SECOND PRINTING IN 1939)

After five years the last chapter of my book was read to me a day or two ago. To take up the story where it left off, I marvel at how little change has occurred in the mental and physical vigor of my life-mate during the interval that has rounded out his fourscore years. There has been even less leisure in these last years than ever, for he feels the necessity of using every possible hour to complete the work he has laid out (and he constantly adds more).

His chief effort has been with a "trilogy" of books, summarizing a philosophy of life he sketched for *More than Gold in California* (Chapter 23 Sunset and Afterglow). One volume, *The California Woodpecker and I*, was published in 1938. This is a comparison of the two "organisms as a whole" both as to their physical and intellectual makeup. The crowning point, to my mind, is the comparison of the "new" and "old" brains. Both creatures respond alike to the motivating centers in the "old" or lower brain. Man has reached the summit in the development of the cerebral cortex, the center of the highest human qualities, reason, judgment, and the moral consciousness. In the bird this "new" brain is very poorly developed. By this "new" upper-brain, man's intellectual and moral actions are, or should be, controlled and inspired. Another volume tentatively entitled *Darwin and the Golden Rule* is largely in manuscript. A third volume is also mostly written, but both must be revamped. Recently, a piece of work in a somewhat different line has occupied him.

From appearances he may remain in the same pleasant quarters, looking out on the same trees for several years, only changing pencils when he wears one out or loses it.

Regarding myself, to my own surprise another half decade has been added to my life-span—years in which I have learned the truth of the biblical dictum, that if one ventures to live past the "three-score and ten" milepost, one's days are filled with more than the usual allotment of tribulations.

This has been true in my case, but there has also been a bright side to the life-story. There are always compensations if we look for them. The book was written in bed in the third year of a physical breakdown which seemed at times destined to end my career, but perhaps prolonged it as a quiescent mode of living was forced upon me. Nearly all outside activities are still prohibited. Although most of the time I can be taken for an afternoon drive.

Immediately after the trying siege of proof-reading my book, I suddenly lost my central eyesight so that reading and writing and the recognition of friends became impossible. This meant bringing a new sense to take the place of the deficient one.

The art of reading had to be acquired by my fore-finger, but having more leisure, I have done more reading than in any preceding five years of my active life. Writing with my finger-tips had also to be acquired, and to be executed by having the typewriter on my lap as I sit bolstered up in bed. Inconvenient as these substitutions are, yet there are advantages. Probably none of you can read in the darkness of the night with your book snugly under the covers. One would not choose these makeshifts for nature's methods, but it is fortunate that such compensations can be made.

With all the deprivations that have come there have been great and unexpected pleasures. The two most unexpected were within the University Circle. One came from the Prytaneans, that Honor Society of women students of the University of California at whose birth I assisted in my own home. Having decided to undertake a dormitory for women students, they gave it the name of Mary Bennett Ritter Hall. The second and greatest honor of my life was the conferring upon me by the Regents and Faculty of the University of the Honorary Degree of an LL.D., with the following tribute by the president, Robert Gordon Sproul:

"First dean of women at the University of California, in fact if not in title; teacher, physician, and friend to the women students of three generations. Always in the forefront of those who seek the general welfare, you have counted as achievement only that which inspired achievement in others. A daughter of the argonauts, you have found and shared more than gold in California."

All in all there is much satisfaction to be found in this eighth decade in spite of the somewhat dreary prognostication by the prophet of old. May all those who traverse this long road through the Valley of the Shadow feel the warm glow of the lowering sun as I do, and may those who are on the sunny slope of Life's upward pathway, and those still in that sunshine, but on the descending slope, join with me in this modern "Psalm of Life:"

"The same God Who causes the trees to grow beautiful and tall; Who inspires the birds to build their nests; Who through the mystery of instinct leads all living things along their way, is also present in my life, calling me to be true, to be honest, to be steadfast and unafraid."

Mary Bennett Ritter

Berkeley, California,
November 19, 1939